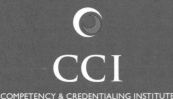

COMPETENCY & CREDENTIALING INSTITUTE

Personal Commitment to Extraordinary Care

Assisting In Surgery

PATIENT-CENTERED CARE

Jane C. Rothrock, PhD, RN, CNOR, FAAN

Patricia C. Seifert, RN, MSN, CNOR, CRNFA, FAAN

Library of Congress Cataloging-in-Publication Data

Assisting in surgery : patient-centered care / [edited by] Jane Rothrock, Patricia Seifert.

   p. ; cm.

  Includes bibliographical references and index.

  ISBN 978-0-9815642-0-3 (pbk. : alk. paper)

  1. Operating room nursing. 2. Operating room technicians. I. Rothrock, Jane C. II. Seifert, Patricia C. III. Competency & Credentialing Institute. IV. Title. [DNLM: 1. Operating Room Nursing. 2. Patient-Centered Care. 3. Surgical Procedures, Operative—nursing. WY 162 A848 2009]

RD32.3.A8655 2009

617'.917—dc22

                       2009031790

ISBN-13: 978-0-9815642-0-3

ISBN-10: 0-9815642-0-8

Printed in the United States of America.

Contributors, Reviewers, Illustrators, and Graphic Designers

CONTRIBUTORS

Robert Blumm, MA, RPA-C, DFAAPA
Adjunct Instructor, Surgery and Emergency Medicine,
Physician Assistant Studies
Hofstra University
Hempstead, NY

Nancy Davis, RN, NP (Retired)
Cascade, ID

Jeanne K. LaFountain, RN, MBA, CNOR, CRNFA
Nursing Program Manager/Perioperative Clinical Educator
Perioperative Services, Richard M. Ross Heart Hospital at the Ohio State University
Columbus, OH

Russell R. Lynn, MSN, CRNA
Associate Program Director,
Nurse Anesthesia Program
University of PA School of Nursing
Philadelphia, PA

James R. McCarthy, RN, CNOR, CRNFA
Perioperative Nursing Services
Temple University Hospital
Philadelphia, PA

Rose Moss, RN, MN, CNOR
Perioperative Nurse Consultant
Del Norte, CO

Julie Mower, RN, MSN, CNS, CNOR
Credentialing and Education Project Manager
CCI
Denver, CO

Denise O'Brien, MSN, RN, ACNS-BC, CPAN, CAPA, FAAN
Clinical Nurse Specialist, Perianesthesia Care Areas
University of Michigan Health System
Ann Arbor, MI

John T. Paige, MD, FACS
Assistant Professor of Clinical Surgery
Louisiana State University School of Medicine
New Orleans, LA

Jane C. Rothrock, PhD, RN, CNOR, FAAN
Professor and Director, Perioperative Programs
Delaware County Community College
Media, PA

Patricia C. Seifert, RN, MSN, CNOR, CRNFA, FAAN
Education Coordinator
Cardiovascular Operating Room
Inova Heart and Vascular Institute
Falls Church, VA
and
Editor-in-Chief
AORN Journal

Tim Snider
Editorial Director
BookMasters, Inc.
Ashland, OH

Elizabeth A. P. Vane, LTC, AN, RN, MS, CNOR
Assistant Professor, Perioperative Clinical Nursing Specialist Program
Graduate School of Nursing, Uniformed Services, University of the Health Sciences
Bethesda, MD

Linda J. Wanzer, RN, MSN, CNOR
Assistant Professor
Director, Perioperative Clinical Nurse Specialist Program
Graduate School of Nursing, Uniformed Services, University of the Health Sciences
Bethesda, MD

Mary K. Weis, RN, MSN, ACNS-BC, CNOR, CRNFA
Clinical Nurse Specialist
Department of Surgery, Centracare Clinic
St. Cloud, MN

Jennifer Welsch
Senior Full Service Project Director
BookMasters, Inc.
Ashland, OH

REVIEWERS

Brian Campbell, BSN, CRNA
Staff Nurse Anesthetist
Winchester Anesthesia Associates
Winchester Hospital
Winchester, MA

Susan Carzo, RN, CNOR, RNFA
Staff Nurse
Winchester Hospital
Winchester, MA

Beverly A. Kirchner, RN, CNOR, CASC
President, Genesee Associates, Inc.
Southlake, TX

Charles Moss, RN, CRNA
Director, Anesthesia Services
San Luis Valley Regional Medical Center
Alamosa, CO

Janette M. Parsons, RN, MSN, RNFA, CNOR
Family Nurse Practitioner
Marjorie K. Unterberg School of Nursing and Health Studies
Monmouth University
West Long Branch, NJ

Joseph H. Viveiros, RN, RNFA, CNOR
Staff Nurse
Winchester Hospital
Winchester, MA

Jennifer L. Zinn, RN, MSN, CNS-BC, CNOR
Clinical Nurse Specialist for Operative Services
Moses Cone Health System
Greensboro, NC

ILLUSTRATORS AND GRAPHIC DESIGNERS

Molly Borman
Biomedical Illustrations
Fort Collins, CO

Larin Zamora
Graphics Designer
Littleton, CO

To Sean, nephew and new high school graduate who has expressed an interest in a nursing career: We need bright, tenacious, bold-thinking young men like you in nursing. Much love to you from Aunt Jane.

—Jane C. Rothrock

To my assisting colleagues—RNs, MDs, PAs, and Technologists: Thank you for all that you have taught me, not the least of which is that there is always so much more to learn.

—Patricia C. Seifert

Table of Contents

Preface

Assisting in Surgery: Patient-Centered Care is specifically designed for healthcare professionals who assist in surgery. The focus of the book—as the title states—is patient-centered care. It is that focus that facilitates achieving positive patient outcomes, a goal embraced by all members of the surgical team.

This book's proud ancestry includes the 1987 textbook, *The RN First Assistant— An Expanded Perioperative Nursing Role,* written by the current book's first editor. Subsequent editions of this groundbreaking textbook reflected the value and exemplary practice of the assistant in surgery.

The current text has been expanded to include a multidisciplinary approach that includes nurses, physicians, physician assistants, and surgical technology assistants. It is appropriate not only that the "real world" of surgery be reflected but also that the importance of communication, collaboration, sharing and improvement of surgical skills, and leadership be highlighted. The book covers a broad spectrum of surgical information which can be used by practicing clinicians as well as students learning the clinical skills of the assistant at surgery.

The editors' personal and professional careers have been enriched by our association with colleagues: nurses, physicians, surgical technologists, and physician assistants. Their generosity in sharing knowledge and experience in the current book illustrates the teamwork exemplified in producing a book and in achieving optimal patient outcomes. Surgery is a team effort, and the contributions of each member of the surgical team produce a whole greater than the sum of its parts. The same can be said for this book. While each chapter focuses on a topic essential to assisting in surgery, the whole of the book focuses on the patient and protecting him or her from vulnerabilities. It may fairly be said that patients undergoing a surgical or other invasive procedure feel vulnerable. It is our intent that the assistant in surgery, whether in an educational program or practicing in a surgical setting, assist in alleviating those vulnerabilities in a manner marked by clinical talent, cognitive acumen, and an approach that is humanistic and caring.

Patient Positioning

Rose Moss

INTRODUCTION

Facilitating access to the structures undergoing surgical repair is one of the primary responsibilities of the First Assistant (FA) for achieving a successful patient outcome. This is accomplished by positioning the patient in a manner that promotes patient safety and creates optimal exposure to the surgical site for the operators.

Patient positioning, the art and science of moving and securing the human body into place, is an interdisciplinary task performed in the operating room (OR) suite on a daily basis. The FA recognizes that positioning is a collaborative effort by all members of the surgical team (i.e., surgeon, anesthesia provider, circulating nurse, FA, surgical technologist, nursing assistant), therefore, everyone must be aware that positioning can profoundly affect the patient in many ways. The patient undergoing surgery presents special concerns, including the inability to relate sensations of discomfort or pain; the need for strange and/or unnatural posturing for various procedures; and the effects of anesthetic agents and other drugs that affect normal physiologic functions. Prevention of injury to the patient (and to staff) is paramount; care must be taken to protect the patient and ensure that his or her physiological status remains as close to preoperative values as possible. While positioning a patient, the FA and other team members need to understand the relationship between certain positions and risks for injuries specific to those positions. It is also important that the FA understand the physiological changes that occur with a change in position.

PATIENT SAFETY

Patient positioning during surgery must provide optimal exposure of the surgical site, while simultaneously allowing access to the patient's airway, intravenous lines, and monitoring devices. Optimal positioning also prevents any potential complications related to the selected surgical position, such as compromise in physiological functions and mechanical stresses of the body parts. The FA knows that a surgical position should not compromise the cardiovascular, integumentary, musculoskeletal, nervous, or respiratory systems, or other vulnerable areas.

One of the expected outcomes related to safety is that the patient is free from signs and symptoms of injury from positioning (Petersen, 2007). Potential position-related injuries range from minor skin abrasions and backache to serious morbidity (Table 1-1); the injuries that may occur may be permanent or only temporary (Seibert, 2009). Complications from these injuries can lead to infection, tissue necrosis, paralysis, loss of limbs, and even loss of life. While most patients recover from minor positioning-related injuries, more

Table 1-1   Potential Position-Related Injuries

System	Potential Injuries
Cardiovascular system	Deep vein thrombosis (DVT) Ischemic injuries Vascular occlusion
Head, eyes, ears, nose, throat	Blindness Corneal abrasion Facial edema Vocal cord edema
Integumentary system	Abrasions Alopecia Decubitus ulcers
Musculoskeletal system	Amputation Backache Compartment syndrome Rhabdomyolysis
Nervous system	Decreased cerebral blood flow Increased intracranial pressure Peripheral neuropathy Quadriplegia
Respiratory system	Atelectasis Endobronchial intubation

Source: Adapted from Seibert, E.M. (2009). Positioning for anesthesia and surgery. In J.J. Nagelhout, & K.L. Plaus (Eds.), *Nurse Anesthesia* (4th ed., p. 428). St. Louis: Saunders Elsevier.

serious injuries, psychological trauma, and permanent disability may result in an increased length of hospital stay and recovery (Seibert, 2009). Therefore, safe and effective positioning of the surgical patient is essential and requires knowledge of the relevant anatomy and physiology, as well as demonstrated competency in proper positioning techniques with the use of positioning equipment.

In order to safely position surgical patients, all members of the perioperative team must be aware of factors that increase the risk for injury. Both perioperative and patient-related factors (Table 1-2) can increase the potential for position-related injuries (Seibert, 2009). Perioperative factors include:

- Positioning devices: straps and braces used to secure or restrain the patient, crutch-type stirrups, and axillary or shoulder rolls can cause pressure and temporary injury if excessively tight or improperly used.

Table 1-2   Perioperative and Patient-Related Factors Associated with Position-Related Injuries

Perioperative Factors	Patient-Related Factors
Positioning Devices	**Body Habitus**
– Axillary roll	– Bulky musculature
– Bolsters	– Malnutrition
– Ether screen	– Obesity
– Fracture bed post	
– Headrests	**Preexisting Conditions**
– Leg holders	– Alcoholism
– Positioning frames	– Anemia
– Shoulder braces	– Diabetes mellitus
– Stirrups	– Limited joint mobility
– Bed straps	– Liver disease
	– Peripheral neuropathies
Length of Procedure	– Peripheral vascular disease
– Greater than 4 hours	– Smoking
Anesthetic Techniques	
– General anesthesia	
– Hypotensive techniques	
– Neuromuscular blockade	

Source: Adapted from Seibert, E.M. (2009). Positioning for anesthesia and surgery. In J.J. Nagelhout, & K.L. Plaus (Eds.), *Nurse Anesthesia* (4th ed., p. 423). St. Louis: Saunders Elsevier.

- Length of the procedure: prolonged operating times (i.e., longer than 4 hours) contribute to postoperative positioning complications, including postoperative visual loss, nerve injuries, and compartment syndrome.
- Anesthetic techniques: patients undergoing general anesthesia cannot move in response to painful stimuli caused by uncomfortable body positions; movement may also be limited when the patient is sedated. Further, the hypotensive effects of general anesthesia may lower perfusion pressures to an unacceptable level in patients with hypertension or other comorbidities. Muscle relaxation caused by neuromuscular blocking agents or volatile anesthetics may lead to stretch injuries by allowing increased joint mobility.

Patient-related factors include:

- Body habitus: extremes of body habitus contribute to the risk of positioning complications. Underweight patients may develop decubiti or nerve damage due to inadequate adipose tissue over bony prominences. Obese patients are at increased risk for morbidity due to positioning because large tissue masses exert increased pressure on dependent body parts. Patients with a muscular physique may also be at a higher risk for compartment syndrome and ulnar nerve injury.
- Preexisting pathophysiology: preexisting conditions, including anemia, alcoholism, hypertension, diabetes mellitus, peripheral vascular disease, and peripheral neuropathies can aggravate the physiologic effects of the various surgical positions.

All members of the surgical team should actively participate in safely positioning the patient. General safety considerations for positioning include, but are not limited to, the following (AORN, 2009a):

- Provisions should be made to provide patient dignity and privacy during transport, transfer, and positioning.
- Movement or positioning of the patient should be a coordinated effort with the surgical team.
- Specific patient needs should be communicated to the perioperative team before initiating transfer or positioning the patient.
- Attention should be given to protecting the patient's airway at all times during patient transfer and positioning.
- Before and during transfer and positioning, members of the perioperative team should communicate with each other regarding securing drains, tubes, and catheters; actions must be taken to support these devices and prevent

them from dislodging; after transfer and positioning, team members should confirm that these devices have maintained patency.

- The patient's body alignment should be monitored and maintained.
- When the patient is on the OR bed, he or she should be attended by surgical team members at all times.
- There should be an adequate number of personnel and required equipment to safely position the patient.
- The patient's tissue integrity should be monitored.
- Positioning equipment should be used to protect, support, and maintain the patient's position.
- Padding should be used to protect the patient's bony prominences.
- The patient's arms should be positioned to protect them from nerve injury.
- The location of the patient's fingers should be confirmed to ensure they are positioned clear of OR bed breaks or other hazards.
- Safety restraints should be applied carefully to avoid nerve compression injury and compromised blood flow.
- The patient's body should be protected from contacting metal portions of the OR bed.
- The patient's head should be placed in a neutral position and placed on a headrest.
- A pillow may be placed under the back of the patient's knees to relieve pressure on the lower back.
- The patient's heels should be elevated off the underlying surface when possible.
- The patient's head and upper body should be in alignment with the hips; the patient's legs should be parallel and the ankles uncrossed.
- If the patient is pregnant, a wedge should be placed under the patient's right side to displace the uterus to the left and prevent supine hypotensive syndrome due to the uterus compressing the vena cava.
- Unless necessary for surgical reasons, the patient's arms should not be tucked at his or her sides when in the supine position.
- Direct pressure to the eye should be avoided in order to decrease the risk of central retinal artery occlusion and other ocular damage, including corneal abrasion and postoperative visual loss; contact lenses should be removed and safely stored.

These general safety considerations will be explored in greater depth in the discussion of specific positions.

There are additional safety considerations for positioning morbidly obese patients (AORN, 2009a). Morbid obesity is associated with patients who have a body mass index (BMI) greater than 40 or who weigh at least 100 lbs over their recommended weight. The pathophysiology of morbid obesity as well as the effects of the various surgical positions can have adverse effects on cardiopulmonary function, such as:

- Airway compromise due to a short, thick neck.
- Risk of difficult intubation.
- Increased risk for hypoxia.
- Increased risk for intra-abdominal pressure on the diaphragm.
- Increased risk of aspiration.
- Decreased cardiac output.
- Increased pulmonary artery pressure.
- Risk of compression to the inferior vena cava.

The following are some of the interventions used to position the morbidly obese patient:

- Ensure the OR bed is capable of articulating and supporting patients who weigh 800 to 1,000 lbs (363.3 to 454 kg).
- Ensure mattresses can provide sufficient support and padding without "bottoming out."
- Use side attachments or stirrups on the OR bed if the patient's legs do not fit on the OR bed.
- Use padded sleds or toboggans to contain the patient's arms at the side of the body if necessary, if they can be used without putting excessive pressure on the arms.
- Use an extra-long, extra-wide safety strap for patients who exceed the length limits for a standard size safety strap; sheets should not be substituted for inadequately sized safety straps.

STAFF SAFETY IN MOVING PATIENTS

While the hazards and associated precautions related to patient safety during transfer and positioning in the perioperative environment are well recognized, less attention is paid to the associated hazards positioning presents to the staff, such as the physical stresses and potential for work-related musculoskeletal disorders (MSDs) and injuries found in healthcare facilities. The Occupational Health and Safety Administration (OSHA, 2009) has studied workplace practices and found that musculoskeletal injuries caused by patient lifting, transferring, and repositioning are numerous, costly, and preventable. The National Institute of Occupational Safety and Health (NIOSH, 2008) has determined the safe maximum lifting limit to be 46 lbs for women and 51 lbs for men. To reduce injuries, an array of equipment and devices is commercially available to help move even the largest, fully incapacitated patients.

Another trend that demonstrates the increasing attention to staff safety during patient transfer and positioning is the recognized need by federal agencies and professional nursing associations for ergonomically healthy work practices. OSHA defines ergonomics as the science of fitting the job to the worker. A mismatch between the physical requirements of the job and the physical capacity of the worker can result in work-related MSDs (OSHA, 2009). The science of ergonomics also includes the design of equipment and work tasks that conform to the capability of the worker and provides a means for adjusting the work environment and work practices to prevent injuries before they occur.

A number of professional organizations have initiated safe patient handling strategies. In 2003, the American Nurses Association (ANA) launched a proactive, multifaceted campaign aimed at promoting safe patient handling. In 2006, the Association of periOperative Registered Nurses (AORN) developed its *Position Statement on Ergonomically Healthy Workplace Practices*, demonstrating its commitment to the attainment and maintenance of an ergonomically healthy workplace to protect all staff members in the perioperative setting (AORN, 2006). Patient handling creates an ergonomic hazard that, if not corrected, can cause injury to perioperative staff members (AORN, 2009b). Given the aging workforce, healthy workplace practices are especially important to reduce work-related injuries.

The following safety measures for all members of the perioperative team are specifically related to transfer and positioning of patients (AORN, 2009a):

- When planning patient care, the positioning equipment needed for the specific operative or invasive procedure should be anticipated.
- During the preoperative assessment, unique patient considerations that require additional precautions for procedure-specific positioning should be identified.
  - Patient needs should be assessed by a registered nurse prior to transport to determine the necessary equipment and both the skill level and number of transport personnel required.
- All members of the perioperative team should use proper body mechanics when transporting, moving, lifting, or positioning patients.
  - An adequate number of personnel should be available to ensure patient and personnel safety when transporting the patient.

- High-risk tasks should be identified and ergonomic solutions implemented to eliminate or reduce the risks for occupational injury.
- The potential hazards associated with patient transport and transfer activities should be identified and safe practices established.
- The patient should be safely positioned under the direction of and in collaboration with the surgeon and anesthesia provider.
  - Four caregivers should be available for a supine-to-prone patient transfer. One anesthesia provider should support the patient's head and maintain the patient's airway while other team members are responsible for the patient's trunk and extremities. Additional team members may be required for patients with a BMI of 40 or greater.
  - Two team members, plus the anesthesia provider, can safely transfer a patient weighing up to 48.5 lbs (22.0 kg) from the supine to prone positions. Three caregivers, plus the anesthesia provider, can safely transfer a patient weighing up to 72.7 lbs (33.0 kg). If a patient weighs more than 73 lbs, it is necessary to use assistive technology and a minimum of four or more caregivers.
- Transport and positioning equipment should be periodically inspected and maintained in proper working condition.
- Positioning equipment should be used in a safe manner, according to the manufacturers' written instructions.
- Perioperative personnel should receive initial education, competency validation, and updated information on patient positioning, new positioning equipment and procedures, and ergonomic safety.

The potential for injury to both patients and staff when transferring patients in the OR, especially in light of the growing population of obese patients, has stimulated the development of surgical bed and patient transport equipment that incorporate innovative and versatile designs (Surgical Products, 2009). Examples of these innovative products include new beds and transport devices that can facilitate the patient's movement throughout the entire surgical journey with minimal need for transfers. These devices ease the transport and transfer of patients by reducing much of the physical strain on the staff.

Innovative features that have been introduced into the health care setting which reduce the physical stress and risk of injury to patients as well as staff members include:

- Systems that provide patient transfer directly from the patient's hospital bed to a mobile OR bed via an automated conveyance system.

- Heated surfaces to enhance the patient's comfort and promote relaxation.
- Mobile, remote-controlled OR beds with an unrestricted 1000-lb patient capacity, thereby increasing stability in both transport and extreme patient positioning.
- Portable OR beds designed to lift and move patients weighing up to 700 lbs without physically moving the lift.
- Integrated safety controls to prevent falls or other injuries to patients and staff.
- Transfer devices using air to lift the patient.
- Interchangeable tabletops that can be docked to a fixed or mobile base via a transporter; OR time can be reduced because intubation and postoperative monitoring can occur outside of the OR.
- Contoured shapes for easier patient loading and unloading, especially in tight areas, as well as anti-pinch hand holds.
- Products designed for bariatric patients such as motorized transfer devices capable of functioning in both chair and stretcher modes; integrated handset control mechanisms for all powered functions (including sit-to-stand lift, chair-to-stretcher articulation, independent elevating swing legs, and vertical lift) facilitate safe patient handling for the staff.
- Wider seats and pressure management cushions enhance safety and ease of transfer of patients for staff.

ANATOMIC AND PHYSIOLOGIC CONSIDERATIONS RELATED TO POSITIONING

Improper positioning and/or failure to properly protect body surfaces and structures can result in harmful physiological effects; therefore, protection of these systems and structures during positioning is vital to prevent positioning-related injuries and promote positive patient outcomes. A systems review of the major anatomical and physiological considerations when positioning surgical patients is presented below.

Cardiovascular System

Alteration of hemodynamic status during surgery occurs to varying degrees due to both anesthesia and the selected patient position. In response to myocardial depression and vasodilation induced by volatile anesthetics, cardiac output and blood pressure are usually decreased under general anesthesia, which results in blood pooling in dependent body areas, thereby reducing preload and decreasing stroke volume (Seibert, 2009). Hemodynamic changes are also affected by the administration of neuromuscular blocking agents, which further decrease venous return due to the interruption of normal muscle tone. Administration of opioids and other volatile agents slows the heart rate to cause additional decreases in cardiac output and blood pressure (Seibert, 2009). Furthermore, normal compensatory mechanisms that increase heart rate when hypotension develops are diminished by general anesthetics, thereby rendering cardiac output and blood pressure more susceptible to gravitational forces (Seibert, 2009).

Hemodynamic changes are generally minimal in the supine and lateral positions; however, cardiac output and blood pressure are usually decreased in the sitting, prone, and flexed lateral positions, in which the lower extremities are placed in a dependent position (Seibert, 2009). The Trendelenburg, or head-down, position usually increases venous return to the heart and may help to elevate blood pressure when necessary. The reverse Trendelenburg position produces an uphill gradient for the arterial blood supply and may therefore decrease blood pressure; this may be helpful to prevent postoperative cerebral edema following brain surgery. The reverse Trendelenburg position also enhances venous blood pooling in the lower extremities; this reduces circulating blood volume to the heart and head. Head-up positions may be helpful in determining a patient's volume status. If the head is elevated to 75 degrees for several minutes and the patient experiences an increase in heart rate with a concomitant decrease in blood pressure compared to the supine position, the patient's circulating volume is significantly decreased.

Venous air embolism (VAE) is a recognized consequence of surgical procedures performed in the sitting position; however, VAE may occur in any position where a negative pressure gradient exists between the right atrium and veins at the surgical site (Seibert, 2009). Complications related to VAE are directly proportional to both the speed and volume of entrained air, ranging from no effect with minimal amounts of air, to hypotension, cardiac arrhythmias and arrest, and death with larger amounts (Seibert, 2009). VAE and its monitoring techniques are outlined in the discussion of the sitting position.

Deep venous thrombosis (DVT) and pulmonary embolus (PE) are also major risk factors for the surgical patient; therefore, prevention of these potential consequences is an important aspect of perioperative care (AORN, 2009c). Intraoperative factors that increase the risk for development of DVT and PE include (Heizenroth, 2007):

- Compression to both deep and peripheral vessels from a safety strap or restraint that is too tight.

- Slowed venous return when legs are placed in a dependent position (i.e., in the sitting position or lowered during knee arthroscopy).
- Hyperabduction of the arms beyond 90 degrees.

In order to reduce the risk, surgical team members should assess the vascular status of the patient's upper and lower extremities preoperatively; take measures to reduce the assessed risk; continue to evaluate vascular status intraoperatively and postoperatively; use compressive antiembolic stockings or sequential compressive devices; and assess radial pulses whenever arms are extended (Heizenroth, 2007).

Integumentary System

The skin is the largest organ of the body and its first line of defense in preventing pressure ulcer development. The skin overlying bony prominences is significantly different from skin elsewhere on the body: it is usually thinner, with little protective subcutaneous tissue; therefore, it requires special care and attention. The three physical forces used to establish and maintain a surgical position—pressure, shear, and friction—can injure the skin and underlying tissue (Heizenroth, 2007):

- Pressure is the force placed on the underlying tissue. Varying degrees of pressure can come from multiple sources, such as:
  - the weight of the body as gravity presses it downward toward the surface of the OR bed;
  - the weight of equipment resting on or against the patient, such as Mayo stands, drills, edges of the OR bed or vertical posts for self-retaining retractors;
  - positioning devices (e.g., stirrup bars, arm or leg holders, that can rest against the patient under tension); and
  - members of the surgical team leaning on the patient.
- Shear is the folding of underlying tissue that occurs when the skeletal structure moves while the skin remains stationary. Shearing can occur when the head of the OR bed is raised or lowered and when the patient is placed in the Trendelenburg or reverse Trendelenburg position. As gravity pulls the skeleton down, the stretching and folding of the underlying tissues as they slide with the skeleton occlude vascular perfusion, leading to tissue ischemia.
- Friction is the force of two surfaces rubbing against one another. Friction can occur when the patient's body is dragged across coarse or rough surfaces such as bed linen, instead of being lifted. Friction can result in denuding of the epidermis, thereby making the skin more susceptible to higher stages of pressure ulcer formation, as well as pain and infection.

Pressure ulcers, regardless of their origin, are negative outcomes for the patient and may result in pain, additional procedures, and increased costs. Because the OR is a high-risk environment for the development of pressure ulcers, this is an especially important concern for the surgical patient (Schultz, 2005). Although preventable in most cases, pressure ulcers are becoming more prevalent; an estimated 2.5 million patients are treated for pressure ulcers in acute care facilities in the United States each year (Duncan, 2007). Pressure ulcer incidence rates range from 0.4% to 38% in acute care settings. Pressure ulcers have also been associated with extended length of stay and increased mortality, as an estimated 60,000 patients die annually from complications due to hospital-acquired pressure ulcers (Duncan, 2007). The estimated cost of managing a single full-thickness pressure ulcer is as high as $70,000, and the total cost for treatment of pressure ulcers in the United States is estimated at $11 billion per year (Duncan, 2007).

Recently, the problem of pressure ulcers has gained greater awareness by federal regulatory agencies and accrediting bodies. Effective October 2008, the Centers for Medicare and Medicaid Services (CMS) identified pressure ulcers as one of the conditions for which it will not reimburse a facility unless it is proven that the patient had the condition upon hospital admission (Beaver, 2008). Pressure ulcers occur in spite of widespread clinical knowledge about how to prevent them. In 2007, CMS reported 257,412 cases of preventable pressure ulcers as secondary diagnoses; the average cost for these cases was $43,180 per hospital stay (Beaver, 2008). The Joint Commission has also addressed the prevention of pressure ulcers. One of its National Patient Safety Goals (NPSG) is to prevent health care-associated pressure ulcers by assessing and periodically reassessing each patient's risk for developing a pressure ulcer and take action to address any identified risks (The Joint Commission, 2008).

In addition to assessing the patient's risk factors for pressure ulcer development, the perioperative team must also use positioning equipment and accessories properly. All positioning equipment should be used in a safe manner, according to the manufacturers' written instructions. The following are some of the specific measures that can be taken to reduce the risk for pressure ulcers (AORN, 2009a):

- Use equipment that is designed to redistribute pressure.
- Select a surface that is able to reduce excessive pressure on bony prominences.
- Pad the patient's bony prominences.
- Elevate the patient's heels off the underlying surface when possible.
- Use a lateral transfer device (e.g., friction-reducing sheets, slider board, air-assisted transfer device) for supine-to-supine patient transfer.

Musculoskeletal System

The human musculoskeletal system provides form, stability, and movement to the human body; it is composed of the skeleton, muscles, cartilage, tendons, ligaments, joints, and other connective tissue. During positioning, the musculoskeletal system may be subjected to unusual stress (Heizenroth, 2007). In the alert patient, normal range of motion is maintained by pain and pressure receptors that warn against over-stretching or twisting of ligaments, tendons, and muscles; however, when anesthetics and/or muscle relaxants depress the pain and pressure receptors, the normal defense mechanisms cannot protect against joint and muscle damage (Heizenroth, 2007).

All members of the perioperative team must be aware of resistance to range of motion and take care not to extend a joint beyond what is essential (Heizenroth, 2007). In addition, maintaining the patient's correct body alignment and support-ing his or her extremities and joints reduces the potential for injury during transfer and positioning (AORN, 2009a). Furthermore, the patient's head and upper body should be in alignment with the hips; his or her legs should be parallel; and the ankles uncrossed (AORN, 2009a).

Compartment syndrome is a potentially serious complication that damages neural and vascular structures due to swelling of tissues within a muscular com-partment (Seibert, 2009). This syndrome is characterized by ischemia, hypoxic edema, and elevated pressure within the fascial compartments of the extremity (Heizenroth, 2007). Positioning factors associated with the development of com-partment syndrome include a tight armboard strap, elevation of an extremity accompanied by systemic hypotension, compression on an elevated extremity due to wrappings that are too tight, pressure from the weight of an extremity against an edge of a leg holder, pressure from the arm of a surgical assistant holding an extremity too tightly, excessive flexion of the knees or hips, and prolonged use of the lithotomy position, especially longer than 5 hours (Heizenroth, 2007). Atten-tion must be paid to the tightness of straps on extremities, the time the patient is in the lithotomy position, and the padding and support for legs positioned in stirrups (Heizenroth, 2007). Fasciotomy is the definitive treatment to release the constricted compartments; if untreated, this syndrome progresses to tissue necrosis and acute renal failure; amputation and death may occur (Seibert, 2009).

Nervous System

The nervous system is composed of two compartments. The central nervous system (CNS), which includes the brain and spinal cord, is the largest part of the nervous system. The peripheral nervous system (PNS) includes the collective nervous structures that do not lie within the CNS. Depression of the nervous system occurs with the administration of anesthetic and other agents; the degree of depression is dependent upon the level of general anesthesia or the type of regional anesthesia (Heizenroth, 2007). When nervous system depression occurs, the body's command system becomes either totally or partially ineffective. Thus, compensatory reactions to changes in physical status no longer respond normally, physiologic adaptive mechanisms are altered, and the stresses of positioning are not automatically compensated (Heizenroth, 2007).

Peripheral neuropathies are common positioning injuries. The brachial plexus is one of the most susceptible and common sites for nerve injuries in almost every surgical position. Its course along the axilla is superficial, and it is easily stretched if the arms are abducted greater than 90 degrees; this is exaggerated if the head is turned to the opposite side (Figure 1-1). The individual nerves of the brachial plexus may be injured when the pressure points at the elbows and wrists are inadequately padded and secured. A poorly cushioned arm can be the cause of compression injury from the sharp edges on the sides of the OR bed.

Brachial plexus injuries are also associated with positioning devices. For example, injuries have been caused by improper placement of shoulder braces or damaged armboards falling off the OR bed (Seibert, 2009). In addition, sternal retraction during cardiac surgery has been implicated as a cause of brachial plexus

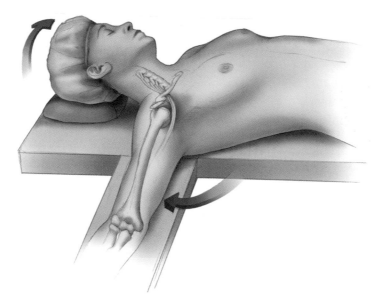

Figure 1-1

Stretching the brachial plexus.

Source: Adapted by M. Borman from Rothrock, J.C. (Ed.). (1999). *The RN First Assistant: An expanded perioperative nursing role* (3rd ed., Fig. 7-3, p. 161). Philadelphia: Lippincott.

injury. Spreading of the sternal retractor leads to pinching of the brachial plexus between the clavicle, which is moved posteriorly, and first rib, which is rotated upward (Seibert, 2009).

Nerves to lower extremities can also be injured by inadequate padding and incorrect positioning. Stretching of the sciatic nerve or direct compression of the common peroneal nerve (at the head of the fibula) against leg supports used in the lithotomy position can easily occur.

Spinal cord injuries, including quadriplegia and paraplegia, are complications of aortic, vascular and thoracic procedures in which the potential for interruption of the blood supply to the spinal cord exists. In rare circumstances, hemiparesis and quadriplegia are associated with surgical procedures performed in the sitting and prone positions (Seibert, 2009).

In order to minimize the risk of injury to the nervous system, safety measures taken by the perioperative team should include but not be limited to the following (AORN, 2009a):

- Attach padded arm boards to the OR bed or procedure bed at less than a 90-degree angle for patients in the supine position.
- Place the palms facing up and extend the fingers when the patient's arms are placed on the arm boards.
- Place the patient's arms in a neutral position when they are placed at the side of the body (i.e., elbows slightly flexed, wrist in a neutral position, palms facing inward).
- Keep patient shoulder abduction and lateral rotation to a minimum.
- Prevent the patient's extremities from dropping below the level of the OR bed.
- Place the patient's head in a neutral position, if not contraindicated by the surgical procedure or any physical limitations of the patient.
- Adequately pad the saphenous, sciatic, and peroneal nerves, particularly when the patient is in a lithotomy or lateral position.
- Place a well-padded perineal post against the perineum between the genitalia and uninjured leg when the patient is positioned on a fracture table.

Respiratory System

Both positioning and anesthesia alter respiratory function. In the alert patient, contraction of the diaphragm and intercostal muscles during spontaneous respiration causes expansion of the thoracic cavity in both anterior-posterior and lateral directions (Seibert, 2009). Gravitational factors affect the distribution of ventilation and perfusion within the lung, the shape of the thoracic cavity, and the movement of the diaphragm and abdominal contents.

In almost every surgical position (except modified sitting and reverse Trendelenburg), the abdominal viscera are shifted upward toward the diaphragm. Consequently, the diaphragm shifts upward and outward, which significantly reduces tidal volume; patients who are obese, pregnant, or have pulmonary disease have additional respiratory compromise in these positions (Heizenroth, 2007). Changes in the patient's posture can significantly affect chest wall compliance and lung volumes, as well as the distribution of ventilation and pulmonary blood flow. In addition, positioning devices may cause mechanical interference with the movement of the chest wall, diaphragm, belly wall, and abdominal contents (Seibert, 2009).

Positional changes that result in redistribution of ventilation and perfusion are least in the sitting position and greatest in the prone and lateral positions (Seibert, 2009). Adult patients can experience a decrease in functional residual capacity (FRC) by 0.5 to 1.0 liters when placed in the supine position. In patients with compromised pulmonary function caused by obstructive or restrictive disease, this can result in a decrease in pulmonary reserve. If the patient is placed in a Trendelenburg position, the abdominal contents move cephalad against the diaphragm, further altering the ventilation/perfusion (V/Q) relationship (Seibert, 2009).

In order to minimize respiratory compromise and keep external chest movement as unrestricted as possible, the surgical team should take the following measures (Heizenroth, 2007):

- Avoid or time-limit the placement of the patient's arms across his or her chest.
- Ensure that straps or tape around the chest area (if required to secure the patient to the OR bed and do not obstruct the surgical site) are not excessively tight.
- Monitor the respiratory status closely with pulse oximetry and arterial blood gas (as needed).

Airway complications that may occur in various surgical positions in the anesthetized patient include endotracheal tube (ETT) displacement, airway edema, and passive regurgitation (Seibert, 2009). When the patient is moved or turned, the ETT may become dislodged, disconnected, or kinked. Widespread edema of the face, tongue, and oropharyngeal structures may occur in the prone, sitting, and head-down positions. The risk for aspiration is increased for patients in the Trendelenburg position because gastric pressure is increased and secretions can accumulate in the oropharynx and nasopharynx (Seibert, 2009).

Other Susceptible Structures

In addition to the major systems discussed above, other anatomic structures are vulnerable to injury and must be protected during positioning (Heizenroth, 2007):

- Breasts: when a female patient is in the prone position, the breasts are compressed between the body weight and the OR bed or chest supports. The medial borders of the breasts can be stretched or injured if the breasts are displaced laterally. Perioperative personnel can place soft ventral supports on the lateral sides of the breasts to reduce the risk of injury.

- Eyes: injuries to the eyes during positioning and surgery can range from corneal abrasions to blindness, as the eyes do not always close during anesthesia and may therefore be susceptible to abrasions from various factors in the OR environment (e.g., sheets, intravenous lines, or drapes). The eyes of unconscious patients should be taped shut; eye shields can be used to provide additional protection. Lacrilube may also be placed in the eyes for corneal protection. In addition, the eyes should be checked to verify that they are not under pressure when the face is in a dependent position (e.g., when the patient is in the prone or lateral position). Contact lenses should be removed preoperatively (even if the lenses are 'extended wear' lenses) in order to reduce the risk of corneal abrasion.

- Fingers: the patient's fingers are at risk for injury during positioning (e.g., when the arms are tucked at the patient's side). The fingers should be straightened with palms facing the patient's body; if the fingers are curled, pressure is exerted on the finger joints, and the fingernails can press into other fingers or body areas. Scissoring injuries to fingers at the leg section of the OR bed, when the patient is in the lithotomy position, can be avoided by wrapping the fingers in towels or having the arms abducted on arm boards at an angle less than 90 degrees. In addition, perioperative team members should never raise the leg section of the OR bed unless the fingers are visualized and secured away from the leg section hinge.

- Genitalia: in certain positions, crushing injuries to the genitalia may occur (e.g., male genitalia can become compressed between the pelvis and frame when in the prone position in a laminectomy frame). Extreme care must be taken to check and prevent compression of male genitalia by adequately padding the post in order to prevent injuries due to extreme pressure.

POSITIONING EQUIPMENT AND ACCESSORIES

Every surgical suite has its own routine supplies and devices that are used for positioning (Table 1-3); these should be clean, in good repair, and used only by personnel who are knowledgeable in the mechanics of the equipment and have demonstrated competency in its use (Spry, 2005). The OR bed may be designed specifically for general, minor, or specialty procedures; all beds have multiple parts and specific functions (Spry, 2005). The OR bed support surface is one of the most consistent and important positioning devices. The material used for the OR bed mattress cover helps prevent pressure ulcers; the traditional firm vinyl covering negates some of the pressure-reducing effect of the foam and has a greater hammock effect. This tough outer cover further reduces the cushioning potential of the mattress and can result in increased pressure and shearing forces. Softer, more pliable covers can provide improved pressure reduction. OR bed cover material should be durable, impervious to moisture and microorganisms, and easily cleaned (Spry, 2005).

TABLE 1-3   Positioning Equipment and Accessories

Equipment	Accessories
Headrests	Blankets, sheets
Anesthesia screen	Donut
Padded armboards	Pillows
Shoulder braces	Sandbags
Kidney braces (lateral positioner)	Surgical vacuum positioning system
Leg stirrups • Candy cane or sling • Knee-crutch • Boot-type	Padding • Sheepskin • Foam • Felt • Cotton • Contoured silicone gel
OR bed safety strap	Tape
Arm straps	Eye pads or shields
Footboard	Pressure-minimizing mattress

OR bed attachments are designed to hold the body part stationary and to facilitate exposure during the procedure; typical OR bed attachments include the following (Phillips, 2007; Spry, 2005):

- Headrests: padded headrests are used for the supine, prone, sitting, or lateral positions. They hold the head securely, but without the pressure that could cause pressure injury to the ears or eyes. Headrests may be shaped like a donut or horseshoe for head and neck procedures; others are flat or concave to stabilize the head and neck in alignment. Nonpadded metal headrests have sterile skull pins that are placed in the patient's head for neurological procedures.
- Anesthesia screen: a metal bar attaches to the head of the OR bed and holds the drapes from the patient's face. It is placed after induction of anesthesia and positioning and is used to separate the nonsterile from the sterile areas at the head of the bed.
- Padded armboards: armboards are used to support the arms if intravenous fluids are being infused, if the arm or hand is the operative site, if the arm placed at the patient's side would interfere with access to the operative site, if space on the OR bed is inadequate to place the arm at the side, or if the arm requires support (e.g., in the lateral position). The armboard is padded to a height level with the OR bed. The patient's arm should be placed palm up, except when the patient is in the prone position, to prevent ulnar nerve pressure and abnormal shoulder rotation. The armboard should never be abducted beyond a 90-degree angle from the shoulder in order to prevent brachial nerve plexus injury from hyperabduction. An armboard with a self-locking mechanism is safest in order to prevent displacement.
- Shoulder braces: shoulder braces or supports are well-padded, adjustable concave metal supports used to prevent the patient from slipping when the head of the OR bed is tilted downward. Braces should be placed over the acromion processes, not over the muscle and soft tissues near the neck. They should be equidistant from the head of the OR bed, with a 1/2-inch (13-mm) space between the shoulders and braces to eliminate pressure against the shoulder. To prevent nerve compression, a shoulder brace should not be used when the arm is extended on an armboard.
- Kidney braces (lateral positioner): kidney braces are also concave metal supports with grooved notches at the base. They are placed under the mattress on the body elevation flexion component of the OR bed and slipped in from the edge of the bed snugly against the body for lateral stability in

the side-lying position. Although the kidney brace is padded, care should be taken so that its upper edge is not pressing too tightly against the body.

- Leg stirrups: metal stirrups are placed in holders on each side of the OR bed to support the legs and feet while in the lithotomy position. Stirrups are available as candy cane or sling stirrups, which have a canvas loop that suspends the legs at right angles to the feet; knee-crutch stirrups, which are special leg holders that can be adjusted for knee flexion and extension; or boot-type stirrups. Knee-crutch stirrups, even if well-padded, can cause some pressure on the back of the knees and lower extremities and may endanger the popliteal blood vessels and nerves. Gel and foam pads may be used for protection when these stirrups are used.
- OR bed safety strap: a wide, sturdy strap composed of a durable material (i.e., conductive rubber, nylon webbing) is placed and secured over the patient's thighs, above the knees, and around the surface of the OR bed in order to restrain leg movement for surgical procedures, except in certain positions. A blanket or other padding should be placed between the patient's skin and the strap. The strap should be placed over, not under, this padding for visualization prior to prepping and draping.
- Arm straps: narrow straps at least 1 1/2 inches (3.8 cm) wide should be placed around the wrists, without pressure, to secure the arms to the armboards. Intravenous lines and other monitoring wires should not be kinked or dislodged by the strap.
- Footboard: a metal footboard can be used as a horizontal extension of the OR bed or raised perpendicular to the OR bed to support the feet. The footboard is padded when the patient is in the reverse Trendelenburg position.

In addition to the OR bed accessories, various positioning accessories are often required in order to achieve certain positions and provide patient comfort; these include (Phillips, 2007; Spry, 2005):

- Blankets and sheets used for patient warmth, to form rolls and bolsters, and as a draw sheet to serve as a patient lift and/or to secure the patient's arms at his or her sides.
- Donut is used as a headrest or to protect the ears and nerves of the head and face. It is composed of foam, contoured silicone gel, or sometimes made from towels. If properly sized, donuts can be used to protect the knees and heels.
- Pillows are used to support and elevate body parts.
- Sandbags are used for immobilization.

- Surgical vacuum positioning system is a waterproof pillow filled with small plastic beads. The patient is first positioned with the beanbag molded to the position; the beanbag is then attached to suction, which withdraws the air from inside the pillow. The beanbag subsequently becomes rigid and maintains the shape to which it was molded.
- Padding may be made of sheepskin, foam, felt, cotton, or contoured silicone gel and is available in various sizes and shapes. Padding is used to protect bony prominences and pressure areas such as elbows, knees, and heels.
- Tape may be used to secure the patient or an extremity in a flexed position. Tape may also be used to securely close the eyelids.
- Eye pads or shields may be used to protect the eyes and maintain them in a closed position.
- Pressure-minimizing mattress may be placed on the OR bed to minimize the pressure over bony prominences, peripheral blood vessels, and nerves during prolonged surgical procedures (i.e., over 2 hours for the average patient; less for a debilitated patient). The pressure-minimizing mattress may be a positive-pressure air mattress, a circulating-water thermal mattress, a foam-rubber mattress with indentations similar to an egg crate, a gel pad, or a dry polymer pad. The manufacturer's instructions should be followed when using any of these devices.

SURGICAL POSITIONS

The intraoperative positions used most frequently are supine, Trendelenburg/reverse Trendelenburg, lithotomy, prone, lateral decubitus, and sitting. A review of these positions, including the related physiological considerations and interventions for patient safety, is presented below.

Supine Position

The supine position is the most commonly used position for procedures on the abdomen, head, neck, extremities, and chest because it allows optimal exposure (Seibert, 2009). In the supine position, also known as the dorsal recumbent position, the patient is positioned lying on his or her back with the head maintained in a neutral position on a small pillow, pad, or donut. The arms are extended on padded armboards and abducted less than 90 degrees in order to prevent injury to the brachial plexus (Figure 1-2). Proper padding at the head improves patient comfort by preventing hyperextension or hyperflexion of the neck, as well as pressure on the occiput. To prevent brachial plexus stretch, the head should not be turned laterally when the arms are abducted on armboards (Seibert, 2009). Rolls

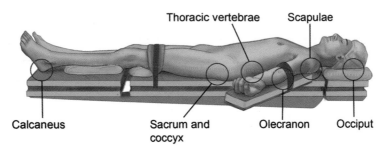

Figure 1-2

Supine position with arms extended.

Source: Courtesy of Phippen, M.L., Ulmer, B.C., & Wells, M.P. (2009). *Competency for safe patient care during operative and invasive procedures* (Fig. 8.2, p. 192). Denver: CCI.

placed under the shoulders may be requested by some surgeons to elevate the thorax for better exposure of the thoracic structures.

Unless it is necessary for surgical reasons, the patient's arms should not be tucked at his or her sides when in the supine position (AORN, 2009a). If there are surgical reasons to tuck the patient's arms at the side with the use of a draw sheet, the sheet should extend above the elbows and be tucked between the patient and the OR bed mattress (AORN, 2009a). If the arms are tucked at the sides, the patient's fingers should be checked to prevent any damage that can be caused by catching them in any part of the OR bed. The fingers should remain in a neutral position (i.e., not hyperflexed or extended). The fingers of each hand may be placed around a hand roll and the hand covered with soft wrapping to maintain the position of the fingers.

Care should be taken to see that the wrists are also in a neutral position. In patients with radial artery blood pressure lines, the FA should ensure that the arterial pressure waveform has not been damped. If the pressure tracing does not illustrate a clear biphasic pattern, the FA or the anesthesia provider should readjust the wrist to improve the pressure tracing. The elbows must be evaluated to determine whether padding is necessary to prevent ulnar nerve compression between the ulnar groove and the side of the OR bed or arm boards.

The FA should ensure that the pressure points from head to toe are well padded. Some patients may need a pillow placed under the knees, slightly flexing the hips and knees to improve the level of comfort. This position is more physiologically neutral and takes extension stress off the knees. The heels are a source of pressure discomfort due to their bony prominences pressing against the operating bed. Damage to the skin and pain at the heel postoperatively can be prevented by the use of foam rubber (egg crate) or other padding. The longer the procedure, the greater is the propensity for problems to arise.

In the supine position, gravity has minimal effects on circulation. Little arterial perfusion gradient is present for the upper or lower part of the body. Venous return to the heart is enhanced by chest excursion during respiration. However, administration of general anesthesia with muscle relaxants inhibits excursion of the diaphragm. In the supine position, the abdominal contents then move cephalad, pressing against the diaphragm and further decreasing functional residual capacity (FRC). Relaxed chest wall muscles are overcome by the elastic recoil of the lungs, further reducing lung volumes. Positive-pressure ventilation partially reverses and improves this picture to decrease the ventilation/perfusion (V/Q) mismatch.

Trendelenburg Position

The Trendelenburg position is a variation of the supine position, with the patient's body tilted head-down (**Figure 1-3**). This position is used during abdominal surgery to improve surgical access to the lower abdominal viscera; this is accomplished with the help of gravity pulling the abdominal contents cephalad. The Trendelenburg position has also been used to increase blood pressure in cases of volume depletion by increasing central blood volume. Patients receiving spinal or epidural anesthesia are prone to sympathectomy and vasodilation, which cause an abrupt decrease in blood pressure. This problem can be minimized with volume repletion, vasoconstriction, and placement in the Trendelenburg position.

The Trendelenburg positioning can also help facilitate the placement of a central line by increasing central venous pressure (CVP). Increased CVP helps to distend the veins to provide an easier target for the initial venipuncture. The Trendelenburg position helps to decrease bleeding at the site of surgery; arterial and venous pressures are decreased by gravity's effect on blood. As the angle of the Trendelenburg

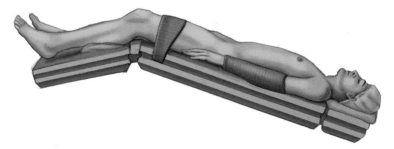

Figure 1-3

Trendelenburg position with knees flexed.

Source: Courtesy of Phippen, M.L., Ulmer, B.C., & Wells, M.P. (2009). *Competency for safe patient care during operative and invasive procedures* (Fig. 8.3, p. 194). Denver: CCI.

position increases, the gravitational effect increases correspondingly, as does the gradient imposed on blood flow.

All pressure points must be protected as for the patient in the supine position. The OR bed is tilted head down, with a 10- to 15-degree head-down tilt, rather than a steep tilt. In the Trendelenburg position, excessive pressure on the clavicle can compress the brachial plexus as it exits the thorax between the clavicle and first rib; therefore shoulder braces should not be used (AORN, 2009a). The arms are vulnerable to injury in the Trendelenburg position, especially if they are positioned on armboards and inadequately restrained, as they can slip off, hyperextend, and abduct above the level of the shoulder, thereby stretching the plexus (Seibert, 2009). Angling the bed downward at the knees and placing a well-padded ankle or chest restraint will maintain the patient in the tilt position without the use of shoulder braces as long as the flexed knee joint is sufficiently caudad of the leg-thigh hinge on the OR bed. This prevents the adjacent firm edge of the depressed leg section of the OR bed from indenting the patient's calf.

Pulmonary mechanics and the V/Q relationship are altered greatly in this position. Abdominal contents pressing against the diaphragm at the base of the lungs decrease FRC and increase the work of breathing in a spontaneously ventilating patient. Under general anesthesia, increased positive inspiratory pressures are required during mechanical ventilation to maintain adequate tidal volume. Blood flow to the head is also increased, raising intracranial pressure. In patients with preexisting intracranial pathology, limited surgical time will help prevent positional sequelae. The aim is to minimize the cerebral edema that can be caused by extended placement in the head-down position.

Reverse Trendelenburg Position

The reverse Trendelenburg position is another variation of the supine position, in which the patient's head is tilted up. It is the opposite of the Trendelenburg position (Figure 1-4). This position is common for laparoscopic procedures of the upper abdomen, where abdominal contents impede visualization of the surgical site. All pressure point considerations are the same, and the patient must be secured on the operating bed by a lightly placed, well-padded restraint across the chest and the use of a padded footboard.

Blood flow to the head is decreased, as are central venous pressure and venous return to the heart. As previously noted, compressive antiembolic stockings or sequential compressive devices may be used to minimize pooling of blood in the lower extremities and the potential for DVT.

In the reverse Trendelenburg position, gravity pulls the abdominal contents away from the diaphragm and helps to improve FRC. Under general anesthesia,

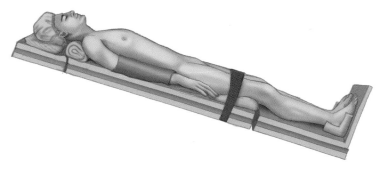

Figure 1-4

Reverse Trendelenburg position.

Source: Courtesy of Phippen, M.L., Ulmer, B.C., & Wells, M.P. (2009). *Competency for safe patient care during operative and invasive procedures* (Fig. 8.4, p. 196). Denver: CCI.

positive inspiratory pressures generated by the ventilator are decreased. Ventilation/perfusion relationships are closer to normal, preferentially increasing blood flow and ventilation to the base of the lungs.

Lithotomy Position

In the lithotomy position, the patient is supine with the legs elevated and flexed at both the hips and the knees (Figure 1-5). The legs are separated to provide surgical access to the perineum. This position is used for portions of colorectal surgery, urological procedures, gynecological procedures, and obstetrics.

Peripheral nerve damage is one of the complications that may occur perioperatively due to placement of the patient in this position. The sciatic nerve can be overly stretched when flexion at the hip is exaggerated and combined with flexion at the knees and external rotation. This is manifested by sensory and motor deficits in the distal lower extremities below the knees. The sciatic nerve bifurcates laterally at the head of the fibula giving rise to the common peroneal and tibial nerves. The common peroneal nerve can be damaged by compression against leg supports that are placed lateral to the knee. Common peroneal nerve damage is manifested by foot drop. The femoral nerve, which supplies motor innervation to the anterior femoral muscles, can be damaged by hyperflexion at the hip. This can be seen when the patient loses the ability to extend at the knee or flex at the hip. Damage to its articular branches may cause sensory loss to the anteromedial portion of the distal lower extremity (the calf). Obturator nerve damage due to hyperflexion at the hip can cause deficits in abduction of the flexed thigh and lateral rotation of the extended thigh. The saphenous nerves need to be protected by adequate padding placed between the distal lower extremity and the stirrups. Sensory deficits will be obvious at points of contact on the leg where nerve compression has occurred against medially placed leg supports.

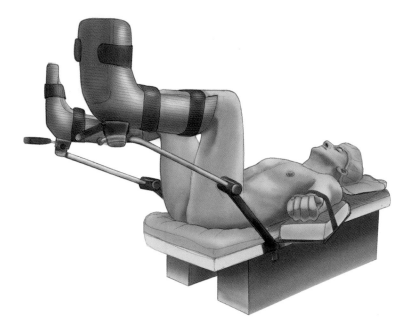

Figure 1-5

Lithotomy position using boot-type stirrups.

Source: Courtesy of Phippen, M.L., Ulmer, B.C., & Wells, M.P. (2009). *Competency for safe patient care during operative and invasive procedures* (Fig. 8.6, p. 198). Denver: CCI.

As in the supine position, FRC is reduced in the lithotomy position. The abdominal contents are compressed when the lithotomy position requires the thighs to be flexed onto the trunk for surgical access to the retropubic space. Diaphragmatic excursion is inhibited and pulmonary compliance is decreased, contributing to any V/Q mismatch that may already exist. Under these circumstances, the patient is usually under general anesthesia and receiving positive-pressure ventilation through a cuffed endotracheal tube (ETT).

Raising and lowering the legs alters hemodynamic status by shifting the blood volume through the effects of gravity. As the legs are raised, venous blood is preferentially shifted to the central core, which increases venous return to the heart. Conversely, as the legs are lowered at the end of the procedure, blood shifts from the central core back to the legs. Hypotension can result in patients who are volume depleted. Volume repletion, vasoconstrictors, and a slow change in position back to supine can minimize this effect.

To reduce the risk of injury when placing a patient in the lithotomy position, the perioperative team should implement the following measures (AORN, 2009a):

- Place stirrups at an even height.
- Position the patient's buttocks even with the lower break of the OR bed in a manner that securely supports the sacrum on the bed surface; confirm proper positioning before the start of the procedure.
- Move the patient's legs slowly and simultaneously into the leg holders to prevent lumbosacral strain.
- Remove the patient's legs from the stirrups slowly and bring them together simultaneously before lowering them to the surface of the OR bed.
- Place the patient's arms on padded armboards, extended less than 90 degrees from the long axis of the OR bed, with the palms facing up and gently secured. Tuck the patient's arms at the sides only if surgically necessary; when necessary to tuck the arms, the elbows should be padded, and the palms should be facing toward the patient's body; the hands should be enclosed and secured with a foam protector.
- Protect the patient's fingers from injury when repositioning the foot of the OR bed.
- Place the patient's heels in the lowest possible position.
- Provide support over the largest surface area of the leg possible.
- Ensure that the patient's legs are not resting against the stirrup posts.
- Ensure that scrubbed personnel are not leaning against the patient's thighs.
- Maintain the lithotomy position for the shortest time period possible.
- Exercise care to avoid shearing when moving the patient to the break in the OR bed during repositioning.

Prone Position

The prone position, in which the patient lies face and chest down on the OR bed, is used for any surgical procedure performed on the dorsal aspect of the body (Figure 1-6). Under general anesthesia, the patient is intubated and the airway is secured while the patient is in the supine position (usually on the transport vehicle). The anesthesia provider remains at the head of the patient, maintaining control of the airway. Other members of the team are positioned at the thorax, hips, and legs, and the transport vehicle is locked in place. Before positioning the patient, all lines, catheters, drains, and tubes (i.e., intravenous, arterial, other monitors) must be freed to prevent tangling. As the patient is turned, the lines should be free and accessible for use by the anesthesia provider. The patient is then slowly turned to the prone position in a coordinated, controlled manner, as directed by

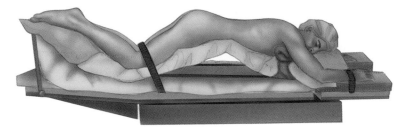

Figure 1-6

Prone position.

Source: Courtesy of Phippen, M.L., Ulmer, B.C., & Wells, M.P. (2009). *Competency for safe patient care during operative and invasive procedures* (Fig. 8.8, p. 203). Denver: CCI.

the anesthesia provider. As the patient is rolled over, he or she is simultaneously received on the far side of the bed. The FA, in collaboration with the anesthesia provider, confirms that all monitoring lines and drainage tubes (e.g., urinary or chest catheters) are intact, secure, and functioning.

Once the patient is prone, many things occur simultaneously. The first, and most important concern, is protecting the airway. To determine that the ETT is still in place and secure, bilateral breath sounds must be auscultated, and a positive end-tidal CO_2 must appear on the capnometer. The patient must then be secured to the OR bed with a gluteal safety restraint. As this is being attended to, the other team members place chest rolls on both sides of the patient that extend from the shoulders to the hips. A pillow may also be placed under the pelvis to allow improved motion of the abdomen and anterior chest wall, improving FRC and pulmonary mechanics. In this position, the viscera can push the diaphragm in an uphill direction. Abdominal contents that may otherwise compress mesenteric and paravertebral vessels are allowed to move more freely, decreasing pressure on the inferior vena cava. Increased intra-abdominal pressure can cause increased intraoperative bleeding.

This position poses many challenges for the surgical team. Pressure point padding and improvement in physiological parameters must be attended to before proceeding with the surgical procedure. General safety interventions when placing the patient in the prone position include, but are not limited to (AORN, 2009a):

- Utilize four caregivers to transfer the patient from the supine to the prone position; one anesthesia provider should maintain the patient's airway and support the patient's head while the other caregivers move the patient's trunk and extremities. Additional caregivers may be required with heavier patients.
- Maintain the patient's cervical neck alignment.

- Provide protection for the patient's forehead, eyes, and chin.
- Use a padded headrest to provide access to the patient's airway.
- Use chest rolls from the clavicle to the iliac crest to allow chest movement and decrease abdominal pressure.
- Place the patient's arms down by his or her sides and safely secure them with the palms of the hands facing in toward the thighs, the elbows and hands protected with padding, and the hands and wrists maintained in anatomical alignment. If this is not possible, place each arm on an armboard with the arms abducted to less than 90 degrees, elbows flexed, and the palms facing downward.
- Position breasts and male genitalia in a way that frees them from torsion or pressure.
- Position the patient's toes so that they hang over the end of the OR bed or are elevated off the bed by placing padding under the patient's shins so that the shins are high enough to avoid pressure on the tips of the toes.

It must be emphasized that close attention must be given to the patient's airway in the prone position. If the ETT becomes dislodged and comes out, it is virtually impossible to reintubate. The patient would have to be placed in either the lateral or supine position emergently in order to resecure the airway.

At the end of the surgical procedure but prior to extubation, the sequence of events may occur in reverse. All lines and monitors are freed and accessible. The ETT is checked and the airway controlled by the anesthesia provider, who directs the placement of the patient into the supine position from the OR bed to the locked transport vehicle. Surgical team members are on both sides of the thorax and hips; another team member is at the feet. The patient is then carefully rolled in a coordinated fashion to the person on the far side of the locked transport vehicle, who accepts the patient. The airway is reconnected to the ventilator and bilateral breath sounds are auscultated. All pressure points are simultaneously checked. The patient may be extubated at this point if extubation criteria are met and then transported to the postanesthesia care unit (PACU).

Lateral Decubitus Position

The lateral decubitus position is used for procedures on the chest or kidneys when the supine position cannot provide sufficient lateral or posterior-lateral exposure. It can also be used for procedures that require access to the lateral or posterior spine or cranium (Seibert, 2009). In the lateral decubitus position the patient's left or right side is down (**Figure 1-7**). The position is designated by which side is down and flush against the OR bed (i.e., left or right lateral decubitus position).

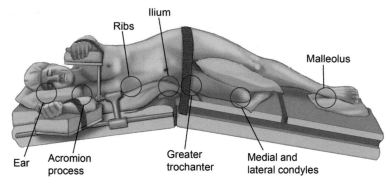

Figure 1-7

Lateral decubitus position.

Source: Courtesy of Phippen, M.L., Ulmer, B.C., & Wells, M.P. (2009). *Competency for safe patient care during operative and invasive procedures* (Fig. 8.7, p. 201). Denver: CCI.

As in all other positions, precautions must be taken to minimize pressure point compression and physiological changes that could compromise the patient's hemo-dynamic status and postoperative outcomes.

After safe anesthesia induction, the first challenge to the surgical team is to safely and properly reposition the supine patient. All team members work together under the direction of the anesthesia provider, who maintains the airway and controls the patient's head. Team members assume positions on both sides of the patient, while another person controls the legs. One team member should place an arm under the patient's thorax while another simultaneously places an arm under the hips and thighs. With the legs also controlled at the ankle, the patient is first positioned on command to the supine position, with the prospective dependent side brought to the midline of the OR bed. The next step is to gently roll the patient into the lateral decubitus posi-tion, with the side at the bed's midline becoming the dependent side. This is also done on command as a coordinated effort. At this time, the patient's airway is immediately checked for patency and resecured if necessary. The head is supported on a headrest or pillow to prevent undue flexion, extension, or side bending in either direction; the cervical spine should be aligned with the thoracic spine. The patient's dependent ear should be padded well and assessed to ensure that it is not folded. The arms are placed at an angle less than 90 degrees anterior to the patient and flexed at the elbow to pre-vent stretching and subsequent damage to the brachial plexus. The nondependent arm may be supported by an arm support that attaches to the bed or a padded Mayo stand. Either device must be sufficiently padded to prevent injury to the skin or ulnar nerve at the elbow. The dependent arm must also be protected with padding at the elbow to prevent compression of the lateral epicondyle against the operating bed.

An axillary roll is placed at the dependent axilla while two team members are positioned on both sides of the patient, gently lifting the thorax. As the airway is being securely held by the anesthesia provider, the axillary roll is placed by the fourth team member. The axillary roll slightly elevates the thorax and enhances excursion of the chest wall and also minimizes compression on the axillary artery. It also decreases pressure and compression at the shoulder and the proximal humerus. A check of the radial pulse in the dependent arm will help determine if compression of the axillary artery has been alleviated.

The legs should be slightly flexed at the hips and knees with a pillow placed between the knees and ankles. The greater trochanter in the dependent femur and the head of the fibula in the dependent lower extremity must be padded adequately to prevent pressure necrosis of the skin and nerve damage. Damage to the common peroneal nerve, which bifurcates at the head of the fibula, causes foot drop (i.e., the inability to dorsiflex the foot at the ankle). Egg crate foam rubber is commonly used for padding of dependent portions of the body.

The patient must be secured to the OR bed with restraints placed across the hips or thighs. Positioning is also maintained with the use of a beanbag device, which is placed on the OR bed prior to the patient's transfer. After the patient is positioned, the beanbag is formed around the patient and suctioned through a special port to retain its molded position around the patient. Because the addition of a beanbag adds height to the bed, care must be taken to ensure that the height of the locked transport vehicle is the same, to facilitate safe patient transfer.

The lateral decubitus position may or may not alter hemodynamic status. If the patient placed in the lateral position is on a level OR bed parallel to the floor, there will be few hemodynamic changes due to positioning. Very few (if any) hemodynamic pressure gradients exist along the length of the body in the long axis. It is important, though, to place pneumatic or compression stockings on the lower extremities to minimize venous pooling. When the kidney rest is raised for urological procedures (e.g., radical nephrectomy), the body is also flexed laterally, which may cause increased pooling of blood in the legs. This causes decreased venous return to the heart and may reduce cardiac output. Therefore, these patients must also have elastic or pneumatic stockings placed on the lower extremities to decrease venous stasis and pooling and to improve venous return to the heart. Lateral flexion can decrease venous return through the inferior vena cava.

Pulmonary relationships and mechanics are altered with the patient in the lateral decubitus position. The dependent hemithorax compresses the lung on that side, decreasing FRC and chest wall compliance. At the same time, mediastinal structures under the influence of gravity further decrease dependent lung volumes. Abdominal viscera press against the diaphragm in a cephalad direction, adding to compression of the lungs. This is a greater concern in mechanically ventilated patients than in spontaneously ventilating patients, whose diaphragmatic movement improves the V/Q relationship.

Gravity effects on pulmonary blood flow preferentially favor the dependent (down side) lung. Less blood flows to the nondependent lung, which is enclosed in the less restricted upper hemithorax. Chest wall compliance of the nondependent (upper) hemithorax is therefore better, allowing more unrestricted mechanical ventilation. Ventilation/perfusion mismatch is magnified by a well-perfused dependent lung that is underventilated and an upper, nondependent lung that is better ventilated with decreased pulmonary blood flow. This is most apparent in patients with pulmonary pathology, particularly those presenting for thoracotomy and subsequent lobe resections or pneumonectomies. Restraining straps should not be placed across the chest wall during nonpulmonary surgery because this can hinder thoracic expansion, contributing to hypoventilation and hypoxemia.

Sitting Position

The term "sitting position" generally refers to any position in which the patient's torso is elevated from the supine position and is higher than the legs. The degree of elevation of the head above the heart can vary greatly, depending on the surgical procedure (Seibert, 2009):

- A true sitting position is one in which the torso is elevated at 90 degrees to the legs.
- A modified sitting position is one in which the torso is elevated 45 degrees, the head is flexed, and the legs are flexed and elevated at the level of the heart. This position is most familiar to the OR team and is also called the lounging, lawn chair, or beach chair position.

Physiologically, gravity's effect on blood flow to the brain occurs by increasing the gradient against which blood must flow. As the sitting angle is increased, the gradient increases. Blood tends to pool in the lower extremities as it shifts away from the head. Baroreceptors in the carotid sinus and aortic arch sense the gravity-mediated shift of intravascular volume from the upper body and act to mediate a sympathetic increase in vascular tone while simultaneously inhibiting parasympathetic response. Venous return to the heart decreases, as does cardiac output, despite an increase in heart rate. Cardiac dysrhythmias (e.g., tachycardia, bradycardia, premature ventricular contractions) are possible during surgery, secondary to retraction on the cranial nerves. If dysrhythmia occurs, the surgeon must be notified, and the dysrhythmia must be treated.

Pulmonary mechanics are more normal in this position than in others. In the sitting position, gravity pulls the abdominal viscera downward, allowing improved excursion of the diaphragm. FRC increases, improving the V/Q relationship at the base of the lungs.

Induction of general anesthesia is conducted in the supine position and the airway is secured once the position of the ETT is confirmed. The position of the patient is then slowly changed to the head-up, sitting position in a controlled, coordinated manner with the anesthesia staff directing the action. All pressure points must be identified and adequately padded. The head is usually placed in head pins in a cervical head holder that is secured to the sides of the operating bed with clamps (Figure 1-8). Padding is placed between the lower thoracic and lumbar spine, adding support to the patient at the lordotic curve. Padding is also placed under the buttocks and the plantar surfaces of the feet, which are placed against a well-padded foot rest to prevent the patient from sliding down during the surgery. The knees are slightly flexed, and the legs are placed roughly at the level of the heart. Arms should be placed across the abdomen with pads under the elbows, which rest against the back of the bed. The torso should be secured with a restraining strap.

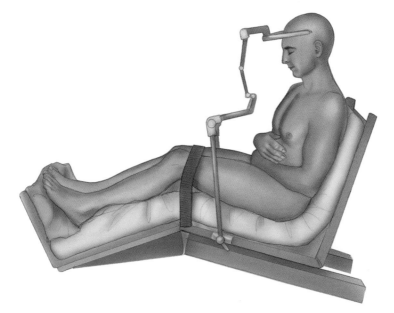

Figure 1-8

Sitting position with cervical head holder.

Source: Courtesy of Phippen, M.L., Ulmer, B.C., & Wells, M.P. (2009). *Competency for safe patient care during operative and invasive procedures* (Fig. 8.9, p. 207). Denver: CCI.

Extremities at the joints should be in as neutral a position as possible to prevent injury from hyperflexion or hyperextension. Pneumatic or compression stockings should be applied to minimize venous pooling and stasis. Use of these stockings also improves venous return to the heart and therefore cardiac output. When all these maneuvers have been completed, a final reexamination of the patient's airway, position, padding, monitors, and intravenous lines should be conducted to ensure patient safety and accessibility for the anesthesia and surgical teams.

For patients undergoing neurosurgery on the posterior fossa, VAE is potentially fatal. If the venous sinuses are opened during the procedure, air can be entrained, leading to eventual circulatory collapse. This is due to the difference between atmospheric pressure and venous pressure at the level of the head in the upright patient. Because atmospheric pressure is greater than venous pressure, air is able to enter the venous sinuses, which are tented open by their attachment to the cranium. The venous sinuses are not collapsible and thus pose a constant threat when the head is elevated above the heart. Air embolism is best monitored with the use of transesophageal echocardiography (TEE) or more commonly by a precordial Doppler monitor that is placed over the right side of the heart to listen for a "millwheel murmur." The FA should review preoperative images to rule out the presence of a cardiac septal defect. Because air can be introduced into the right side of the heart via a central venous pressure line, the air can pass through the defect into the left side of the heart and be ejected into the systemic circulation, potentially embolizing to the brain.

If observation of monitors, unstable hemodynamic status, and a drop in end-tidal carbon dioxide levels suggest an air embolus, the surgeon must be notified immediately. At that time the surgery stops as the surgeon floods the operative site with sterile normal saline solution. The patient is simultaneously lowered to a position in which the head is at least at the level of the heart. Air should be aspirated via a central venous pressure monitor line that is placed at the junction of the superior vena cava and the right atrium prior to the beginning of surgery.

CONCLUSION

Surgical procedures are performed on all parts of the human body, requiring the body to be positioned into various configurations. The optimal position provides the best possible access and exposure to the surgical site, while preventing physiologic compromise. The safety and comfort of the patient must be considered, while focusing on minimizing the risk of injury to major body systems and other vulnerable areas. Positioning is a multidisciplinary task confronted by the surgical team on a daily basis. Through effective teamwork and communication, knowledge of the anatomic and physiologic considerations associated with positioning, and demonstrated competency in the use of positioning equipment and accessories, all members of the surgical team must work together to safely and efficiently position their patients to optimize surgical intervention, while reducing the risk of injury and complications, ultimately promoting positive patient outcomes.

GLOSSARY

Body habitus: physique or body build; the general physical appearance of an individual human body.

Deep vein thrombosis (DVT): development of a thrombus, or clot, in one of the deep veins of the body, usually the iliac or femoral veins or major upper extremity veins. These clots can break off from the vein, travel through the heart, and lodge in the arteries of the lungs, causing a potentially fatal pulmonary embolism (PE).

Ergonomics: practice of designing equipment and work tasks to conform to the capability of the worker; it provides a means for adjusting the work environment and work practices to prevent injuries before they occur.

Friction: force of two surfaces rubbing against one another.

Functional residual capacity (FRC): amount of air remaining in the lungs at the end of a normal expiration.

Ischemia: deficiency of blood in a body part due to constriction or obstruction of a blood vessel.

Pressure: force placed on underlying tissue.

Pulmonary embolism (PE): thrombus that breaks free from a vein, then travels through the veins, reaches the lungs, and lodges in a pulmonary vessel. A PE is a potentially fatal condition; death may result within minutes to hours.

Shear: the folding of underlying tissue when the skeletal structure moves while the skin remains stationary.

Venous air embolism (VAE): entry of gas into the peripheral or central vasculature. VAE results when a pressure gradient favors the entrance of air into the venous system. Upon entry into the venous system, air is transported to the right atrium and ventricle; from there, it has the potential to continue on to the pulmonary arteries where it may cause interference with gas exchange, cardiac arrhythmias, pulmonary hypertension, and even cardiac failure and arrest.

Volatile anesthetics: liquid anesthetics that volatilize to a vapor at room temperature. When inhaled, they are capable of producing general anesthesia.

Work-related musculoskeletal disorders (MSD): conditions that affect muscles, nerves, tendons, ligaments, joints, cartilage, or spinal discs. Work-related musculoskeletal disorders, also referred to as cumulative trauma disorders or repetitive strain injuries, do not include injuries resulting from slips, trips, falls, or similar accidents.

REFERENCES

1. American Nurses Association (ANA). (2003). *ANA launches 'Handle with Care' ergonomics campaign* (9/17/03). Retrieved May 18, 2009 from http://www.nursingworld.org/FunctionalMenu Categories/MediaResources/ PressReleases/2003 /HandleWCarePress-Release.aspx

2. Association of periOperative Registered Nurses (AORN). (2006). *AORN position statement on ergonomically healthy work-place practices.* Retrieved May 18, 2009 from http://www.aorn.org / PracticeResources/AORNPosition Statements/Position_Ergonomics/

3. Association of periOperative Registered Nurses (AORN). (2009a). Recommended practices for positioning the patient in the perioperative practice setting. In *Perioperative standards and recommended practices* (pp. 525–548). Denver: AORN, Inc.

4. Association of periOperative Registered Nurses (AORN). (2009b). Recommended practices for a safe environment of care. In *Perioperative standards and recommended practices* (p. 416). Denver: AORN, Inc.

5. Association of periOperative Registered Nurses (AORN). (2009c). AORN guide-line for prevention of venous stasis. In *Perioperative standards and recommended practices* (pp. 165–182). Denver: AORN, Inc.

6. Beaver, M. (2008). *CMS to put pressure on providers for decubitus ulcer prevention.* Retrieved April 28, 2009, from http://www.infectioncontroltoday.com/articles/decubitus-ulcer-prevention.html

7. Duncan, K.D. (2008). *Preventing pressure ulcers: The goal is zero.* Retrieved April 28, 2009, from http://www.ihi.org/NR/rdonlyres /CCAF8C31-CE3B-46A6-826 -28CBA3D5C087/0/PreventingPres-sureUlcers.pdf

8. Heizenroth, P.A. (2007). Positioning the patient for surgery. In J.C. Rothrock (Ed.), *Alexander's care of the patient in surgery* (13th ed., pp. 131–157). St. Louis: Mosby, Inc.

9. National Institute of Occupational Safety and Health (NIOSH). (2008). *Preventing back injuries in healthcare settings.* Retrieved May 24, 2009 at http://www.cdc.gov /niosh/blog/nsb092208_lifting.html

10. Occupational Safety & Health Administration (OSHA). (2009). *Ergonomics.* Retrieved May 18, 2009 from http://www.osha.gov/SLTC/etools/hospital/hazards/ergo/ergo.html

11. Petersen, C. (2007). Positioning injury. In *Perioperative nursing data set: The perioperative nursing vocabulary* (2nd ed., pp. 43–44). Denver: AORN, Inc.

12. Phillips, N. (2007). Positioning, prepping, and draping the patient. In N. Phillips (Ed.), *Berry & Kohn's operating room technique* (11th ed., pp. 500–504). St. Louis: Mosby, Inc.

13. Schultz, A. (2005). Predicting and preventing pressure ulcers in surgical patients. *AORN Journal, 81*, 986–1006.

14. Seibert, E.M. (2009). Positioning for anes-thesia and surgery. In J.J. Nagelhout, K.L. Plaus (Eds.), *Nurse anesthesia* (4th ed., pp. 420–440). St. Louis: Saunders Elsevier.

15. Spry, C. (2005). *Essentials of perioperative nursing* (3rd ed., pp. 139–143). Boston: Jones & Bartlett Publishers.

16. Surgical Products. (2009). *The new rules of travel for the modern OR.* Retrieved May 18, 2009 from http://www.surgical-productsmag.com/scripts/ShowPR~PUB CODE~0S0~ACCT~0000100~ISSUE~06 07 ~RELTYPE~PR~PRODCODE~4900~ PRODLETT~A.asp

17. The Joint Commission. (2008). *Strategies for preventing pressure ulcers.* Retrieved April 28, 2009 from http:// www.jointcommission.org/NR/ rdonlyres/677EC466-DD6D-43FE-945E-83B8FDD0BC5B/0/Strategiesfor PreventingPressureUlcers.pdf

2 Prepping and Draping

Linda J. Wanzer

Elizabeth A. P. Vane

SKIN PREPARATION

Postoperative surgical site infections (SSIs) are the third most commonly reported hospital-acquired infections in the United States (APIC, 2002; Barnard, 2002). However, Medicare no longer reimburses costs associated with SSIs as of October 1, 2008; thus health care institutions are taking a critical look at practices that place the patient at risk for infections. According to the Deficit Reduction Act of 2005 Section 6081 (USHHS, 2008), the costs associated with hospital-acquired infections or SSIs will now be absorbed solely by the health care institutions. This legislative act places strategic importance on practices supporting aseptic technique, basic infection control, and prevention strategies for the entire surgical team. Identifying factors that place the surgical patient at risk for a surgical site infection forms a focal point for the First Assistant (FA) to implement interventions aimed at preventing infections within the perioperative setting (Akridge, 2004; Vaiden, 2005).

All surgical patients are at risk for infection from endogenous and exogenous sources of contaminates. Adherence to strict aseptic technique while preparing the patient's skin for surgery can minimize this risk and support the goal of reducing the risk of postoperative surgical site infections. When the surgical incision is made or mucous membranes are breached, tissue is exposed and at risk for contamination. Because endogenous microbes (e.g., the patient's own microbial flora) are associated with most wound infections, preparing the patient's skin before surgery is essential to ensuring successful surgical outcomes (APIC, 2002; Gruendemann & Stonehocker, 2001; Mangram et al., 1999). Exogenous microbes (e.g., contaminates from the environment including members of the surgical team, operating room environment, and surgical instruments) also place the patient at risk for surgical site infection (Gruendemann & Stonehocker, 2001; Mangram et al., 1999). Protecting the patient from serious SSI complications requires that the FA has knowledge of the contaminate origin as well as containment strategies for endogenous and exogenous microorganisms.

Vitalized (intact) tissue has enormous resistance to infection and creates a protective barrier for disease prevention, requiring a significant microbial deposit in the tissue to cause an infection (Phillips, 2007). Moist areas of the axilla, mouth, and perineum are ideal incubators for microbial growth. Body areas such as the trunk and extremities have negligible numbers of microbes; however, exposed body parts such as the face, hands, and feet can routinely harbor up to 10^3 microorganisms per gram. As long as the skin surfaces in these regions remain intact, the skin should provide a sufficient barrier to prevent disease at these levels of microbial growth. However, when bioburdens (microbial counts) on the skin surface greater than 10^5 microorganisms per gram are introduced into wounds (through breaches in the skin or surgical incisions), wound infection rates increase dramatically (Mangram et al., 1999; Meakins, 2008). Therefore an effective antimicrobial chemical agent for surgical skin preparation is critical to ensure that microbial destruction occurs on the skin before surgery. Through proper skin antisepsis, the FA can minimize the microbial count of superficial (endogenous) microorganisms (Gruendemann & Stonehocker, 2001).

Anatomy and Physiology of the Skin

Intact skin and mucous membranes form the body's first line of defense against infection by providing the following barriers of protection: (1) anatomical—intact epithelium; (2) chemical—stratified epithelium [sweat (sudoriferous) and oil (sebaceous) glands] that possess a natural biochemical substance with bactericidal properties; and (3) desquamation process and low pH properties—inhibits bacterial colonization (Phillips, 2007). The skin has two distinct layers: the outer epidermis and the deeper dermis (Figure 2-1).

Microorganisms are prevalent on all skin layers and are categorized as either transient or resident flora. The transient flora are those microorganisms that are in loose contact with the skin, such as those in grease, sweat, and oil particles. Because they are in loose contact with the skin, these organisms are easily removed by gentle mechanical friction. Resident flora, on the other hand, usually colonize around a particular body site (e.g., around the glands and hair follicles). They are carried to the surface layer of the skin and shed with perspiration and dead skin cells. Examples of resident flora include *Staphylococcus epidermidis,* aerobic and anaerobic diphtheroid bacilli, aerobic spore-forming bacilli, aerobic and anaerobic

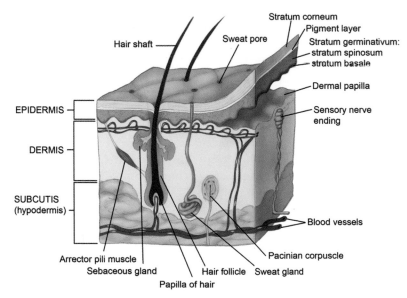

Figure 2-1

Anatomy of the skin.

Source: Courtesy of Phippen, M.L., Ulmer, B.C., & Wells M.P. (2009). *Competency for safe patient care during operative and invasive procedures* (Fig. 9.33, p. 250). Denver: CCI.

streptococci, and gram-negative rods (Mangram et al., 1999). Because the surgical incision breaks the continuity of the skin, skin preparation must be directed at removing transient flora and suppressing the activity of resident flora.

Goals of Skin Preparation

Although skin preparation is commonly performed by the Registered Nurse (RN), all members of the surgical team—especially the FA—should be familiar with skin preparation. The Association of periOperative Registered Nurses' (AORN) Recommended Practices (RP) are widely recognized guidelines (ACS, 2007; AORN, 2009a). According to AORN's RP for Preoperative Patient Skin Antisepsis, the goal of preoperative skin preparation is to:

1. Remove soil, dirt, oil, and transient microorganisms from the epidermis;
2. Reduce the resident microbial count to minimal levels (subpathogenic) within the shortest amount of time;
3. Minimize tissue irritation; and
4. Prevent regrowth/rebound and multiplication of the dermal microbes (AORN, 2009a).

Preoperative Assessment   To accomplish the above goals, the FAs assessment of the patient becomes critical. An analysis of potential risks includes:

1. Infection: include discussion on immunocompromised patients, nutritional status (both over- and underweight), steroid use, and diabetes;
2. Injury: including preexisting breaks in skin integrity, rashes, lesions, and allergies to prepping solutions;
3. Impaired skin integrity: a state in which the skin condition is changed between admission and discharge from the operating room;
4. Delayed surgical recovery: include signs and symptoms of postoperative infection; and
5. Anxiety related to loss of privacy during skin preparation procedures; patient's privacy must be maintained during prep. Often the patient can complete at least part of the initial prep in privacy of own home.

A comprehensive patient assessment must be completed in which the FA compares patient risk factors with physiological findings, clinical data, and psychological indicators to complete the plan of care (Dunscombe & Pasaka, 1999). Examples of assessment elements needed to guide intervention activities related to skin preparation of the surgical patient include:

1. Location of the proposed surgical site;
2. Condition of the skin at or near the surgical site (e.g., skin integrity or presence of body piercings, hair, lesions, localized infections);
3. Numbers and kinds of contaminants present on the skin surface (e.g., debris, soil);
4. Overall skin condition/characteristics (e.g., cleanliness, hair, skin integrity, lesions such as moles or warts, rash, skin eruptions, or abrasion);
5. Previous surgeries/presence of fragile tissue (e.g., scars, keloids);
6. Patient's age, medical condition, and overall physical and nutritional health (e.g., diabetes, nicotine use, steroid use, malnutrition, obesity, prolonged preoperative hospital stay, colonization with microorganisms, coexistent infections at a remote body site, perioperative transfusion, altered immune system);
7. Patient allergies to antimicrobial products;
8. Selection of effective antimicrobial agent(s) for the anatomical location of the surgical site;
9. Infection predictors (e.g., procedure length, procedure type, presence of other devices or instruments); and

10. Patient education in preparing the skin before surgery (e.g., showering or bathing the night before surgery, and preferably the morning of surgery, with chlorhexidine gluconate [CHG]), removal of all cosmetics, removal of all jewelry including body jewelry [e.g., body piercing ornaments], removal of nail polish and/or artificial nail surfaces if in the surgical area (AORN, 2009a; Gruendemann & Stonehocker, 2001; Mangram et al., 1999; Peterson, 2007).

Similar information may be provided also by staff in the surgeon's office prior to admission to the surgical setting.

Two-Phase Process for Preparing the Surgical Site

Policies and procedures governing the process for achieving skin antisepsis vary according to institutional protocol, practice setting, clinical situations, and physician preference. Nonetheless, the broad general principles of reducing the microbial count in the shortest time, suppressing regrowth, using aseptic technique, and attending to patient safety and privacy are applicable to any practice setting (AORN, 2009a).

Preparing the skin for surgery is a two-phase process: (1) precleansing phase—accomplished before arrival to the surgical setting (e.g., the night before and/or the morning of the surgical procedure) to remove organic debris and transient microorganisms on and around the intended surgical site; and (2) surgical site cleansing phase—application of antiseptic agent(s) directly to the surgical site after the patient is positioned for the surgical procedure.

Phase I: Precleansing

Skin Preparation with Showers or Baths   Preoperative showers or baths with an antimicrobial agent(s) are recommended to minimize microbial flora on the skin prior to a surgical procedure and thus reduce the risk for SSI. This recommendation supports two preoperative showers or baths with an antimicrobial agent to cleanse the surgical site of soil and debris and to reduce the number of microorganisms on the skin surface (AORN, 2009a; Gruendemann & Stonehocker, 2001; Mangram et al., 1999). At a minimum, the Centers for Disease Control and Prevention (CDC) recommends that one shower or bath be performed with an antimicrobial agent the night before surgery. However, CDC and AORN also state that unless it is contraindicated, two showers or baths should be performed to achieve maximum benefit from the precleansing process (AORN, 2009a; Mangram et al., 1999).

In a study described in CDCs *Guideline for Prevention of Surgical Site Infection* (Mangram et al., 1999), chlorhexidine gluconate (CHG)-containing products "reduced skin microbial count ninefold while povidone-iodine or triclocarban medicated soap reduced microbial counts 1.3- to 1.9-fold respectively" (Mangram et al., 1999, p. 106). Likewise, studies highlighted in AORN's 2009 Recommended Practices for Preoperative Patient Skin Antisepsis also support the use of CHG as the preferred antimicrobial agent during preoperative showers or baths to reduce microbial counts (AORN, 2009a).

Management of Hair in the Operative Area   The purpose of preoperative skin preparation is to reduce the number of existing microorganisms on skin surfaces at or directly adjacent to the surgical site and to prevent their entry into the surgical wound. The recommendation that hair not be removed preoperatively is supported by a broad, heterogeneous body of research (Meyer, 1995; Mishriki et al., 1990; Tanner et al., 2007). The results from this body of research support the conclusion that preoperative hair shaving causes skin damage (surface abrasion) and has been associated with a relatively high incidence of wound infection (AORN, 2009a; Meyer, 1995; Mishriki et al., 1990; Tanner et al., 2007). Consequently, The Joint Commission (TJC) added a new element to the 2009 National Patient Safety Goals focused on best practices for preventing surgical site infections. Within this new guideline is the expectation that as of January 1, 2010, shaving will no longer be an acceptable method for hair removal. When hair removal is absolutely necessary, clippers or depilatories will be used (Joint Commission, 2008). If hair removal is absolutely necessary because the hair at or in the immediate area of the incision site will interfere with the operation or accurate approximation of wound edges, adhering to the following guidelines may help reduce the risk for surgical site infections:

1. Before beginning the hair removal process, the FA (or the individual performing hair removal) should assess the patient's general skin condition, ensuring that the skin is dry and healthy;
2. When performing the activity, good hand-washing technique and wearing of gloves should prevent cross-contamination;
3. If depilatory creams are used for preoperative hair removal from the surgical site, skin testing should be performed following manufacturer's recommendation. In general, depilatory creams for preoperative hair removal are not recommended because they place the patient at risk for altered skin integrity (e.g., skin reaction, rash) which could result in surgical case cancellation;
4. If hair clipping is the method chosen for preoperative hair removal from the surgical site, it should be performed using sterile, single-use electric or battery-powered clippers (or clippers with a disinfected head);

5. Meticulous care should be taken with the clippers to minimize trauma and irritation to the skin surface;

6. Hair clipping should be performed the day of surgery and in a location outside of the surgical room in which the procedure will take place; and

7. Minimize the amount of hair removed by clipping only the hair that interferes with the surgical procedure (AORN, 2009a; Gruendemann & Stonehocker, 2001; Mangram et al., 1999; Tanner et al., 2007).

Phase II: Surgical Site Cleansing

Preparation for Surgical Site Cleansing   Before initiating skin preparation procedures in the operating room, the FA should:

1. Verify the correct site/side and the presence of the correct site marking per institutional policy and document this activity. Participation in this verification process applies to all members of the surgical team;

2. Identify landmarks denoting skin preparation boundaries supporting the intended surgical procedure (e.g., determine the extent of the area to be included in the prep);

3. Inspect the patient's skin, noting any irritation, rashes, abrasions, localized infection, or presence of body jewelry (e.g., body piercing ornaments) within the surgical preparation area and/or near active electrode sites;

4. Remove all jewelry before cleansing the skin and secure per institutional guidelines;

5. If body jewelry (body piercing ornaments) is removed, cleanse the pierced area thoroughly before beginning the surgical skin preparation;

6. If preoperative showers were not performed, the surgical site should be washed to remove transient microorganisms; this should take place in the preoperative area or in the operating room itself immediately before applying the antiseptic agent for the surgical prep;

7. If the umbilicus is within the surgical prep area, cleanse this area before performing the surgical prep (e.g., instill antiseptic solution into the umbilicus to soften the detritus for ease of removal with cotton applicators);

8. If surgery is to be performed in the area of the feet, hands, or wrists, nails should be short and natural (e.g., without nail polish, or artificial enhancements/extensions, wraps);

9. Select the appropriate antimicrobial agent(s) to be used for skin antisepsis; and

10. Prepare a separate table for skin preparation to confine and contain these instruments and supplies and minimize the potential for transfer

of contaminated items from the prep table to the sterile instrument table (AORN, 2009a; Gruendemann & Stonehocker, 2001; Phillips, 2007).

Surgical Skin Preparation Processes   Cleansing the surgical site to reduce or suppress transient microorganisms and resident flora can be accomplished using a two-step or one-step prep process. Regardless of the process chosen for surgical skin preparation, the following preliminary steps are consistent:

1. Select antiseptic solution(s) based on patient's allergies, proposed surgical incision location, and skin condition;
2. Use and dilute antiseptic solution(s) based on manufacturer's published instructions;
3. Place impervious pads at patient's sides and/or under extremities prior to skin preparation to prevent pooling of solutions and minimize potential risk for chemical irritation/burns;
4. Use impervious drape(s) with an adhesive strip to protect devices such as electrodes, electrosurgical unit dispersive pads, and tourniquets from coming in contact with antiseptic agents; and
5. Don sterile gloves and border the surgical prep site with sterile towels (AORN, 2009a; Peterson, 2007; Phillips, 2007).

Two-Step Skin Preparation Process   The two-step surgical skin preparation process involves the use of an antiseptic solution used in combination with mechanical action to remove loosely attached bacteria, followed by the application of another antiseptic solution to provide a persistent barrier to minimize rebound/regrowth to the surgical site (AORN, 2009a). After the above preliminary steps are completed, the two-step skin prep process continues as follows:

1. Two prep solutions are utilized for this process: soapy antiseptic solution and paint antiseptic solution;
2. Several sponges are placed in the soapy antiseptic solution, and several are placed in the paint antiseptic solution;
3. If the incision site is near the umbilicus, the umbilicus is considered potentially contaminated. Cotton-tipped single-use applicators are dipped into the soapy antiseptic solution to cleanse the umbilicus and then discarded into the trash;
4. The soapy antiseptic sponges are applied in a circular fashion from the proposed incision site to the peripheral boundaries of the defined surgical prep area to mechanically and chemically cleanse the skin (i.e., no backtracking over already prepped areas);

5. The prep sponges/applicators are to be used for a single application only and discarded after reaching the periphery of the designated skin preparation site;

6. A towel is used to blot the antiseptic soap from the surgical prep site;

7. Paint-type antiseptic solution is applied in a circular motion from the proposed incision site to the peripheral boundaries of the defined surgical prep area (using one sponge per application, then discarding);

8. Paint-type antiseptic solution is allowed to air-dry (not blotted or wiped off);

9. Finally, the surgeon may desire to have one sponge dipped in 70% alcohol and applied in a circular motion from the proposed incision site to the peripheral boundaries to complete the prep procedure. If this step is used, time must be allowed for the prepped area to completely dry before drapes are applied to minimize the risk of fire from trapped vapors; and

10. Remove sterile drapes/impervious pads from sides of patient/under extremities after the prep procedure to minimize skin contact with chemicals (AORN, 2009a; Phillips, 2007).

One-Step Skin Preparation Process   In some instances, only antiseptic paint-type solution is applied. This single application may be sprayed on or sponge forceps used for the application. Additional commercial one-step surgical skin preparation products are available as self-contained units complete with cotton-tipped applicators. The process for application is the same as that for the two-step process (e.g., applied in a circular fashion from the proposed incision line to the periphery, no retracing of prepped area, allowing to dry completely before beginning surgical procedure). Number of applications of the antiseptic paint-type solution should be based on manufacturer's published instructions (Phillips, 2007).

Exceptions to Standard Skin Preparation Principles

There are some exceptions to the standard skin preparation principles. Infected or draining wounds, open trauma, body orifices, or ostomy sites are considered potentially contaminated areas. For surgical interventions that involve these types of potentially contaminated sites, the skin preparation technique is reversed, with skin antisepsis beginning with the peripheral areas and moving circularly toward the open wound/contaminated site (i.e., scrub the most contaminated area last) (Phillips, 2007). If a skin graft is being performed, the recipient site is considered the contaminated site (Phillips, 2007). If more than one incision is being made, it is safest to use separate prep trays for each surgical site to minimize cross-contamination.

Documentation of Interventions Supporting Skin Preparation

Although the RN circulating nurse is responsible for documentation of interventions performed, the FA who writes a postoperative note should include documentation of the skin preparation. It is the surgeon's legal responsibility to verify patient identification as well as the correct side/site before the skin preparation process is initiated. Presence of the correct site marking must be documented per institutional policy (Phillips, 2007). In regard to skin preparation, documentation not only establishes accountability but aids surveillance activities in tracing adverse reactions or surgical site infections. At a minimum, the following documentation elements should be addressed in the patient's medical record:

1. Preoperative instruction;
2. Patient report of compliance with preoperative showering instructions;
3. Removal and disposition of any jewelry;
4. Condition of the skin at the surgical site (e.g., presence of rashes, skin eruptions, abrasions, redness, irritation, burns);
5. Hair removal, if performed, including method, time, area;
6. Antiseptic agent(s) used;
7. Area prepped;
8. Name(s) of person(s) performing skin preparation;
9. Precautions taken when flammable agents used (e.g., agent allowed to completely dry);
10. Removal of prepping agent peripheral to the demarcated prep site(s), (e.g., no pooling of solutions noted); and
11. Postoperative skin condition, including any skin irritation or hypersensitivity (allergic) response to preparation solutions (AORN, 2009a).

Antimicrobial Agents for Skin Preparation

The risk of surgical site infection is based on the number and strength of the contaminants and the resistance of the patient. When choosing an antimicrobial product to use for surgical preparation of the skin, the FA must consider the product's characteristics of effectiveness as well as select an agent appropriate for the location of the surgical incision (AORN, 2009a). Characteristics of effectiveness of antimicrobial products to be used for surgical preparation of the skin must, at a minimum, meet the following criteria:

1. Act rapidly;
2. Have a residual/persistent effect;

3. Reduce resident microbes;
4. Contain a non-irritating antimicrobial preparation;
5. Inhibit rebound growth of microbes;
6. Affect a broad spectrum of microbes; and
7. Be nontoxic (AORN, 2009a).

The antimicrobial agent(s) selected must be FDA-approved or cleared, and approved by the institution's infection control personnel. Additionally, to minimize adverse outcomes, final selection of the antimicrobial agent(s) must be individualized and based on the completion of a patient assessment, with consideration given to:

1. Patient allergies or sensitivity to antimicrobial agents;
2. Skin condition (e.g., skin irritation, open wounds);
3. Location of skin preparation site—identification of contraindications for use of specific antimicrobial agents (e.g., alcohol-based agents can cause tissue trauma in neonates and mucous membranes; chlorhexidine gluconate is neurotoxic to nonintact tympanic membranes and causes corneal irritation with eye contact);
4. Review of manufacturer's written information to ensure use follows manufacturer's recommendations; and
5. Surgeon preference (AORN, 2009a; ACS, 2007).

A summary of the characteristics of common skin antiseptic agents used for skin preparation of the surgical patient is outlined in Table 2-1.

DRAPING THE OPERATIVE SITE

Surgical drapes and drape accessories are barrier materials that promote infection control practices by imperviously covering the patient and surrounding area; defining the sterile field; isolating the surgical site from the rest of the patient's body to reduce the risk of surgical site infection; extending the sterile field to hold instruments and supplies; providing a barrier between nonsterile and sterile areas; and helping to protect both the surgical team and the environment from fluids, microorganisms, and bloodborne pathogens (AAMI, 2006a; AAMI, 2006b; AORN, 2009b; APIC, 2002; AST, 2008; Gruendemann & Stonehocker, 2001).

Combining proper draping techniques with the use of proper barrier materials reduces the introduction of endogenous and exogenous sources of infection into the surgical incision (Mangram et al., 1999). Endogenous flora from the patient's skin, mucous membranes, and hollow organs can be a major source of surgical site

Table 2-1 Activity and Considerations for Preoperative Skin Preparation Antiseptics

Antiseptic agent	Mechanism of action	Gram + bacteria	Gram – bacteria	Viruses	Rapidity of action	Persistent/ residual activity	Use on eye or ear
Alcohol	Denatures proteins.[1]	Excellent[1]	Excellent[1]	Good[1]	Excellent[1]	None[1]	No. Can cause corneal damage or nerve damage.[1]
Chlorhexidine gluconate	Disrupts cell membrane.[1]	Excellent[1]	Good[1]	Good[1]	Moderate[1]	Excellent[1]	No. Can cause corneal damage. Can cause deafness if in contact with inner ear.[1]
Povidone-iodine	Oxidation/ substitution with free iodine.[1]	Excellent[1]	Good[1]	Good[1]	Moderate[1]	Minimal[1]	Yes. Moderate ocular irritant.
Chlorhexidine gluconate with alcohol	Disrupts cell membrane and denatures proteins.[1,2]	Excellent	Excellent	Good	Excellent	Excellent	No. Can cause corneal damage. Can cause deafness if in contact with inner ear.
Iodophor with alcohol	Oxidation/ substitution by free iodine denatures proteins.[1,3,4]	Excellent[1,3,4]	Excellent	Good	Excellent	Moderate	No. Can cause corneal damage or nerve damage.

(continued)

Table 2-1 (*Continued*)

Activity and Considerations for Preoperative Skin Preparation Antiseptics

Antiseptic agent	Mechanism of action	Gram + bacteria	Gram – bacteria	Viruses	Rapidity of action	Persistent/ residual activity	Use on eye or ear
Parachoroxylenol (PCMX)	Disrupts cell membrane.[1]	Good[1]	Fair[1]	Fair[1]	Moderate[1]	Moderate[1]	Yes[5]

Antiseptic agent	Use on mucous membranes	Contraindications	Cautions
Alcohol	No		Flammable. Does not penetrate organic material. Optimum concentration is 60% to 90%.[1]
Chlorhexidine gluconate	Use with caution.[2]	Known hypersensitivity to drug or any ingredient.[2] Lumbar puncture and use on meninges.[2]	Prolonged skin contact may cause irritation in sensitive individuals. Rare severe hypersensitivity reactions have been reported.[2] Use with caution on mucous membranes.
Povidone-iodine	Yes	Sensitivity to povidone-iodine. (Shellfish allergies are not a contraindication.)[6]	Prolonged skin contact may cause irritation. May cause iodism in susceptible individuals; avoid use in neonates.[3,4] Inactivated by blood.[7,8]

Chlorhexidine gluconate with alcohol	No	Known hypersensitivity to drug or any ingredient. Lumbar puncture and use on meninges.	Flammable.
Iodophor with alcohol	No	Sensitivity to povidone-iodine. (Shellfish allergies are not a contraindication.)	Flammable.
Parachoroxylenol (PCMX)	Yes[5]	Known hypersensitivity to PCMX or any ingredient.[5]	Minimally effective in the presence of organic matter. The FDA has classified PCMX as Category III (data are insufficient to classify it as safe and effective). The FDA continues to evaluate PCMX.[5]

[1] Mangram, A., Horan, T., Pearson, M., Silver, L., & Jarvis, W. (1999). Guideline for prevention of surgical site infection. *American Journal of Infection Control, 27,* 97–132.

[2] Denton, G. (2001). Chlorhexidine. In S. Block (Ed.), *Disinfection, Sterilization and Preservation* (5th ed., pp. 321–336). Philadelphia, PA: Lippincott Williams & Wilkins.

[3] Bryant, W. & Zimmerman, D. (1995). Iodine-induced hyperthyroidism in a newborn. *Pediatrics, 95,* 434–436.

[4] EnviroSystems, Incorporated (2008). *Technical overview, Biocides.* Retrieved November 7, 2008 from http://www.envirosi.com/technical.shtml

[5] Smerdely, P., Lim A., Boyages, S., Waite, K., Roberts, V., et al. (1989). Topical iodine-containing antiseptics and neonatal hypothyroidism in very-low-birth weight infants. *Lancet, 2,* 661–664.

[6] American Academy of Allergy Asthma and Immunology. (2004). *Academy position statement: The risk of severe allergic reactions from the use of potassium iodide for radiation emergencies.* Retrieved November 7, 2008 from http://www.aaaai.org/media/resources/academy_statements/position_statements/potassium_iodide.asp

[7] Gottardi, W. (2001). Iodine and iodine compounds. In S. Block (Ed.), *Disinfection, sterilization and preservation* (5th ed., pp. 159–183). Philadelphia, PA: Lippincott Williams & Wilkins.

[8] Zamora, J., Price, M., Chuang, P., & Gentry, L. (1985). Inhibition of povidone iodine's bactericidal activity by common organic substances: An experimental study. *Surgery, 98,* 25–29.

infection; thus, strict adherence to proper skin preparation prior to surgery is essential (AST, 2008; Mangram et al., 1999). Exogenous sources of contamination from the surgical team members, environment, and surgical instruments can also contribute to contamination leading to surgical site infections. However, this potential risk can be controlled with the proper selection and application of barrier materials (AST, 2008).

The act of draping in surgery is focused on covering the patient and surrounding areas with a sterile barrier to create and maintain an adequate sterile field during surgery. The role of barrier materials used in operating room gowns and drapes has received considerable attention in the literature, especially with the development of new synthetic and reusable materials. With a goal to "prevent the penetration of microorganisms, particulates, and fluids" (Gruendemann & Stonehocker, 2001, p. 273), the physical and bacteriological characteristics of draping materials need to be considered when selecting barrier materials for use in the perioperative environment (Belkin, 2002). Environmental considerations in the disposal of biohazardous waste and/or business practices associated with the handling of reusable drapes (practices) are other important concerns.

Examples of drapes used as protective barriers for patients undergoing surgery include towels, laparotomy sheets, thyroid sheets, chest sheets, hip sheets, perineal sheets, laparoscopy sheets, split sheets, minor sheets, medium sheets, single sheets, leggings, stockinettes, impregnated adhesive incise sheets, eye/ear sheets, breast sheets, and extremity sheets. Not only is the surgical patient covered with a protective barrier prior to surgery, but furniture and equipment used in surgery are also covered (e.g., chairs, ring stands, Mayo stands, lasers, robots, c-arms, x-ray cassettes, cords, cameras, foot pedals, light handles, tourniquets, and endoscopes) (Gruendemann & Stonehocker, 2001; Phillips, 2007).

When performing draping procedures, give consideration to providing a sterile, safe environment for surgical intervention, as well as one that is comfortable and private for the awake patient (Table 2-2, 2-3). The risk for infection, possible loss of dignity, and potential anxiety are patient problems for which interventions might be developed (Peterson, 2007).

Reusable Drapes

Reusable barrier drapes and products should ensure appropriate barrier protection. Reusable drape characteristics should be:

1. Porous to eliminate heat buildup;
2. Steam sterilizable and able to withstand multiple steam sterilization cycles;
3. Free of discolorations and toxic substances such as allergens, dyes, and laundry detergent residues;

Table 2-2   AORN Recommended Practices for Surgical Drape Selection

1. Surgical drapes should be evaluated according to the AORN recommended practices for product selection in perioperative practice settings.
2. Materials used for surgical drapes should be resistant to penetration by blood and other body fluids as necessitated by their intended use.
3. Surgical drapes should maintain their integrity and be durable.
4. Materials used for surgical drapes should be appropriate to the methods of sterilization.
5. Surgical drapes should resist combustion.
6. Surgical gowns and drapes should be comfortable and contribute to maintaining the wearer's desired body temperature.
7. Surgical drapes selected for use should have a favorable cost-benefit ratio.
8. Policies and procedures for selecting and using surgical gowns and drapes should be developed, reviewed regularly, revised as necessary, and readily available in the practice setting.

Source: Association periOperative Nurses (AORN). (2009). Recommended practices for selection and use of surgical gowns and drapes. In R. Conner (Ed.), *2009 AORN perioperative standards and recommended practices* (pp. 361–365). Denver: AORN, Inc.

4. Free of holes, punctures, tears, or thinned/stretched areas (i.e., from towel clips or sharp instruments) prior to sterilization;
5. Able to track number of uses, launderings, and sterilizations as well as having a method to monitor the fabric's barrier effectiveness after repeated processing's. Repeated laundering and steam sterilization gradually disrupt the integrity of the fabric, and repeated drying and ironing render the fabric moisture–permeable. Useful life of reusable drapes is considered to be 75 washes for treated cotton and 30 washes for untreated cotton;
6. Repairable (i.e., holes must be covered with heat-sealed patches made of the same type of material as the drape. Stitching is not allowed because it compromises the barrier of the drape);
7. Able to be fan-folded or rolled and arranged, based on sequence of use for sterilization and packaging;
8. Sufficiently impermeable to prevent moisture from soaking through the drapes and potentially exposing the patient to the migration of microorganisms, or it should be treated with chemicals to render fabrics nonwicking and liquid resistant) (AST, 2008; Gruendemann & Stonehocker, 2001; Phillips, 2007).

Table 2-3   Analysis of Drape Properties

Drape Properties	Performance Characteristics	Methods for Barrier Testing (see glossary for test details)	Manager's Analysis of Drape Properties
Barrier Performance	**Level 1:** • Surgical drapes (inclusive of critical zones) and drape accessories that pass **one laboratory test** designed to measure how well the material will perform when fluids fall or splash onto the fabric.[1,2]	**AATCC 42 test:** *Water resistance: Impact Penetration test/Spray Impact test.*[3]	• Results from *Impact Penetration test:* blotter weight gain of ≤4.5 g to achieve Level 1 classification. • When interpreting the AATCC 42 test, the lower the number the higher the resistance to fluid penetration.[3,4] • All surgical drapes should, at a minimum, meet the Level 1 barrier performance requirements for liquid resistance.[3]
	Level 2: • Surgical drapes (inclusive of critical zones) and drape accessories that pass **two laboratory tests** designed to simulate the different types of liquid exposures occurring in surgery: spraying, splashing, or soaking in conjunction with leaning and pressing.[1,3,5]	**AATCC 42 test:** *Water Resistance: Impact Penetration test/Spray Impact test.*[3,5] **AATCC 127 test:** *Water Resistance: Hydrostatic Pressure (Hydrohead test).*[3,5]	• Results desired from *Impact Penetration test:* blotter weight gain of ≤1.0 g to achieve Level 2 classification from the AATCC 42 test.[3,5] • Results desired from *Hydrostatic Pressure test:* a hydrostatic pressure of at least ≥20 cm to achieve Level 2 classification from the AATCC 127 test.[3,5] • At this level, the higher the hydrostatic pressure, the more resistant the material is to liquid penetration. A higher number means the material has better resistance.[5]

Level 3:

- Surgical drapes (inclusive of critical zones) and drape accessories that pass the same **two laboratory tests** as in level 2 but at a higher level of performance.[1,3]

AATCC 42 test:
Water Resistance: Impact Penetration test (Spray impact test).[3,5]

AATCC 127 test:
Water Resistance: Hydrostatic Pressure (Hydrohead test).[3,5]

Level 4:

- Surgical drapes and drape accessories that demonstrate the ability to resist liquid penetration in a quantitative laboratory test from the American Society for Testing and Materials.[3]

ASTM F1670 test:
Synthetic Blood Resistance test.[5]

Strength:

- Surgical drapes and drape accessories must demonstrate a level of strength required to withstand the stresses encountered during typical surgical procedure, when exposed to both wet and dry conditions.[5]

Breaking strength tests:
Grab Tensile Strength test, Strip Tensile Strength test, and Burst Strength test.[5]

Tear strength tests:
Elmendorf Tear Strength test, Trapezoidal Tear Strength test, and Tongue Tear Strength test.[5]

- Results desired from *Impact Penetration test:* blotter weight gain of ≤1.0 g to achieve Level 3 classification from AATCC 42 test.[3]
- Results desired from *Hydrostatic Pressure test:* a hydrostatic pressure of at least ≥50 cm to achieve Level 3 classification from AATCC 127 test.[3]

- Results desired from *Synthetic Blood Resistance test:* **Pass:** no visible liquid penetration after 60 minutes within all critical zone components to achieve Level 4 classification from the ASTM F1670 test.[3,5]
- Level 4 drapes offer impervious protection and are designed for fluid-intensive surgical procedures.

- Results desired from *Breaking strength tests:* the greater the force required to cause a puncture, rupture, or breakage in the fabric under increasing pressure or pulling stress, the greater the strength of the material.[5]
- Results desired from *Tear tests:* the greater the force required to tear the fabric under controlled force, the greater the material's resistance to a continuation of a tear when a tear in the fabric occurs in the sterile field.[5]

(continued)

Table 2-3 *(Continued)*

Drape Properties	Performance Characteristics	Methods for Barrier Testing (see glossary for test details)	Manager's Analysis of Drape Properties
		Puncture and tear resistance tests: *Puncture Propagation Tear method.*[5]	• Results desired from *Puncture and tear resistance tests*: the greater the force required to snag/tear under typical use in surgery (e.g., stress to fabric by contact with sharps/pointed instruments), the greater the strength of the material.[5]
Linting	**Abrasion, cut, & tear resistant:** • Integrity of the surgical drapes and drape accessories should not change during normal use under wet or dry conditions even when material is rubbed against another material (e.g., stomach area of gown rubbing against the drape on the surgical table).[5]	**ASTM D4966:** *Martindale Abrasion test.*[5]	• Results desired from the *Martindale Abrasion test*: the abrasion rating/number of cycles the fabric endured continuous rubbing without showing signs of a change in appearance from the original fabric (e.g., breaks, pilling, holes) should be ≥3 (on a scale of 1–5).[6] • Abrasion-prone material could weaken/thin during normal use, adversely affecting barrier properties and causing the material to tear or generate lint.
	Low linting: • Surgical drapes and drape accessories should be lint-free to minimize the introduction of aerosolized particles into the surgical wound.[9]	**Gelbo Lint test, Flexing in Air test, Twisting in Air test, or Shaking in Water test.**[5,7,8] **ASTM F50-83 test:** *Helmke Drum test.*[5]	• Results desired from *Gelbo Lint test, Flexing or Twisting in Air tests and Shaking in Water tests*: the smaller the number of loose fibers (lint) released from nonwoven fabric subjected to repetitive flexing, twisting, and compression cycles within an air test chamber or immersed in water indicates the fabric's lower propensity to generate lint when used in the clinical setting.[5]

Flammability	**Combustion/flame resistant:**	National Fire Protection Association—**NFPA 702–1980:** *Standard for Classification of the Flammability of Wearing Apparel.*[1,10]	• Documentation exists that identifies surgical drapes as a source for lint particle generation made up of cellulose and cotton fibers. These particles, when introduced into surgical wounds, can cause foreign body reactions (granulomatous peritonitis) or even embolize within arteries.[2,5]
	• Surgical drapes and drape accessories should be flame-resistant and able to self-extinguish quickly once the ignition source is removed.[2]		• Results desired from *Helmke Drum test:* Category I indicates the lowest particle density taken from air samples while the material is rotated in a drum. The smaller the particulate count, the lower the propensity to generate lint.[5]
	• Ignition sources at the surgical field that pose high risk for combustion include lasers, electrosurgical units, and other high-energy devices.[2]	Consumer Product Safety Commission's **16 CFR 1610:** *Standard for the Flammability of Clothing Textiles.*[11]	• Results desired from *NFPA 702–1980 test:* the longer it takes the flame to spread, the more flame resistant the material.
			Class 1: slow burning/flame spread > 20 seconds.
			Class 2: moderately flammable/flame spread 8 to 19 seconds.
			Class 3: Relatively flammable/flame spread 3 to 7 seconds.[1,10]
			• NFPA 702-1980 test is still cited in the literature but was officially removed as an active standard in 1987.[1,5]
			• Results desired from *16 CFR 1610 test:* the longer it takes the flame to spread the more flame resistant the material.
			Class 1: normal flammability/textiles with no nap or pile with flame spread ≥ 4 seconds; textiles with a nap or pile with flame spread ≥ 7 seconds **are** acceptable for use.

(continued)

Table 2-3 (*Continued*)

Drape Properties	Performance Characteristics	Methods for Barrier Testing (see glossary for test details)	Manager's Analysis of Drape Properties
			Class 2: Intermediate flammability/textiles with nap or pile with flame spread between 4–7 seconds **may** be acceptable for use. Class 3: Rapid and intense burning/flame spread <4 seconds **may not** be used.[11] • Surgical drape packages should be labeled with a flammability rating identifying the fabric meets *Class 1 Flammability Requirements for 16 CFR 1610.*[1] • 16 CFR 1610 measuring ease of ignition and speed of flame spread is the national standard currently used for testing and rating flammability of textiles.[11]
	Electrostatic-resistant: • Surgical drapes and drape accessories should be able to accept or dissipate electrical charge given the challenges inherent in the operative environment (relative humidity/temperature, length of surgical case, material exposure to abrasion/rubbing/friction/[5]	**Electrostatic clinging of fabrics:** *Fabric-to-Metal test.*[5] **Should flammable anesthetics be used, the following test methods should be used:** *Electrostatic Decay test and Surface Resistivity test.*[5]	• Results desired from *Fabric-to-Metal test:* the lower the electrical charge generated, the shorter the cling time, which results in material with greater antistatic properties (decreased tendency of fabric to cling).[5,12,13] • Results desired from *Electrostatic Decay test:* 0.5 seconds is the criterion set for drapes charged with 5000 volts of static electricity to effectively discharge all but 500 volts.[5] • Results desired from *Surface Resistivity test:* an electrical resistivity of $\leq 1 \times 10^{11}$ ohms/sq.[5]

- Testing the electrostatic properties of drapes to be used in areas where anesthesia is delivered is no longer a requirement in the United States because flammable anesthetics are no longer used. A warning label against the use of these products may still be present on drape products in the event that flammable gases might be encountered.[5]

- Results desired from *Shrink test*: the percentage of shrinkage after washing, drying, and sterilizing the fabric indicates the material's resistance to shrinking.[5]

- Results desired from *Biocompatibility test*: Materials should be free of chemicals or toxic ingredients that could irritate tissue or adversely affect the patient or end user.[1,5]
- In an effort to enhance barrier properties (e.g., fluid, flame, or stain resistance), additives or permanently bonded chemicals may be used that could be toxic or cause irritation to tissues (e.g., dermatitis, allergic reactions).[5]

pressure/compression) in the presence of electrical devices and alcohol-based prep solutions.[5]

Ease of Use

Shrinkage:
- Reusable surgical drapes and drape accessories should maintain their original dimensions when subjected to repeated washing, drying, and sterilization for a designated period of uses.[5]

Shrink test.[5]

Biocompatibility:
- Surgical drapes and drape accessories are Class II medical devices and as such must undergo cytotoxicity, sensitization, and irritation testing to ensure that they are free of chemicals or toxic ingredients that may pose a potential hazard to the patients' organs or tissues (e.g., laundry residues and nonfast dyes).[2,5,14]

ANSI/AAMI/ISO 10993 series: *Biological evaluation of medical devices.*[5]

(continued)

Table 2-3 (*Continued*)

Drape Properties	Performance Characteristics	Methods for Barrier Testing (see glossary for test details)	Manager's Analysis of Drape Properties
	Drapeability: • Surgical drapes and drape accessories should be made of a material that conforms easily to the patient and other related equipment in the surgical environment, and allows for the placement and manipulation of instruments.[1,2,5]	**Handle-o-Meter test.**[5] **Cantilever Stiffness test.**[5] **Cusick Drape test.**[5] **Cup Crush test.**[15]	• Results desired from *Handle-o-Meter test:* a lower reading (lower force required to manipulate the material through a designated space) equates to a more drapeable product.[5] • Results desired from *Cantilever Stiffness test:* the shorter the length of material needed to extend over the edge of a horizontal surface to achieve a predetermined bend in the fabric, the more drapeable (less stiff) the material is determined to be.[5] • Results desired from *Cusick Drape test:* a lower drape coefficient equates to a more drapeable product (less stiff).[5] • Results desired from *Cup Crush test:* a lower cup crush value (total energy required to crush the material through to the peak load point) indicates a softer material.[15] However, a higher value may indicate better drapeability, as in the case of polypropylene fabric.[4] • There is currently no test method that directly correlates the perception of a material's softness to its drapeability.[5]

Ease of Use:

- The level of comfort of surgical drapes and drape accessories can be influenced by the sensitivity of the patient's skin, the properties of the drape (e.g., design, fit, breathability, softness, weight/strength, surface slickness, electrostatic properties, color, glare, and odor), and environmental conditions typical of an operative environment (e.g., workload, stress, room temperature, relative humidity, and air changes).[5]

- Results desired: surgical drapes should be—
  1. Dull/nonglaring to minimize color distortion from reflected light,[2] and
  2. Porous, to maintain an isothermic environment that supports the patient's normal body temperature but eliminates heat buildup.[1]

[1] Gruendemann, B., & Stonehocker, S. (2001). *Infection prevention in surgical settings.* Philadelphia: W. B. Saunders Co.

[2] Phillips, N. (2007). *Berry & Kohns operating room technique* (11th ed.). St Louis: Mosby/Elsevier.

[3] Association for the Advancement of Medical Instrumentation (AAMI). (2006a). ANSI/AAMI PB70:2003 Liquid barrier performance and classification of protective apparel and drapes intended for use in health care facilities. In *AAMI standards and recommended practices. Sterilization Part 1: Sterilization in health care facilities* (pp. 911–942). Arlington, VA: AAMI.

[4] Kimberly-Clark (2004). A guide to the guidelines. *OR Today.* Retrieved September 26, 2008 from www.mdpublishing.com/ORToday/PDFs/KimberlyClark_chart.PDF

[5] Association for the Advancement of Medical Instrumentation (AAMI). (2006b). ANSI/AAMI TIR11:2005 Selection and use of protective apparel and surgical drapes in health care facilities. In *AAMI Standards and recommended practices. Sterilization Part 1: Sterilization in health care facilities* (pp. 943–990). Arlington, VA: AAMI.

(continued)

[6] Truscott, W. (2006). Lint and particle contamination during diagnostic and interventional procedures in the cardiac catheterization lab. *Cath Lab Digest*. Retrieved September 30, 2008 from http://www.cathlabdigest.com/article/6211

[7] Schraag, J. (2006). Barrier protection, gowns and drapes. *Infection Control Today*. Retrieved October 1, 2008 from http://www.infectioncontroltoday.com/articles/691feat3.html

[8] Kimberly Clark Glossary. (2008). *Gelbo lint test definition from the Kimberly Clark Glossary*. Retrieved October 30, 2008 from http://www.kchealthcare.com/LrnGlossary.asp

[9] Association of Surgical Technologists (AST). (2008). *AST recommended standards of practice for surgical drapes*. Retrieved September 26, 2008 from www.ast.org/pdf/Standards_of_Practice/RSOP_Surgical_Drapes.pdf

[10] National Fire Protection Association (NFPA). (1980). Standard for classification of the flammability of wearing apparel. In NFPA 702 (1980 ed.) (pp. 702-1–702-10).

[11] Consumer Product Safety Commission (CPSC). (2004). National archives and records administration, the code of federal regulations, title 16 – Commercial practices, Chapter II – *Consumer product safety commission, Part 1610 – Standard for the flammability of clothing textiles*. Retrieved September 26, 2008 from http://www.access.gpo.gov/cgi-bin/cfrassemble.cgi?title=200416

[12] Schindler, W., & Hauser, P. (2004). Antistatic finishes. In *Chemical finishing of textiles*. Manchester, England: Woodhead Publishing. Retrieved October 30, 2008 from http://books.google.com/books?id=4jkUpC1OtuwC&dq=chemical+finishing+of+textiles&printsec=frontcover&source=bl&ots=mVhsZp06sv&sig=BYqWKBDheXP1bRWJiR9PgnZOPQ&hl=en&sa=X&oi=book_result&resnum=28ct=result#PPP1,M1

[13] American Association of Textile Chemists and Colorists (AATC). (2005). AATC 115 electrostatic clinging of fabrics: Fabric-to-metal test. *IHS*. Retrieved October 30, 2008 from http://engineers.ihs.com/document/abstract/ACUUTAAAAAAAAAAA

[14] Wallin, R., & Upman, P. (1998). A practical guide to ISO 10993-11: Systemic effects. *Medical device & diagnostic industry (MDDI)*. Retrieved November 1, 2008 from http://www.devicelink.com

[15] US Patent 6936554. (2005). Nonwoven fabric laminate with meltblown web having a gradient fiber size structure. *Patent storm*. Retrieved October 30, 2008 from http://www.patentstorm.us/patents/6936554/fulltext.html

These materials are considered advantageous in terms of institutional cost. However, they do have a number of disadvantages. Consideration must be given to the amount of time, personnel, and equipment needed to reprocess reusable drapes (e.g., they must be inspected for holes, washed after every use, refolded, sterilized, and stored). When reusable drapes are heavily soiled, they present contamination hazards to personnel because they must be handled multiple times from the point of use until the laundry process has been completed. Processing reusable woven materials "is a complex process requiring specialized equipment, adequate space, qualified personnel who are provided with ongoing training, and continuous monitoring for quality assurance" (AAMI, 2006c, p. 876). A system must also be devised for tracking the number of times these drapes are reprocessed because the barrier effectiveness can diminish with repeated sterilization (Gruendemann & Stonehocker, 2001). If a facility decides to launder the reusable woven materials in-house, their equipment must be effective in reducing the pathogenic organisms that colonize the surface and interstices of cotton drapes (OSHA, 1992). Additionally, the manufacturer's standards must be strictly adhered to in regard to defining barrier quality and reprocessing limitations. Commercial companies do exist that perform this function for hospitals and can eliminate the need for "in-house" processing and quality controls.

Single-Use Drapes

The evolution of synthetic, disposable draping systems has resulted in the production of lightweight, soft, lint-free, nonirritating, static-free, flame-resistant, and moisture-resistant single-use drapes. Some disposable drapes have antimicrobial reinforcements and attached troughs and pouches to collect fluids; others have drain ports and nonskid instrument pads built into the design (Gruendemann & Stonehocker, 2001; Phillips, 2007). Although easy to use, disposable drapes have disadvantages in terms of environmentally safe disposal, cost, inventory levels, and storage space.

Draping Techniques

Preparing the patient's skin for surgery (prepping the skin with antimicrobial agent[s]) reduces the number of microorganisms present at the surgical site but does not render the skin sterile. Surgical drapes complete the process of preparing the surgical field by providing a physical protective barrier to prevent microbial contamination of the surgical site. Surgical drapes also establish a "margin of safety" in and around the surgical field for ease of movement by the surgical team, and for the placement of instruments and sterile supplies (Gruendemann

& Stonehocker, 2001). The process of draping the surgical patient and the surgical field is the same whether using reusable cotton drapes or disposable synthetic drapes. The variance exists with the various types of drapes needed to support the variety of surgical procedures performed within the perioperative environment. In either case, the process of draping is a procedure in which the FA must be an expert.

Demarcate the Operative Parameters

Towel Drapes   One of the first steps is to allow the prep solution to completely dry prior to draping the patient. The draping process often begins with the application of the towel drape as a mechanism to demarcate and identify the operative parameters. The conventional four-towel method uses four surgical towels placed around the operative site. These may be fully opened or folded in half lengthwise and placed next to the skin (**Figure 2-2**). If reusable towels are used, the towel should be secured with nonperforating towel clamps. The disposable draping towel typically has an adherent sticky strip for fixation.

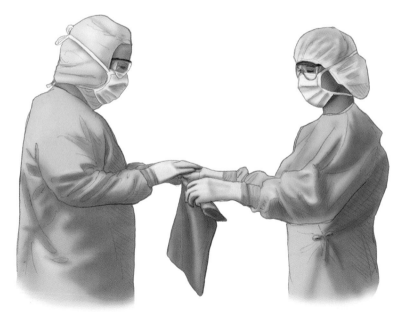

Figure 2-2

Handing the drape towel to the surgeon.

Source: Courtesy of Phippen, M.L., Ulmer, B.C., & Wells M.P. (2009). *Competency for safe patient care during operative and invasive procedures* (Fig. 9.59, p. 273). Denver: CCI.

Plastic Incise Drapes Some surgeons prefer a plastic incise drape to the use of four towels. If a plastic incise towel drape is used, two sterile team members are required (Figure 2-3). The drape, made of impermeable polyvinyl with adhesive on one side, is carefully applied and pressed firmly into place with a sterile rolled towel or lap sponge to minimize air pockets and wrinkles. The self-adhering draping materials may be used:

1. instead of the towel drape,
2. in combination with the towel drape,
3. as an aperture drape, or
4. as a plastic sheet.

The use of plastic incise impermeable polyvinyl drapes to inhibit microbial infection is controversial. Advocates of this type of drape claim that its advantage

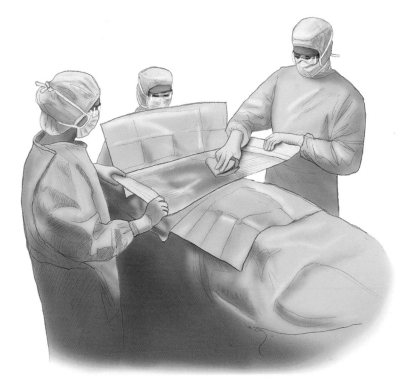

Figure 2-3

Incise drape.

Source: Courtesy of Phippen, M.L., Ulmer, B.C., & Wells M.P. (2009). *Competency for safe patient care during operative and invasive procedures* (Fig. 9.60, p. 274). Denver: CCI.

is in preventing lateral migration of skin microorganisms. Others claim that the heat and moisture buildup under the draped area actually promotes microbial growth. Some of the larger plastic drapes are available impregnated with anti-microbial agents. Plastic incise drapes are commonly used in orthopedics and implant surgery, where their usefulness is apparent in keeping the implant from any contact with skin surfaces. These drapes are also helpful in isolating surgical anatomy where a high occurrence of microorganisms is expected, such as with stomas.

Application of Fenestrated Sheet   Following application of towels or plastic incise drapes, a large fenestrated sheet may be applied. Fenestrated sheets are most commonly used in surgical interventions of the abdomen, chest, flank, and back. The length and width of the fenestration can vary to accommodate approaches to the abdomen, thyroid, breast, kidney, hip, and perineum. The fenestrated sheet is placed over the towels and incision site (Figure 2-4). The drape should be large enough to provide a wide margin of sterility between the operative site and surrounding unsterile areas.

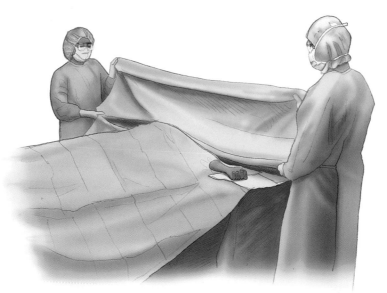

Figure 2-4

Fenestrated sheet.

Source: Courtesy of Phippen, M.L., Ulmer, B.C., & Wells M.P. (2009). *Competency for safe patient care during operative and invasive procedures* (Fig. 9.66, p. 276). Denver: CCI.

Principles of Aseptic Technique in Draping

The procedures for draping the patient are rooted in the principles of basic aseptic technique. The following guidelines are established to create a sterile field by establishing a protective barrier that prevents microorganisms, particulates, and fluids from contaminating the surgical incision.

1. Place drapes on a dry area (allow prep solution to dry before draping).
2. Allow sufficient time to permit careful application.
3. Allow sufficient space to observe sterile technique.
4. Drapes should be handled as little as possible.
5. The sterile field should be kept in view throughout the draping procedure.
6. Never reach across the operating bed to drape the opposite side—go around the bed.
7. Protect the gown and gloves from contact with unsterile, undraped areas.
8. Take towels and towel clips to the side of the operating bed from which the surgeon is going to apply them before handing them to him or her.
9. Carry folded drapes to the operating bed:
   a. Maintain an adequate distance from unsterile areas.
   b. Watch the front of the sterile gown for potential to bulge and inadvertently touch the nonsterile operating bed during the draping procedure.
   c. Hold drapes above waist level to avoid touching nonsterile areas, but avoid touching the overhead operating light.
   d. Hold a drape high until it is directly over the proper area, and then lay it down where it is to remain. Once a sheet is placed, do not adjust it.
   e. Protect gloved hands by cuffing the end of the sheet over them. Do not let gloved hands touch the skin of the patient.
10. The drape must be prevented from unfolding or flipping down during the draping process by being held in its compact shape. While unfolding a sheet from the prepped area toward the foot or head of the operating bed, protect the gloved hand by enclosing it in a turned-back cuff of sheet provided for this purpose. Keep hands at bed level.
11. Once the drape is placed on the patient, the drape is unfolded from center to periphery with care taken not to slide the sheet out of place when opening the folds.
12. Once the drape is placed, it cannot be moved or repositioned.
13. The edges of the drape that fall below bed level are considered unsterile.

14. If a drape becomes contaminated, do not handle it further. Discard it without contaminating gloves or other items:
    a. If the end of a sheet falls below waist level, do not handle it further. Drop it, and use another.
    b. If sterility is in doubt, consider the drape contaminated. Do not handle it further. Drop it, and use another.
    c. If a drape is incorrectly positioned, do not handle it further. The circulating nurse peels it from the operating bed without contaminating other drapes or the prepped area.
15. A towel clip that has been fastened through a drape has its points contaminated. Remove it only if absolutely necessary, and then discard it from the sterile setup without touching the points. Cover the area from which it was removed with another piece of sterile draping material.
16. If a hole is found in a drape after it is placed, the hole must be covered with another piece of draping material or the entire drape discarded.
17. A hair found on a drape must be removed, and the area must be covered immediately. Although hair can be sterilized, the source of a hair found on a sterile drape is usually unknown. If the hair were to migrate into the surgical wound, it could cause a foreign body tissue reaction; therefore, remove the hair with a hemostat and hand the instrument off the sterile field.
18. The sterile field should be continually monitored and maintained to ensure that the sterile field remains intact (AST, 2008; Phillips, 2007).

All members of the surgical team are responsible for maintaining the integrity of the sterile field during the operative procedure. As the patient's advocate, the FA monitors this integrity along with circulating and scrub personnel, surgeon, and anesthesia providers. As such, movements of team members are carefully coordinated because the team provides a method of confining and containing supplies and instruments used in the care of the surgical patient.

CONCLUSION

Because infections that develop in clean surgical wounds are caused primarily by exogenous microbial sources, proper preparation of the patient's skin before making the surgical incision is one of the most important ways to decrease infection in clean operations. The most commonly used antimicrobial agents for skin antisepsis are the iodophors; however many more agents with the same efficacy are available. The FA must be aware of all products used to prepare the skin for surgical intervention. In addition, the FA must be able to guide the selection process to ensure that the appropriate agent is chosen for the type of procedure and surgical site, taking into account the complete patient assessment, patient risk factors, and surgeon preference. Proper technique in the surgical preparation of the skin is essential to prevent chemical injury and maintain skin integrity. Sterile drapes are then applied to define and maintain the sterile field, inclusive of the patient, the equipment, and the surgical instruments, during the operative procedure. Drapes (woven or unwoven) should preserve their barrier characteristics and protect the patient, the environment, and the surgical team from bloodborne pathogens, fluids, and microorganisms. It is the responsibility of the FA to select the appropriate barrier level needed for a surgical case, based on experience and potential exposure risks. Prevention of surgical site infection is a multifaceted, ongoing process that requires the FA to pay particular attention to details of technique in preparing the surgical site for the procedure, as well as closely and continually monitor the barrier drape integrity throughout the procedure. The FAs commitment to preventing potential adverse consequences for the patient makes meticulous prepping, draping, and adherence to aseptic technique a natural component of skill proficiency.

GLOSSARY

ASTM F1670 test: standard test method for resistance of materials used in protective clothing to penetration by synthetic blood. Measures the strike-through of synthetic blood while under constant contact pressure. The test begins with synthetic blood on the drape sample at atmospheric pressure for 5 minutes, then changes to 2.0 psi for 1 minute, and then reverts back to atmospheric pressure for 54 minutes. Test results are reported as a "pass" or "fail". To pass the test, there is to be no visible liquid strike-through seen on the drape sample after 60 minutes (AAMI, 2006b). Surgical drapes that pass this test are considered impervious, and rated by AAMI as a Level 4 barrier protection category, designed for fluid-intensive surgical procedures (Gruendemann & Stonehocker, 2001).

Barrier protection: ability to resist liquids and the microorganisms that travel in liquids, from striking through a surgical drape. AAMI has defined four levels of liquid barrier protection for surgical drapes: Level 1 offers the least fluid protection and Level 4 offers the most fluid protection. It is up to the end user to determine the level of liquid barrier protection needed for the surgical case (AAMI, 2006a; AAMI, 2006b).

Coatings: semiliquid urethane or silicone layers used on one side of a surgical drape to protect against fluid and microorganism strike-through (AAMI, 2006b).

Comfort: a subjective term for surgical drapes that depends on many details including: design, weight, draping ability, softness, color, glare, odor, breathability, surface slickness, and electrostatic properties. Other surgical environmental factors that affect drape comfort include: workload, stress, room temperature, relative humidity, and air changes. "Comfort" is a term that is difficult to scientifically test for objectively, and is best determined while actually using the drapes in surgical procedures. Additionally, skin sensitivity to drape material can influence the perception of comfort (AAMI, 2006b).

Drapeability: the ability to cover and conform to an object. Surgical drapes and drape accessories should be made of a material that conforms easily to the patient and related equipment in the surgical environment and allows for the placement and manipulation of instruments (AAMI, 2006b; Gruendemann & Stonehocker, 2001; Phillips, 2007). Drapeability tests include the Cup Crush test, Handle-O-Meter test, Cantilever Stiffness test, and the Cusick Drape tests (AAMI, 2006b). There is currently no test method that correlates the perception of a material's softness with its drapeability (AAMI, 2006b).

Nonskid surfaces: application of a brushed texture or a coating around the drape fenestration to prevent sliding when laying down surgical instruments (AAMI, 2006b).

Nonwoven fabrics: common fabric for single-use surgical drapes. These nonwoven fabrics contain natural fibers (e.g., wood pulp, cotton) and synthetic fibers (e.g., rayon, polyester, nylon) but are not manufactured by weaving or knitting (AAMI, 2006b; Gruendemann & Stonehocker, 2001; Phillips, 2007). Common surgical nonwoven drape fabrics are spunlace, spunbond/meltblown, wet-laid, and composite (AAMI, 2006b).

Puncture and Tear Resistance test: measures a drape sample's ability to resist a snagging and tearing type of puncture. Surgical drapes should be resistant to puncture and tearing by typical use of surgical instruments and equipment. The greater the force needed to snag and tear, the greater the strength of the material (AAMI, 2006b).

Surface Resistivity test: used when flammable anesthetics will be present in the operating environment. Testing the electrostatic properties of drapes to be used in areas where anesthesia is delivered is no longer a requirement in the United States because flammable anesthetics are no longer used. A warning label against the use of these products may still be present on drape products in the event that flammable gases might be encountered (AAMI, 2006b). This test method equilibrates a drape sample to specific temperature and humidity conditions and tests for electrical resistance using a resistance meter. The results desired from this test are an electrical resistivity of $\leq 1 \times 10^{11}$ ohms/sq (AAMI, 2006b).

Surgical drape and drape accessories: described by the FDA as a medical device "made of natural or synthetic materials intended to be used as a protective patient covering, such as to isolate a site or surgical incision from microbial and other contamination" (AAMI, 2006b, p. 955; FDA, 2008).

Tear Strength test: performed under specified conditions in which an initial tear is made intentionally and more tests are done to continue that tear. Surgical drapes should be resistant to tearing by typical use of surgical instruments and equipment. Three commonly used tear tests are Elmendorf Tear Strength, Trapezoidal Tear Strength, and Tongue Tear Strength tests (AAMI, 2006b). The greater the force required to tear the fabric under controlled force, the greater the material's resistance to a continuation of a tear that occurs in the sterile field (AAMI, 2006b).

Woven fabrics: common fabric for reusable surgical drapes; manufactured by weaving or knitting two yarns that cross at right angles (AAMI, 2006b). These multiple-use fabrics can be made of polyester (e.g., a tightly woven, fine filament yarn, chemically finished fabric) or from composite materials (e.g., knitted fabric laminated with a film or coat) to increase the barrier properties (AAMI, 2006b).

REFERENCES

1. Akridge, J. (2004). Raising the bar on surgical gowns and drapes. *Healthcare Purchasing News*. Retrieved November 3, 2008 from http://findarticles.com/p/articles/mi_m0BPC/is_9_28/ai_n6199932/pg_7?tag=artBody;col1

2. American Academy of Allergy Asthma and Immunology. (2004). *Academy position statement: The risk of severe allergic reactions from the use of potassium iodide for radiation emergencies.* Retrieved November 7, 2008 from http://www.aaaai.org/media/resources/academy_statements/position_statements/potassium_iodide.asp

3. American Association of Textile Chemists and Colorists (AATC). (2005). AATC 115 electrostatic clinging of fabrics: Fabric-to-metal test. *IHS.* Retrieved October 30, 2008 from http://engineers.ihs.com/document/abstract/ACUUTAAAAAAAAAAA

4. American College of Surgeons (ACS) (2007). *ACS surgery: Principles & practice.* W. Souba, M. Fink, G. Jurkovich, L. Kaiser, W. Pearce, J. Pemberton, & N. Soper (Eds.). Hamilton, Ontario: BC Decker. See www.acssurgery.com

5. Association for the Advancement of Medical Instrumentation (AAMI). (2006a). ANSI/AAMI PB70:2003 Liquid barrier performance and classification of protective apparel and drapes intended for use in health care facilities. In *AAMI standards and recommended practices. Sterilization Part 1: Sterilization in health care facilities* (pp. 911–942). Arlington, VA: AAMI.

6. Association for the Advancement of Medical Instrumentation (AAMI). (2006b). ANSI/AAMI TIR11:2005 Selection and use of protective apparel and surgical drapes in health care facilities. In *AAMI standards and recommended practices. Sterilization*

Part 1: Sterilization in health care facilities (pp. 943–990). Arlington, VA: AAMI.

7. Association for the Advancement of Medical Instrumentation (AAMI). (2006c). ANSI/AAMI ST65:2000 Processing of reusable surgical textiles for use in health care facilities. In *AAMI standards and recommended practices. Sterilization Part 1: Sterilization in health care facilities* (pp. 849–909). Arlington, VA: AAMI.

8. Association of periOperative Registered Nurses (AORN). (2009a). Recommended practices for preoperative patient skin antisepsis. In R. Conner (Ed.), *2009 AORN perioperative standards and recommended practices* (pp. 549–567). Denver: AORN, Inc.

9. Association of periOperative Registered Nurses (AORN). (2009b). Recommended practices for selection and use of surgical gowns and drapes. In R. Conner (Ed.), *2009 AORN perioperative standards and recommended practices* (pp. 361–365). Denver: AORN, Inc.

10. Association for Professionals in Infection Control and Epidemiology (APIC). (2002). Surgical services. In *APIC test of infection control and epidemiology* (2nd ed., pp. 53, 1–11). Washington, DC: APIC, Inc.

11. Association of Surgical Technologists (AST). (2008). *AST recommended standards of practice for surgical drapes.* Retrieved September 26, 2008 from www.ast.org/pdf/Standards_of_Practice/RSOP_Surgical_Drapes.pdf

12. Barnard, B. (2002). Fighting surgical site infections. *Infection Control Today.* Retrieved October 1, 2008 from http://www.infectioncontroltoday.com/articles/241feat1.html

13. Belkin, N.L. (2002). A historical review of barrier materials. *AORN Journal, 76,* 648–653.

14. Bryant, W., & Zimmerman, D. (1995). Iodine-induced hyperthyroidism in a newborn. *Pediatrics, 95,* 434–436.

15. Consumer Product Safety Commission (CPSC). (2004). National archives and records administration, the code of federal regulations, title 16—Commercial practices, Chapter II—*Consumer product safety commission, Part 161—Standard for the flammability of clothing textiles.* Retrieved September 26, 2008 from http://www.access.gpo.gov/cgi-bin/cfrassemble.cgi?title=200416

16. Denton, G. (2001). Chlorhexidine. In S.S. Block (Ed.), *Disinfection, sterilization and preservation* (5th ed., pp. 321–36). Philadelphia, PA: Lippincott Williams & Wilkins.

17. Dunscombe, A., & Pasaka, L. (Eds.). (1999). *CRNFA study guide.* Denver: Certification Board Perioperative Nursing.

18. EnviroSystems, Incorporated (2008). *Technical overview, biocides.* Retrieved November 7, 2008 from http://www.envirosi.com/technical.shtml

19. Gottardi, W. (2001). Iodine and iodine compounds. In S.S. Block (Ed.), *Disinfection, sterilization and preservation* (5th ed., pp. 159–183). Philadelphia, PA: Lippincott Williams & Wilkins.

20. Gruendemann, B., & Stonehocker, S. (2001). *Infection prevention in surgical settings.* Philadelphia: W. B. Saunders Co.

21. Joint Commission (2008). *The Joint Commission Hospital Accreditation Program 2009 chapter: National patient safety goals.* Retrieved Nov 3, 2008 from http://www.jointcommission.org/NR/rdonlyres/31666E86-E7F4-423E-9BE8-F05BD1CB0AA8/0/HAP_NPSG.pdf

22. Kimberly-Clark. (2004). A guide to the guidelines. *OR Today.* Retrieved September 26, 2008 from www.mdpublishing.com/ORToday/PDFs/KimberlyClark_chart.PDF

23. Kimberly Clark Glossary. (2008). *Gelbo lint test definition from the Kimberly Clark Glossary.* Retrieved October 30, 2008 from http://www.kchealthcare.com/LrnGlossary.asp

24. Mangram, A., Horan, T., Pearson, M., Silver, L., & Jarvis, W. (1999). Guideline for prevention of surgical site infection. *American Journal of Infection Control, 27,* 97–132.

25. Meakins, J.L. (2008). Prevention of postoperative infection. In *ACS surgery: Principles*

& practice. W. Souba, M. Fink, G. Jurkovich, L. Kaiser, W. Pearce, J. Pemberton, & N. Soper (Eds.). Hamilton, Ontario: BC Decker. See www.acssurgery.com

26. Meyer, G. (1995). Recommendation for surgical skin preparation: An integrative review of the literature. *Online Journal of Knowledge Synthesis for Nursing, 2,* 73–79.

27. Mishriki, S. F., Law, D. J., & Jeffrey, P. J. (1990). Factors affecting the incidence of postoperative wound infection. *Journal of Hospital Infection, 16,* 223–230.

28. National Fire Protection Association (NFPA). (1980). Standard for classification of the flammability of wearing apparel. In *NFPA 702* (1980 ed., pp. 702-1–702-10).

29. Peterson, C. (Ed.). (2007). *Perioperative nursing data set: The perioperative nursing vocabulary* (2nd ed.). Denver: AORN, Inc.

30. Phillips, N. (2007). *Berry & Kohn's operating room technique* (11th ed.). St Louis: Mosby/Elsevier.

31. Schindler, W., & Hauser P. (2004). Antistatic finishes. In *Chemical finishing of textiles.* Manchester, England: Woodhead Publishing. Retrieved October 30, 2008 from http://books.google.com/books?id=4jkUpC1OtuwC&dq=chemical+finishing+of+textiles&printsec=frontcover&source=bl&ots=mVhsZp06sv&sig=BYqWKBDheXP1IbRWJiR9PgnZOPQ&hl=en&sa=X&oi=book_result&resnum=2&ct=result#PPP1,M1

32. Schraag, J. (2006). Barrier protection, gowns and drapes. *Infection Control Today.* Retrieved October 1, 2008 from http://www.infectioncontroltoday.com/articles/691feat3.html

33. Smerdely, P., Lim, A., Boyages, S., Waite, K., Roberts, V., Leslie, G., Arnold, J., & Eastman, C. (1989). Topical iodine-containing antiseptics and neonatal hypothyroidism in very-low-birth weight infants. *Lancet, 2,* 661–664.

34. Tanner, J., Moncaster K., & Woodings, D. (2007). Perioperative hair removal: A systematic review. *Journal of Perioperative Practice, 17,* 118–121, 124–132.

35. Truscott, W. (2006). Lint and particle contamination during diagnostic and interventional procedures in the cardiac catheterization lab. *CathLab Digest.* Retrieved September 30, 2008 from http://www.cathlabdigest.com/article/6211

36. U.S. Department of Health and Human Services. (2008). *Deficit reduction act.* Retrieved October 1, 2008 from http://www.cms.hhs.gov/MedicaidGenInfo/08_DRASection.asp

37. U.S. Department of Labor, Occupational Safety & Health Administration (OSHA). (1992). *Bloodborne pathogens, regulations (standards-29CFR 1910.1030).* Retrieved November 3, 2008 from http://www.osha.gov/pls/oshaweb/owadisp.show_document?p_table=STANDARDS&p_id=10051

38. U.S. Food and Drug Administration. (FDA). (2008). Title 21: Food and drugs, Chapter 1: Food and drug administration of health and human services, subchapter H: medical devices, part 878: general and plastic surgery devices, section 878.4370 *Surgical drape and drape accessories.* Retrieved November 3, 2008 from https://www.accessdata.fda.gov/scripts/cdrh/cfdocs/cfCFR/CFRSearch.cfm?fr=878.4370

39. US Patent 6936554. (2005, August 30). Nonwoven fabric laminate with melt-blown web having a gradient fiber size structure. *Patent Storm.* Retrieved October 30, 2008 from http://www.patent-storm.us/patents/6936554/fulltext.html

40. Vaiden, R. (2005). *Core curriculum for the RN First Assistant* (4th ed.). Denver: AORN, Inc.

41. Wallin, R., & Upman, P. (1998, July). A Practical guide to ISO 10993-11: Systemic effects. *Medical device & diagnostic industry (MDDI).* Retrieved November 1, 2008 from http://www.devicelink.com

42. Zamora, J., Price, M., Chuang, P., & Gentry, L. (1985). Inhibition of povidone iodine's bactericidal activity by common organic substances: An experimental study. *Surgery, 98,* 25–29.

3

Tissue Handling

John T. Paige

INTRODUCTION

In the late 19th Century, two major advances in the field of surgery occurred, laying the foundation for modern practice: the discovery of anesthesia and the adoption of principles of asepsis. William Steward Halsted, a legendary figure in American surgery, was one of the first surgeons to recognize the immense benefits that could arise from these innovations when they were combined with precise surgical technique. In doing so, he helped create a "school for safety in surgery" that emphasized gentle tissue handling, meticulous hemostasis, sharp dissection, aseptic practice, and attention to detail. His theories eventually won out over the then popular concept of completing a procedure as speedily as possible. His success in lowering surgical infection rates and improving patient outcomes demonstrated the merits of this "safety in surgery" approach. Today, many of the surgical principles he advocated are still commonly employed.

Just as in Halsted's era, the contemporary surgical assistant (referred to in this book as "first assistant," or FA) is an integral member of the operating room (OR) team. In the highly complex, dynamic environment of the modern OR, the FA plays a crucial role in providing safe, effective care to the patient. A well-prepared, knowledgeable, technically dexterous FA who has a firm grasp of the operative plan and can anticipate the next step in the procedure can enhance a surgeon's abilities, making a good surgeon look great. By contrast, an unprepared, naive, technically challenged FA with a poor understanding of the operative plan can hamper a surgeon, causing even a gifted surgeon to struggle. A talented FA is able to provide exposure effectively, handle tissues appropriately, and attain hemostasis efficiently in close coordination with the surgeon and without impeding the progress of the operation. He or she makes possible the safe, efficient completion of the procedure and works to help the team as a whole function more effectively. To do so, the FA must master important teamwork skills. He or she must know each team member's role, communicate openly and clearly, maintain constant awareness of the overall situation, manage resources, and monitor continually for potential problems. Although complex, these interactive skills contribute to optimal teamwork, improving both efficiency and safety (Halverson et al., 2009).

This chapter focuses on tissue handling techniques commonly used in the surgical care of the patient. It begins with a brief overview of the wound healing process, which is also discussed in Chapter 8. Next, it discusses fundamental surgical principles important to the proper handling of tissues in surgery, followed by a brief discussion of patient positioning (see also Chapter 1) and preparation. It then reviews five essential tissue handling techniques (i.e., incision, dissection, retraction, hemostasis, and suturing/stapling), discussing principles and instruments. Finally, it discusses the challenges and special considerations of tissue handling in the setting of laparoscopic surgery.

OVERVIEW OF WOUND HEALING

From the moment of injury to any tissue, the healing process begins, initiating a cascade of biochemical and microscopic events invisible to the naked eye (Table 3-1). This first phase of wound healing, known as the *inflammatory phase*, involves the release of vasoactive substances such as serotonin, histamine, and bradykinin to promote initial capillary constriction and hemostasis, followed by dilation to increase blood flow to the injured tissue. The body mobilizes platelets and initiates the coagulation cascade to promote hemostasis and seal the wound through the deposition of fibrin and clot. Next, waves of white blood cells (i.e., polymorphonuclear leukocytes, monocytes, and then macrophages) enter the wound to clean it of cellular debris and foreign material. During this process, the wound appears red, edematous, and warm to the touch. Finally, fibroblasts migrate to the wound in preparation for the next phase of healing. The inflammatory phase may last up to five days.

The *proliferative phase* is the subsequent phase in wound healing. In this phase the fibroblasts that have migrated into the wound begin to produce collagen, rapidly increasing the wound's tensile strength. Fibrin and fibronectin are released to create the substance to which the fibroblasts adhere. In addition, new blood vessels are created, which help to nourish the fibroblasts. The squamous epithelium begins to restore the surface anatomy of the skin through

Table 3-1   Phases of Wound Healing

Phase	Length of Time	Events
Inflammatory (lag or exudative phase)	1 to 5 days	Initial vasoconstriction. Platelet aggregation and formation of platelet plug, then clot. Phagocytosis of debris from damaged tissue and blood clot.
Proliferative (also called fibroblastic or connective phase)	Up to 3 weeks	Collagen is produced. Wound tensile strength increases. Granulation tissue forms.
Remodeling (also called maturation, differentiation, resorptive, or plateau phase)	21 days to months	Collagen fibers reorganize and tighten to reduce scar. Tensile strength increases.

Source: Modified from Competency and Credentialing Institute. (2009). *CRNFA study guide and practice resource* (Table 1, p. 40). Denver, CO: Author; and Rothrock, J.C. (Ed.). (1999). *The RN First Assistant: An expanded perioperative nursing role* (3rd ed., Table 11-1, p. 261). Philadelphia: Lippincott.

replication and migration at the basal cell level. Damp dressings at this phase preserve moisture, aiding in squamous epithelial migration and preventing desiccation of newly formed cells. Any significant drying impedes the epithelialization process and delays wound healing. The proliferation phase lasts up to three weeks.

The transition from the proliferative phase to the final *remodeling phase* of wound healing is gradual. The wound's tensile strength increases with cross-linking of collagen. Scar formation occurs with the creation of fibrous connective tissue and myofibroblasts promote wound contraction. Scar maturation and remodeling of the wound may last for years. External forces such as pressure dressings can help during this phase. Since contraction and remodeling tend to take the path of least resistance, the appropriate use of splints is necessary to prevent contractures and deformities over flexion creases, such as in the neck, elbow, or axilla. For skin wounds, maximal wound tensile strength is achieved about six weeks after the initial injury and recovers typically to about 80% of its preinjury value.

Both local and systemic factors can influence wound healing. Important local factors include concentrations of ascorbic acid (Vitamin C), oxygen, zinc, amino acids, and other nutrients and vitamins. Adequate blood flow to the injured tissue is also crucial for repair. Local tissue exposure from prior radiation therapy can negatively impact healing. Systemic factors that can impede wound healing include older age, obesity, chronic disease state (e.g., malignancy, anemia, diabetes), immunosuppression (e.g., use of corticosteroids, HIV, recent chemotherapy), and dehydration.

Surgical wounds are classified into four categories, based on the risk of infection for each wound type (Box 3-1). This assessment is completed at the time of the surgical procedure. *Clean wounds* comprise approximately three quarters of all surgical wounds. They are created under sterile conditions without any break in aseptic technique. Clean wounds are also made without entering epithelial lined structures (i.e., the respiratory, alimentary, or genito-urinary tracts). *Clean-contaminated wounds* have usual and normal flora from incisions on epithelial-lined structures. Any controlled entry into a viscus is considered a clean-contaminated wound. *Contaminated wounds* have sufficient microorganism contamination to cause infection after a period of incubation (i.e., within about six hours). They include fresh traumatic wounds, wounds with acute inflammation, wounds with gross spillage of gastrointestinal contents, wounds exposed to infected bile or urine, and wounds involving procedures with a major break in aseptic technique. *Dirty wounds* are wounds that are severely contaminated or infected prior to operative intervention. Old traumatic wounds with devitalized tissue, abscess wounds, and wounds exposed to contents from a perforated viscus fall into this category.

Caring for Traumatic Wounds in the Emergency Department

It is not uncommon for the FA to accompany the surgeon to the ED to assess the patient and care for traumatic wounds. As mentioned, traumatic wounds are either contaminated or dirty by definition. As such, several important questions should be asked by the FA before closing such a wound in the ED: What is the time inter-val from injury? What is the mechanism of injury? Where is the wound located? What is the patient's overall condition? The risk of infection increases with the time interval between injury and wound closure. In general, most fresh traumatic wounds can be closed (i.e., sutured, stapled, or wound edges approximated with a skin tape/"glue") up to six to eight hours after injury. Whenever doubt exists about safe closure, however, the wound should be left open to heal by "second-ary closure." The area of tissue loss in the wound will gradually fill with granula-tion tissue. Crush wounds containing devitalized tissue and wounds contaminated with feces, saliva, soil, or clothing have increased infection risk. Before any closure is attempted, all dead tissue and foreign material must be removed. Mechanical cleansing of the wound using saline irrigation can help to reduce infection. Care must be taken, however, to avoid overzealous scrubbing during mechanical cleans-ing, which might further damage tissue.

Box 3-1	Classification of Surgical Wounds

Wounds can be classified according to the likelihood and degree of microbial contamination at the time of the surgical procedure. The importance of adhering to principles of asepsis and sterile technique is noted by "no break in technique." When a break in technique occurs, the wound is reclassified. A widely accepted classification scheme, based on early work of the CDC, is listed below:

Clean Wound (Class I): nontraumatic; no inflammation; no break in technique; respiratory or gastrointestinal (GI) tracts not entered; primary wound closure; drains in surgical site, if placed, accomplished with closed drainage system. These are uninfected operative wounds in which no inflammation is encountered and the respiratory, alimentary, genital, or uninfected urinary tracts are not entered. In addition, clean wounds are primarily closed and, if necessary, drained with closed drainage. Operative incisional wounds that follow nonpenetrating (blunt) trauma should be included in this category if they meet the criteria. Clean wounds have a 1% to 5% risk of infection. *Examples:* craniotomy; coronary artery bypass surgery.

Clean-Contaminated Wounds (Class II): no spillage when entering GI (includes biliary tract), genitourological (GU), or respiratory tracts; primary closure; drains placed in surgical site; minor but not major break in technique occurred. These are operative wounds in which the respiratory, alimentary, genital, or urinary tract is entered under controlled conditions and without unusual contamination. Specifically, operations involving the biliary tract, appendix, vagina, and oropharynx are included in this category, provided no evidence of infection or major break in technique is encountered. Clean-contaminated wounds have an 8% to 11% risk of infection. *Examples:* cholecystectomy; appendectomy.

Contaminated Wounds (Class III): fresh, traumatic wound (less than 4 hours old); gross spillage from GI (includes biliary tract) or GU tract; major break in technique; acute inflammation present. These include open, fresh, accidental wounds, operations with major breaks in sterile technique or gross spillage from the GI tract, and incisions in which acute, nonpurulent inflammation is encountered. Contaminated wounds have a 15% to 20% risk of infection. *Examples:* colon resection with gross spillage of bowel contents; open fracture (less than 4 hours old).

Dirty or Infected Wounds (Class IV): acute inflammation; traumatic wound (more than 4 hours old); wound with retained devitalized tissue; perforated viscera; microbial contamination prior to surgical procedure. These include old traumatic wounds with retained devitalized tissue and those that involve existing clinical infection or perforated viscera. This definition suggests that the organisms causing postoperative infection were present in the operative field before the operation. Dirty or infected wounds have a greater than 27% risk of infection. *Example:* ruptured appendix.

Sources: Garner, J.S. (1995). *Guideline for prevention of surgical wound infection, 1985.* Retrieved February 22, 2009 from wonder.cdc.gov/wonder/prevguide/p0000420/p0000420.asp; Price, P., & Smith, C. (2008). Wound healing, sutures, needles and stapling devices. In K.B. Frey (Ed.), *Surgical technology for the surgical technologist—A positive care approach* (3rd ed., pp. 279–280). Clifton Park, NY: Delmar Cengage Learning; Roche, J. (2004). The RNFA in the intraoperative phase. In S.A. Allen (Ed.), *CRNFA study guide.* Denver, CO: Competency and Credentialing Institute.

BASIC SURGICAL PRINCIPLES

In order to master common tissue handling techniques, a strong understanding of basic surgical principles is useful. These principles are fundamental for the surgical care of the patient, and they can serve as a guide for the FAs approach to aiding the surgeon. They include the following:

1. First, do no harm—this is the foremost principle, dating back to Hippocrates, reminding all health care professionals that their primary goal is to help heal.
2. Ensure adequate exposure—a clear, unobstructed operative field with enough room to maneuver is essential for success.
3. Minimize tissue damage—this goal can be achieved by adhering to these principles:
   a. Handle all tissue gently.
   b. Approximate, do not strangulate tissue when suturing and tying knots.
   c. Favor sharp dissection over blunt dissection.
   d. Preserve blood supply and functional tissue as much as possible.
4. Maintain two-point traction—using this principle in sharp dissection and incisions aids with accuracy.
5. Ensure hemostasis through direct pressure, proximal/distal vessel control, and precise clamping and ligating.
6. Employ economy of time and motion—excess or extraneous movement should be minimized in order to proceed as quickly and safely through an operation as possible.

By keeping the above principles in mind, the FA will be able to approach new operative situations and challenges in a more systematic and deliberate manner. As a result, the FA will contribute to the safe, efficient care of the surgical patient.

PATIENT PREPARATION IN THE OPERATING ROOM

Before starting any operative procedure, the FA should prepare for it in several ways. First, he/she should come mentally prepared. Such mental preparation should include a review of the patient's medical history and illness (See Chapter 7 for a full discussion of preoperative assessment of the surgical patient). The FA should also know the type of procedure scheduled as well as the critical steps that such a procedure will entail. Finally, the FA should know who will be on the OR team for the procedure and what roles each person will assume (Haynes et al., 2009; Paige et al., 2008).

The FA should also help to prepare the patient for the operation. This preparation includes making sure that the proper prophylactic regimens have been followed to improve the delivery of care. These regimens include antibiotic (Whitman et al., 2008), thromboembolic, and antiemetic protocols. The FA should also assist in placing the patient in the proper position for the planned operative procedure. Typically, patients are placed in the supine position, lying flat on the OR bed for most abdominal procedures. The lithotomy position, in which the legs are placed in stirrups with the patient lying on his/her back, is used when access to the vagina or anus is desired. The prone jack-knife position, in which the patient lies on the stomach with slight flexion at the hips, allows access to the anus and/or back. Finally, the lateral decubitus position, in which the patient lies on the side with arms outstretched, permits access to the flank. In any position, care must be taken to protect against neurologic and skin injury by padding pressure points. The patient's extremities should also be placed in the proper position and secured. (Chapter 1 provides a full discussion of positioning the surgical patient). After proper positioning and padding, the operative site itself is prepared through anti-microbial cleansing of the surgical site ("prepping"). A sterile field is created by draping (Chapter 2 provides a full discussion of skin preparation and creating and maintaining a sterile field).

Once the patient has been properly prepped and draped, the FA assists in pre-paring the operative environment to maximize ergonomics for the surgeon and him/herself. Since most surgeons are right-handed, operations tend to be done from the patient's right side to make it easier for the surgeon to use his/her right hand. Occasionally, the surgeon will stand on the left side of the patient. The FA should position him/herself opposite the surgeon. Other assistants stand at the head or foot of the patient with their body perpendicular to the surgeon's body. The height of the OR bed (commonly referred to as the "OR table") should reach the surgeon's elbows. The FA should attempt to be in a similar position relative to the height of the OR bed. This height places the wrist in its desired position by allowing it to be in slight extension in the operative field. If the OR bed is too high, the result can be compensatory flexing of the wrists that may reduce small muscle control in the hands by elongating the long extensors and shortening the long flex-ors. As a result, the FA can become more easily fatigued.

For procedures in deep cavities such as the mouth or depressed body spaces, the OR bed should be lowered below the level of the surgeon's elbows. This posi-tion allows the wrists to remain in slight dorsal extension in order to improve dexterity and finger strength. Generally, wrist flexion should be avoided. Finally, in certain cases, such as microsurgical procedures, both the surgeon and FA should be seated. By sitting, the arms can rest on the OR bed, minimizing gross motor movement.

Optimal illumination of the operative field should also be verified before starting a procedure. ORs typically have two overhead lights (one large and one small) mounted on movable booms above the operating bed. In general, the OR bed should be placed in position so that it is centered under the lights before the patient is anesthetized. For most surgical procedures, the best position for the lights is along the vertical axis of the patient (i.e., one light at the head of the patient and one at the foot). Lights placed behind the surgeon and FA can interfere with illumination through shadowing, although it is desirable in certain situations (e.g., in the mouth for cleft palate repair). Shadowing can also be minimized by overlapping light fields and by the use of a headlight in cases where the incision is narrow (e.g., thoracotomy) or the structures are deep (e.g., abdominal aorta surgery).

COMMON TISSUE HANDLING TECHNIQUES

Each surgical procedure unfolds as a series of discrete steps designed to fulfill a particular goal. Each step's successful completion is often aided by skillfully employing one or more of five common tissue handling techniques: incision, dissection, retraction, hemostasis, and suturing/stapling. Mastery of these five techniques requires not only a familiarity with the necessary manipulations, but an in-depth knowledge of the instruments and accessories used. This section discusses technical features of each of these five tissue handling techniques and briefly reviews key instruments and accessories commonly used with them.

Incision

Since obtaining access to the region of interest is required for every operation, knowing the proper technique to create a skin incision is crucial. The FA should give thoughtful consideration to the placement and size of an incision beforehand. This precaution can profoundly impact the ease with which an operation proceeds. The primary goal of any incision is to provide safe access to underlying structures. A proper incision should also be the appropriate size to allow adequate exposure as well as space for manipulation. When possible, it should avoid any anatomic obstacles and should be done in a manner that promotes the best cosmetic result. Three guiding principles determine the location of an incision: 1) the accessibility the incision will provide; 2) the flexibility of the incision, so that it can be extended if more exposure is needed; and 3) how securely it can be closed.

The instrument most commonly used for making an incision is the scalpel. Of the various blades available, the general purpose Nos. 10 and 20 blades are used most frequently for skin. These two blades are designed with a wide blade and a straight cutting surface. Long skin incisions, such as a midline laparotomy, are best made

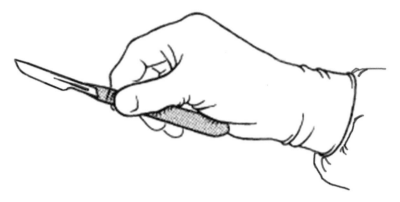

Figure 3-1

Long skin incisions, such as the abdominal midline incision, are best made with the scalpel held between the thumb and first two fingers like a violin bow. Holding the scalpel in this position allows the balance point to pivot on the middle finger while lateral movement is controlled by the index finger and thumb.

Source: Adapted from Rothrock, J.C. (Ed.). (1999). *The RN First Assistant: An expanded perioperative nursing role* (3rd ed., Fig. 8-2, p. 188). Philadelphia: Lippincott.

with the scalpel held between the thumb and the first two fingers, similar to holding a violin bow (Figure 3-1). This position allows the middle finger to serve as a pivot point for balancing, while the index finger and thumb control lateral movement of the instrument. It also enables the arm to move as a unit from the shoulder. The weight and force of the arm are used to control downward pressure and, thus, incision depth. Alternatively, the index finger can be placed on the back of the handle, and incision depth controlled by added pressure applied to the top of the handle.

When grasping the scalpel for incision, the handle is forced against the thenar muscles of the hand. The wrist controls lateral and vertical movement. One single controlled movement is made through the skin and subcutaneous tissues, as the scalpel blade is held perpendicular to the skin (Figure 3-2). This position is preferable to the blade held at an angle to the skin. A smooth, perpendicular cut prevents beveling of the skin and sharply transects blood vessels, allowing effective retraction. Also, this technique allows rapid, controlled entry into a body cavity in an emergency situation (e.g., midline laparotomy for ruptured abdominal aortic aneurysm or thoracotomy for cardiac compression).

Specialty blades are available for specific situations and purposes. For example, the No. 15 blade is used for small skin incisions or incising fine structures. The smaller curve of this scalpel blade means the cutting surface is concentrated at the tip. When using this blade, the scalpel should be held like a pencil with the heel of the hand resting firmly on adjacent tissue for stability. With this technique,

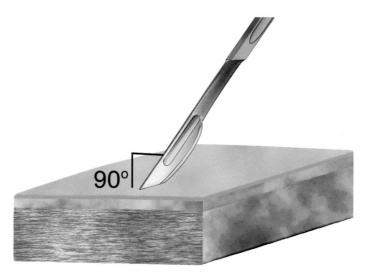

Figure 3-2

Proper scalpel angle.

Source: Courtesy of Phippen, M.L., Ulmer, B.C., & Wells, M.P. (2009). *Competency for safe patient care during operative and invasive procedures* (Fig. 16.14, p. 495). Denver: CCI.

finger movement allows fine control, allowing pinpoint cutting accuracy. For stab incisions, the No. 11 blade, which has a sharp tapered point, is ideal. It is commonly employed to puncture abscesses or vessel walls. It is also used for full-thickness excision of small lesions. When cutting with it, a sawing motion may be necessary.

The electrosurgical unit (ESU) is an accessory that helps make an incision. Typically, a skin incision is begun with a scalpel, and the underlying tissues are then divided using the ESU. One randomized study comparing scalpel versus use of electrosurgery in abdominal incisions demonstrated that electrosurgery is significantly superior for reducing incision time, blood loss, and postoperative pain (Kearns et al., 2001). When a monopolar ESU is used (ESUs are discussed in detail in Chapter 5), the cut mode is used to divide tissue when little or no hemostasis is desired. It produces a great amount of heat over a short period of time. The FA should hold the active electrode (i.e., the ESU pencil) just over the tissue to be cut and then activate it; the tissue effect is achieved through vaporization (Figure 3-3).

To prepare for skin incision, the FA should use the principle of traction/countertraction to stretch and fix the skin. Sponges are a useful accessory to perform this maneuver on a moist skin surface. Once proper skin tension is attained, it should not be relaxed, unless the surgeon pauses in making the incision or lifts the scalpel. Steadily increasing traction as the incision begins helps with division of tissue. Inadvertent tightening or relaxing during the cutting may result in misdirection

Figure 3-3

Vaporization of
tissue using the cut
waveform.

Source: Courtesy of Phippen,
M.L., Ulmer, B.C., & Wells,
M.P. (2009). *Competency
for safe patient care during
operative and invasive
procedures* (Fig. 17.3,
p. 513). Denver: CCI.

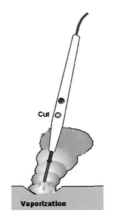

or beveling of the incision. A beveled skin edge increases the risk of necrosis and uneven closure of skin margins. Uneven pulling as an incision is deepened also causes each sweep of the scalpel/electrosurgical device to fall into a different line, terracing the wound and impeding healing. The FA may need to reset his/her hands several times during a long incision in order to maintain proper traction. The FA should inform the surgeon of the need for an impending hand rest. To avoid inadvertent scalpel injury, the FA must also pay attention to the surgeon's movements.

Incisional Approaches to the Abdomen   Since the abdominal cavity is opened more frequently than any other area in general surgery, the FA must be familiar with the various incisional approaches used to enter the abdomen. Generally, abdominal incisions can be classified into four categories, based on incision orientation on the skin: midline, paramedian, oblique, and transverse (Figure 3-4). A brief overview of each type of abdominal incision with examples ensues.

Midline Incisions   The midline incision is the standard approach to entering the abdomen. This vertical incision has several advantages over other types of abdominal incisions. First, it provides excellent access to every region in the peritoneal cavity and, consequently, each intraperitoneal structure. Second, it provides quick access to the abdomen with minimal dissection. In fact, the surgeon can open the skin and subcutaneous fat safely as well as divide the linea alba and peritoneum rapidly in an emergency. Third, the incision can be extended quickly, either within the abdomen or into the chest via a median sternotomy. By lifting the walls of the abdomen, such extension in the abdominal cavity is made easier. Fourth, since the linea alba is without either blood vessels or nerves above the umbilicus, entry into the peritoneum in this region is relatively bloodless and causes little injury to nerves. Below the umbilicus, the linea alba is more difficult to locate because it becomes a fine line between the abdominal muscles.

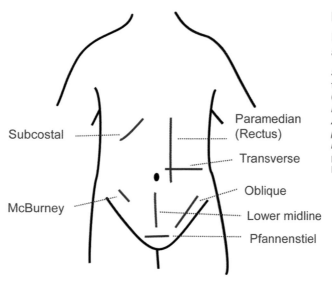

Figure 3-4

Incisions of the abdomen.

Source: Adapted from Rothrock, J.C. (Ed.). (1999). *The RN First Assistant: An expanded perioperative nursing role* (3rd ed., Fig. 8-1, p. 184). Philadelphia: Lippincott.

Subcostal

McBurney

Paramedian (Rectus)

Transverse

Oblique

Lower midline

Pfannenstiel

When incising around the umbilicus, care must be taken to avoid beveling the edges of the incision to reduce risk of ischemia to the skin. This result is achieved by keeping the blade perpendicular to the skin at all times. The umbilicus is best circumnavigated by making a curvilinear incision around it. Alternatively, the FA can place traction on the skin around the umbilicus aimed toward his/herself and pull it out of the way—allowing for a linear cut in the midline. Finally, care must be taken when entering the peritoneum to avoid injury to abdominal contents. By grasping a fold of peritoneum with forceps, palpating the fold to ensure that it is free of underlying structures, and sharply incising the peritoneum to create a small opening, injury can be avoided. The peritoneal incision can be safely extended by placing two to three fingers through the opening between the peritoneum and its underlying contents and then cutting the peritoneum over the fingers.

Paramedian Incisions   Paramedian incisions are vertical incisions made lateral to the midline over the region of the rectus muscle. Like midline incisions, they can extend the entire length of the abdomen from the xiphoid to the level of the symphysis pubis. They are, however, time consuming. These incisions fall into three categories. *Medial paramedian incisions* are made at the medial border of the rectus muscle just to the right or left of the midline. Since the rectus muscle is retracted laterally, both muscle and nerve damage is limited. Care must be taken when extending this incision below the umbilicus because the inferior epigastric artery emerges from the peritoneal cavity at the semicircular Line of Douglas, midway between the umbilicus and symphysis pubis. Often, the epigastric artery requires ligation. *Transrectus paramedian incisions* split the medial aspect of the rectus muscle instead of retracting it. As a result, these incisions can create greater blood loss and nerve injury than medial paramedian incisions. Finally, *lateral paramedian incisions* (also known as pararectus incisions) involve an incision on the anterior rectus sheath laterally. The rectus muscle is then retracted laterally, and an incision is made on the medial aspect of the posterior rectus sheath, similar to medial paramedian incisions. Although paramedian incisions are theoretically stronger because they buttress the rectus muscle, prospective randomized studies have not demonstrated any clear advantage of this type of incision compared to midline incisions (Cox et al., 1986; Ejlersen et al., 1990).

Oblique Incisions   Oblique incisions tend to follow Langer's lines of tension on the skin, allowing for a better cosmetic result. They are typically angled and can be straight or curved in form. Nerve injury is limited with these incisions as well. Three common oblique incisions used in abdominal surgery are the McBurney incision, the Kocher incision, and the lower oblique incision.

The *McBurney incision* is the standard incision used for open appendectomy. It is made perpendicular to an imaginary line extending from the umbilicus to the anterior superior iliac crest in the right lower quadrant and located at the junction of the middle and outer thirds of its length. In this manner, the incision is made in the direction of the external oblique muscle fibers. It is usually 4 to 5 inches long (10.16–12.70 cm). The underlying muscle layers are then sequentially split in the same direction of their fibers to minimize muscle damage and postoperative weakness at the incision. Due to the mobility of the skin and subcutaneous tissues, the incision can be placed below the bikini line and skin retracted cephalad.

The *Kocher incision* (also known as the "right subcostal incision") is used in open gallbladder and biliary tree operations. It starts approximately one third the distance between the xiphoid and the umbilicus in the midline, and extends parallel to the costal margin about 1 inch (2.5 cm) below. The rectus muscle is divided, and branches of the superior epigastric artery are ligated. A left-sided version of the Kocher can be used for splenectomy. The two can be combined to create a chevron or bucket handle incision, which provides excellent exposure to the upper abdomen. Subcostal incisions are more time consuming than midline incisions.

The *lower oblique incision* is typically used for transplant, urological, and certain types of vascular surgery. They require transection of the abdominal wall and flank muscle, and electrocoagulation is often used to minimize bleeding of the muscles. The lower oblique incision provides access to retroperitoneal structures such as the aorta and kidneys, and it can be extended to the chest for superior access, creating a thoracoabdominal incision. The retroperitoneal approach to the aorta can decrease the rate of postoperative pulmonary problems compared to the midline incision.

Transverse Incisions   Transverse incisions are horizontal skin incisions, although they can curve to varying degrees. They are similar to oblique incisions since they also follow Langer's lines of tension and produce minimal nerve and vessel damage. The fascia is then typically divided in the midline. An *infraumbilical transverse incision* can provide very good exposure to the pelvis and lower abdomen. Exposure of the entire abdomen, however, is limited with this type of incision. The *Pfannenstiel incision* is commonly used in gynecological surgery. A curvilinear incision is made approximately 2 inches (5 cm) above the symphysis pubis down to the rectus muscles, which are then divided transversely. They are dissected up superior to the umbilicus, and retracted laterally. A vertical incision is then made in the fascia midline, providing excellent exposure to the pelvic organs. The skin incision is below the bikini line, allowing for an excellent cosmetic result. Care must be taken to avoid injury to the bladder when entering the abdomen using the Pfannenstiel incision.

Dissection

Dissection is an essential tissue handling technique in any surgical procedure. Careful and accurate dissection allows the surgeon and FA to delineate the structures of interest in a safe, efficient manner that minimizes damage to adjacent tissue and organs. Key components of any dissection technique include *adequate exposure* of the region or structure being dissected, *good illumination* of the surgical field, *meticulous hemostasis*, and *two-point traction* of the tissue being dissected. Often, two-point traction can be established using a fixed anatomical structure as one point. For example, the gallbladder can be dissected off the liver bed by gently pulling it down and using the liver as the fixed anatomical point. In any dissection, inadvertent injury is avoided by clearly defining the anatomy through exposure and good surgical lighting. Of the two, sharp dissection is preferred over blunt in most circumstances because of its precise, accurate nature.

The most common instrument used in dissection is the scissors, although a scalpel is utilized by some surgeons. Scissors are of varied shapes (e.g., straight or curved) and lengths (i.e., long or short), with different types of tips (e.g., blunt or sharp) (Figure 3-5). The two most commonly used in general surgery are the Mayo and Metzenbaum scissors, both of which have curved tips. These curves allow versatility in the angle of dissection. In addition, they provide the ability to lift and palpate tissue. The Mayo scissors is heavier and reserved for cutting large or thick structures. The Metzenbaum is finer and is used for most sharp dissection.

Scissors should be held with the thumb and ring fingers placed through the instrument rings. The distal joints of the index and long fingers should curl beneath the scissor's shank. With this technique, the instrument has three points of fixation against

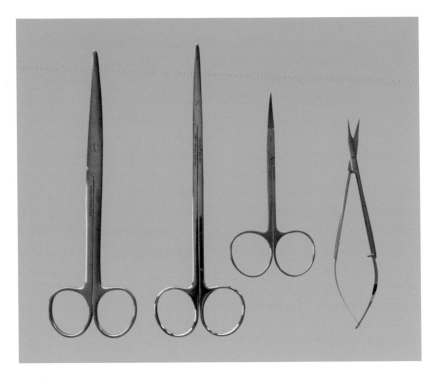

Figure 3-5

Scissors. *Left to right*: Mayo dissecting scissors, straight; Metzenbaum dissecting scissors; Iris scissors, straight; and Westcott tenotomy scissors, straight.

Source: Provided courtesy of Tighe, S.M. (2007). *Instrumentation for the operating room: A photographic manual* (7th ed., Fig. 1-2, p. 15). St. Louis: Mosby. Reprinted by permission.

the hand. The index and long fingers provide stability and can control the direction of the blade tips. When dissecting through very dense tissue, further downward pressure on the tips and blades is achieved by extending the index finger along the shanks, beyond the fulcrum of the scissors, and pressing the thumb on one handle through the ring hole. Finally, during dissection, the FAs body should be turned so as to maintain an axial relationship between the forearm and the scissors.

Dissection with a curved scissors such as a Metzenbaum allows for a variety of blade tip positions when the scissors are rotated along the axis of the forearm. The most natural manner for dissecting with scissors is by cutting away from oneself from right to left. Left to right cuts may require rotating the body and cocking the wrist. A forearm in a supinated position can make fine hand control more difficult, because it causes added strain and fatigue.

A clean cut is necessary when performing *sharp dissection*. If the scissors are blunt, a clean cut can be achieved by squeezing the blades together. Two-point traction also allows for clean cuts. Finally, cuts should be made with a single, smooth motion. When dissecting an object from surrounding tissue, the tip of the curved scissors should follow the curve of the object (e.g., the curve of the scissors should follow the curve of a cyst).

Blunt dissection can be used to create a tunnel that follows the shape of the structure of interest or to define a tissue plane. To accomplish these maneuvers, gentle pressure is applied to the Metzenbaum scissors with the blades firmly apposed. The blades are then gently spread to open with only enough room to make a cut. The scissors are then removed, the blades rotated 90 degrees, the lower blade inserted into the space, and the cut made. Dissection should occur one tissue layer at a time. Do not cut with scissors beyond the clearly defined area that was bluntly dissected.

Retraction

Retraction is a key component in gaining adequate exposure in any surgical procedure. In addition, retraction is often employed to help with dissection through the use of two-point traction. When retracting tissue, gentleness is crucial. Prolonged, excessive pressure can damage tissues, resulting in unwanted complications. Improper retraction techniques can cause problems such as nerve praxis, organ injury (e.g., liver or spleen tears), and decreased blood flow from inadvertent vena cava compression. Constant yet adequate controlled force, therefore, is best for retraction. Several different instruments have been developed to assist with retraction in surgery. They range from simple hand-held devices for grasping or holding structures to more complex self-retainers. Chapter 4 provides a full discussion of retraction. A brief description of some more commonly used devices follows.

Grasping Instruments   Grasping instruments are useful to provide two-point traction for dissection or to hold structures. Clamps or forceps are the most common grasping instruments. Clamps have ratchets that permit them to be locked into a position. The *Kocher clamp* is a toothed instrument useful to retract fibrotic or heavily scarred areas for dissection. This clamp provides a firm grip on such tissue, lessens hand fatigue and minimizes slippage. Frequently, the Kocher clamp is used during opening or closing an abdomen to lift and hold the peritoneum, allowing underlying abdominal contents to fall away. Its small jaws apply great pressure to a small area. Because of this capability, it is considered a crushing instrument. Care must be taken, therefore, to ensure that it is not mistakenly given to an FA or surgeon in lieu of another instrument such as a Kelly clamp. To avoid this problem, the FA or surgeon should always note the type of clamp before applying it to any tissue. If the Kocher clamp is used to clamp across bowel, a cuff of tissue should be left distal to it to prevent slippage.

The *Allis clamp* is a fine-toothed instrument used to retract more delicate tissue, such as transected bowel. It too applies a large amount of pressure to a small area. Therefore, minimal pressure is needed to hold it since the jaws are unlikely to slip. The type of tissue for which an Allis clamp can be used depends on the number and fineness of its teeth. The *Babcock clamp*, unlike the Allis and Kocher clamps, is considered a nontraumatic clamp. It does not have teeth, and it is broad and thin-bladed. It is typically used to encircle tubular structures such as the appendix or fallopian tube and allows these structures to be gently retracted. A Babcock should be ratcheted only enough to hold the tissue adequately. Finally, the *tenaculum* is a heavy toothed clamp designed for holding tougher, heavier tissues such as the cervix or thyroid. The teeth cause less metal to come into contact with the tissue.

Thumb forceps are an extension of the surgeon's or FAs fingers and allow for precise handling of tissue. In addition to retraction, forceps are used in a variety of other tissue handling techniques (e.g., as an adjunct in suturing or hemostasis). In general, they are commonly used by the nondominant hand to assist with maneuvers done by the dominant hand. The FA will often use forceps to assist with dissection by providing two-point traction or by helping provide exposure. Forceps can be smooth or have teeth. Toothed forceps are good for grasping fibrotic or scarred tissue (Figure 3-6). The *Adson forceps* is also particularly useful for grasping skin. It is a

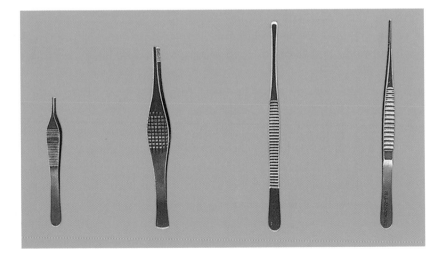

Figure 3-6

Forceps. *Left to right*: Adson tissue forceps; Ferris Smith tissue forceps; Russian tissue forceps; DeBakey vascular tissue forceps.

Source: All figures for 3-6 provided courtesy of Tighe, S.M. (2007). *Instrumentation for the operating room: A photographic manual* (7th ed., Fig. 3-6, p. 27). St. Louis: Mosby. Reprinted by permission.

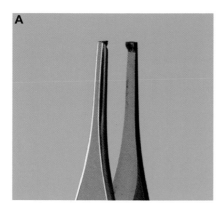

Figure 3-6A

Adson tissue forceps, tip.

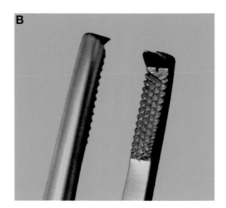

Figure 3-6B

Ferris Smith tissue forceps, tip.

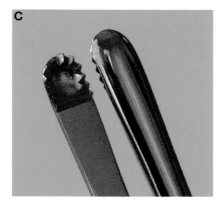

Figure 3-6C

Russian tissue forceps, tip.

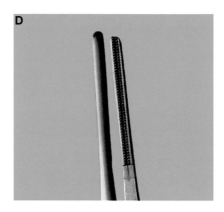

Figure 3-6D

DeBakey vascular tissue forceps, tip.

small-toothed forceps that has longitudinal rows of teeth that allow for firm fixation and distribution of force without trauma to the tissue. Smooth, nonpuncturing forceps are best to hold delicate structures such as bowel or peritoneum.

Forceps should be grasped as if holding a pencil (or by using a modified pencil grip) in order to give the greatest maneuverability (Figure 3-7). In this manner, one blade of the forceps becomes an extension of the thumb while the other is an extension of the opposing fingers. The grip on the forceps should be gentle and balanced. If the FAs hand becomes fatigued when holding the forceps, or if the tissue cannot be adequately grasped, another forceps or clamp should be used.

When not in active use, the forceps may be tucked in the palm (referred to as "palmed") and supported by extending the ring and little finger. The straight middle finger remains free for use. Palming while alternately grasping with forceps or fingers

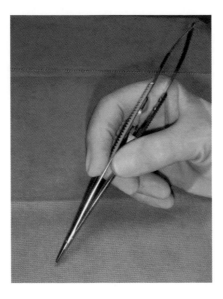

Figure 3-7

Pencil grip. Forceps should be held as if holding a pencil.

Source: Photo courtesy Winchester Hospital, Winchester, MA.

can save time. If the little finger or ring finger is required to complete a one-handed tie, the forceps can be temporarily pinched in the web between the thumb and index finger. To move the forceps back into a position of use, the palm is turned down, and the thumb and index finger are used to grasp the forceps in the desired place.

Hand-Held Retractors   Hand-held retractors are used to retract tissues for exposure. They can be used to retract superficial or deep structures. The FA should become familiar with the various types of specialty retractors. They have been designed for specific purposes and situations. When using any hand-held retractor, a constant force should be applied in the direction and with the force prescribed by the surgeon.

The *Deaver retractor* has a curved handle and is designed to be held palm up. In this manner, the retractor tip is kept "toed-in," reducing the force needed to provide retraction. The *Kelly-Richardson retractor* comes in various sizes. It is used to hold back the wound edge during fascial incision or closure. An *"army-navy" retractor* is smaller with one short blade and one long blade that can be used to retract more superficial tissues at varying depths. A *malleable retractor* is a straight blade that can be bent into any desired position to assist with retraction. It is often used to keep abdominal contents away from the fascia during closure of the abdomen.

A sponge may also be used to retract abdominal contents. The organs to be retracted are held with the spread fingers of an open hand. The opened sponge is placed over the hand by the second hand or with long forceps. The deep edge of the sponge is curled under the organs to be retracted at the level of the retroperitoneum. The upper edge of the sponge is tucked under the incision, between the organs and the anterior abdominal wall. During a procedure, it is useful for the FA who places sponges to announce how many have been used. This measure helps to ensure sponge retrieval when the count is performed. Foreign objects unintentionally left in patients (often referred to as a "retained foreign object" or RFO) are a significant surgical safety issue and are considered an avoidable error or "never event" by the Centers for Medicare and Medicaid (CMS) (please refer to Chapter 8 for a more complete discussion of "never events") (Price, 2008; NQF, 2009; Retzlaff, 2009).

Self-Retaining Retractors   Self-retaining retractors are designed to retract tissue without the need for a person to constantly hold the device. In this manner, self-retaining retractors can free the FA to assist with other aspects of the procedure while exposure is maintained. The *Weitlaner retractor* is a self-retaining device used for superficial procedures such as inguinal herniorrhaphy. Deep self-retaining retractors include the *Balfour retractor* that can be used to retract abdominal contents during laparotomy (**Figure 3-8**). Adjustable blades of varying depths

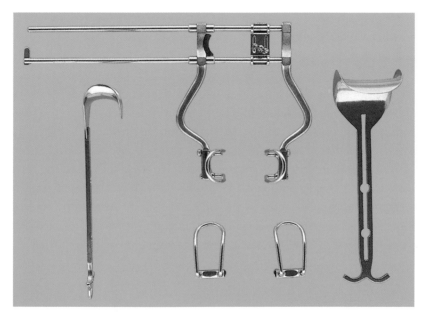

Figure 3-8

Balfour retractor: *Top to bottom, left to right*: Balfour abdominal retractor: retractor frame with two detachable shallow fenestrated blades; one shallow center blade; two deep fenestrated blades; and one deep center blade.

Source: Provided courtesy of Tighe, S.M. (2007). *Instrumentation for the operating room: A photographic manual* (7th ed., Fig. 4-8, p. 33). St. Louis: Mosby. Reprinted by permission.

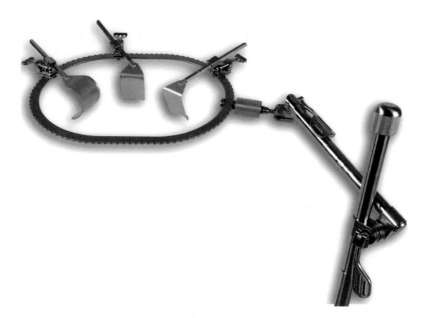

Figure 3-9

Omni Flex Post: Omni retractor.

Source: Courtesy of Omni-Tract® Surgical. Reprinted by permission.

permit retraction of the abdominal wall itself or deeper structures. When opening such a device, care must be taken to avoid trapping tissue between the blades and the abdominal wall, causing damage. The hand should be placed between the blade and tissues to avoid trapping structures. Also, moist, double-folded sponges are used to cover underlying tissues to protect them. Another self-retaining retractor is the *Omni* (**Figure 3-9**), also known as the *"iron intern."* It has large articulating arms that are secured to the OR bed and provide a constant retraction. Other devices, such as the *Bookwalter retractor*, have large metal rings that are secured to the OR bed via a post. Retractors are then placed on the ring to provide exposure.

Hemostasis

Ensuring hemostasis during a surgical procedure is crucial for its safe, efficient completion. Without adequate hemostasis, exposure can be compromised and dissection made more difficult. In addition, suturing can be negatively affected and wound healing impaired. Precision in identifying and controlling a bleeding point is essential. Direct pressure, using either a gloved finger or moistened sponge, over the site of bleeding often can provide temporary control in preparation for definitive hemostasis. For example, during skin incision, the FA may place a moistened sponge against the open ends of transected vessels. In cases of oozing in localized regions, sponges can be packed in the desired location. In deep recesses, a "sponge on a stick" (a sponge grasped in a packing forceps) may be required to gain temporary hemostasis via direct pressure. The FA should maintain pressure with this device until the surgeon is ready to control the bleeding site. The sponge is then slowly rolled off the vessel to expose it. Gaining proximal control of a large bleeding vessel via a vascular clamp may be necessary in order to ensure hemostasis. Finally, directly grasping the vessel with an instrument can provide temporary hemostasis.

Definitive hemostatic techniques include ligation, electrocoagulation, and suturing. Bleeding from individual vessels or rapid, extensive loss of blood from hemorrhage is best controlled by ligation. Ligation often requires identification and clamping of the vessel. The *hemostat* or *Kelly* clamp is used (one technique for using a hemostat is shown in **Figure 3-10**). A vessel can be clamped using either the tip or jaw technique. In the tip technique, the tip of the instrument points toward the vessel. In the jaw technique, the tip of the instrument points away from the vessel. The vessel is grasped in the greater curve of the instrument, allowing its tip to extend beyond the structure. Although more tissue is clamped within the jaw, the extended tip allows a ligature to be more easily trapped as it is passed. The jaw technique is especially useful when clamping between uncut structures prior to transection (e.g., vascular pedicles, omentum, or the falciform ligament). The reason is that knot tying is easier if the tip is pointing in the direction of the cut (i.e., away from the vessel).

When a ligature is being placed, the FA should hold the hemostat with the fingers outside the loops of the rings. This technique permits optimal rotation of the instrument for tie placement without twisting the vessel. The handles of the clamp should be held away from the wound to allow the hands of the person tying the knot to obtain access. The clamp tip should be exposed without pulling on the vessel once the first loop of the tie is in place. The clamp is then gently removed in one of two ways after the first tie is thrown. Using the three-point grasp technique, the thumb and index fingers are placed in the rings of the instrument. The tip is then rested on a firm surface and the index finger pressed on the closed shanks to "push" the clamp away. In the second method for removal, the fingers are not placed in the instrument rings (see **Figure 3-10B**). The thenar eminence of the thumb grasps the instrument finger ring on the left. The ring is then pinched between the thumb and the ring finger. The index finger is then pressed on the instrument finger ring to disengage the clamp.

Electrocoagulation can also be used to control bleeding definitively. Typically, it is used for smaller vessels or bleeding points. A thumb forceps or hemostat can be used to grasp the bleeding vessel precisely, and the current can be applied to the

Figure 3-10

Hemostat technique.

A

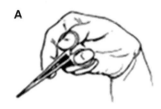

B

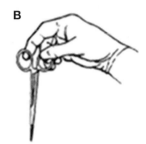

Figure 3-10A

In grasping a bleeder, the method shown in A is the most sure. Only the very tip of the instrument is used to capture the smallest amount of tissue containing the bleeder. Consequently, the smallest amount of tissue is devitalized by ligature or electric current.

Figure 3-10B

Once the hemostat is placed, however, the fingers should be withdrawn from the rings, and the hemostat should be grasped as in B. The ring closest to the FA is grasped between thumb and middle finger, and the index finger is kept mobile enough to release the ratchet of the instrument by pressure against the ring. In this maneuver, the whole instrument is firmly stabilized with the ring that is held between the thumb and third finger. This technique also allows the FA to manipulate the point of the instrument through an almost 360-degree arc, which would not be possible if the fingers were still placed through the rings, as shown in the original position in A. Performing the recommended technique will require practice and expertise to develop smooth manual dexterity.

C

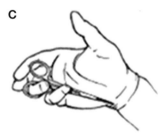

Figure 3-10C

Once the hemostat has performed its function, it may be carried for immediate reuse as indicated in C. The lower ring is hooked by the distal end of the fourth finger, and the body of the instrument is then held to the palm of the hand by the fifth finger. This allows the thumb, middle, and third fingers to be mobile. The FAs ability to continue to assist is not limited, inasmuch as an entire surgical procedure can be expertly handled with just these three digits. Any time the hemostat is to be used again, it can be flipped out as shown in A and then returned to the position shown in C again when its duty has been accomplished. This maneuver is not limited to the use of the hemostat. It can be used with scissors or any comparable ringed instrument that is not too long.

Source: Adapted from Rothrock, J.C. (Ed.). (1999). *The RN First Assistant: An expanded perioperative nursing role* (3rd ed., Fig. 12-1 A,B,C, p. 289). Philadelphia: Lippincott.

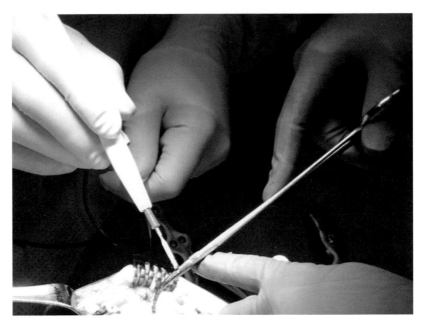

Figure 3-11

Buzz hemostat. Applying current from the active electrode of the ESU to a surgical instrument. When preparing to apply current, hold the hemostat with a full grip to disperse current over a wider surface area. Touch the hemostat (or other clamp) before activating the ESU pencil.

Source: Photo courtesy of Winchester Hospital, Winchester, MA.

instrument to desiccate the site (Figure 3-11). Pinpoint application of high current for short bursts is also useful. Desiccation of large areas, however, should be avoided because of the extensive tissue damage it can cause.

Finally, suturing can be used to provide definitive hemostasis. It may involve the closure of a small hole in a vessel, the oversewing of a cut vessel edge, or the application of a figure of eight suture to tie off a bleeding vessel that has retracted into tissue.

The FA must keep the operative field clear of blood and clot during a procedure. The use of suction to prevent pooling of blood within the operative field using quick, smooth movements is helpful. Clot can be removed from a wound by taking a moistened sponge, pressing it firmly against the clot, and lifting it away using a slight grasping of the fingers. Heavy rubbing should be avoided to prevent rebleeding. When using a sponge to remove liquid blood, a gentle blotting action should be employed.

Suturing/Stapling

Suturing and stapling are core tissue handling techniques for any anastomosis or wound closure. When performing either technique, creating a tension-free approximation of the involved structures without inducing tissue ischemia is critical for success. As with other tissue handling techniques, adequate exposure, meticulous hemostasis, and proper illumination are essential for efficient, safe suturing or stapling.

A needle holder and thumb forceps are required for suturing. As with other ringed instruments, the needle holder is held with the index and middle fingers supporting the shank. The thumb and ring finger are inserted into the instrument rings. The thumb can also be removed from the instrument ring and the ring supported by the MP joint of the thumb. When suturing, a curved needle should be grasped proximally between its junction with the suture and the middle of the needle. It should enter the tissue at a right angle with the forearm in pronation (Figure 3-12). The forearm is then placed in a supine position to complete the throw. The needle is then removed by grasping it proximal to its point with the forearm pronated. Finally, the needle is extracted from the tissue easily with the forearm placed in the supine position.

Stapling devices come in varying sizes and shapes, each designed for a particular function (Figure 3-13). They are commonly used to transect structures or create anastomoses and may be designed for specific purposes such as use on the small

Figure 3-12

Inserting needle. When inserting a needle through tissue, it should enter the tissue at a right angle.

Source: Courtesy of Phippen, M.L., Ulmer, B.C., & Wells, M.P. (2009). *Competency for safe patient care during operative and invasive procedures* (Fig. 16-13, p. 491). Denver: CCI.

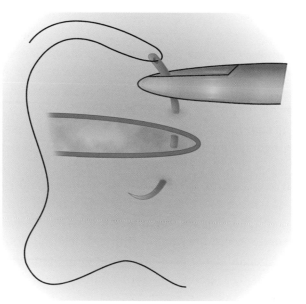

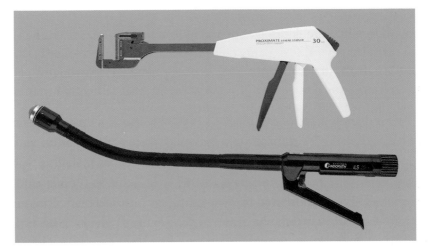

Figure 3-13

Linear and circular endo stapler: *Top to bottom*: linear stapler, 30 mm; endoscopic circular stapler.

Source: Provided courtesy of Tighe, S.M. (2007). *Instrumentation for the operating room: A photographic manual* (7th ed., Fig. 14-6, p. 61). St. Louis: Mosby. Reprinted by permission.

bowel or for completion of a large bowel anastomosis near the anus (e.g., left colon to lower rectum). Before firing any stapler when making an anastomosis, care must be taken to ensure that tissue is properly apposed and that the staple jaws are free of any outside tissues that may have inadvertently become caught in them. One advantage of stapling devices is the time saved in performing anastomoses and closing wounds. The FA must be thoroughly acquainted with the many numerous stapling devices available for use, and he or she must be familiar with their mechanisms of action.

The FA must also have a keen understanding of the many types of suture material available, so that he or she can be effective in aiding the surgeon. Suture is available in a broad array of sizes and lengths with equally varying types of needles. Though such variety can seem overwhelming, suture material can be divided into two broad categories: absorbable and nonabsorbable. This division is useful in determining which suture to choose and in classifying the relative tensile strength and tissue reactivity of each type of suture (suture and suturing techniques are more fully discussed in Chapter 6). Within each category, the suture may come from synthetic or natural sources. A suture may be composed of multiple (i.e., braided or twisted; referred to as "multifilament") or single (i.e., monofilament) strands. In general, braided sutures are easier to tie, but they can produce more tissue reaction. Ideally, a suture should provide maximal strength during wound healing with minimal tissue reactivity.

Wound Closure: The Abdomen

Prior to closing an open abdomen, drain placement may be necessary. In general, abdominal drains are placed to drain a localized region of infection (i.e., an abscess cavity) or localized fluid leak (e.g., bile leakage). They should not be used for generalized drainage of peritonitis or as a substitute for hemostasis (i.e., to control bleeding). When placing a drain, the shortest, most direct route to the skin should be selected. A small stab wound placed away from the main incision should be just large enough to allow the drain to come out. The drain is secured to the skin with nonabsorbable suture after skin closure. A dressing is applied at the end of the procedure to prevent maceration of the surrounding skin. The dressing should not pull on the drain when removed.

Proper fascial closure is critical to prevent dehiscence. When closing fascia, nonabsorbable sutures of the appropriate gauge (e.g., size 0 or 1 Nylon) should be used. Stitches should be placed 3/8 inch to 3/4 inch (1.0 to 1.5 cm) back from the fascial edge at 3/8 inch (1.0-cm) intervals. A continuous or running suture is quicker than interrupted suture placement (see Chapter 6). Care must be taken to prevent fraying or other damage to the suture with the needle holder, because this problem can cause eventual rupture and wound disruption. *A mass closure that includes muscle increases strength.* When using monofilament suture, multiple knots must be tied to prevent slippage. Finally, the fascia should be approximated when tying the knots. The tissue need not be strangulated. A closure that is too tight can lead to tissue ischemia and suture pull-through with dehiscence.

Skin can be closed using absorbable subcuticular sutures, nonabsorbable sutures that can be pulled out, or skin staples. Stapling devices are quicker and designed to evert and appose the skin automatically. To prevent scarring, nonabsorbable sutures or staples can be removed within three to five days, although they are typically left in place for seven to ten days. Care must be taken to ensure that fascial and subcutaneous closures are strong enough to prevent any wound breakdown before removing skin sutures or staples.

The dressing chosen to cover a wound should provide an optimal environment for epithelialization. Dressings should create a moist environment without causing maceration or damage to granulation tissue or surrounding skin (van Winterswijk & Nout, 2007). Semipermeable, transparent membranes are one dressing example. For wounds that are draining, the dressing should prevent exudate from coming into contact with healthy skin by wicking and absorbing the exudate effectively.

TISSUE HANDLING CONSIDERATIONS IN LAPAROSCOPY

The laparoscopic revolution has transformed general surgery. Patients are now able to undergo operations adapted to the minimally invasive technique. These procedures produce less pain, shorten hospital stays, and have better cosmetic outcomes compared to open procedures. Patients can also return to work more easily and quickly. Not surprisingly, laparoscopy has become an integral part of the general surgeon's practice, and the FA is frequently called upon to assist in these operations. Given laparoscopy's unique character, however, the skill sets required to perform and assist in laparoscopy are different from those for open surgery. The FA needs to understand these differences fully in order to adapt the tissue handling techniques used in open surgery.

Laparoscopy differs from open surgery in three key aspects. First, visualization of the abdomen occurs via the use of a camera scope, and participants view the surgical procedure on a two-dimensional monitor instead of in three-dimensional space. As a result, both surgeon and FA must conduct surgery without depth perception. Second, the abdominal wall trocars used to access the abdomen create a fulcrum effect by which any movement outside the abdominal cavity translates into movement in an opposite direction within the abdominal cavity. For example, external movement of an instrument by the hand to the right outside the abdomen will make the instrument's tip move to the left within the abdomen and vice versa. Movement upward will make the tip of the instrument move downward and vice versa. Lastly, the long instruments used in laparoscopy decrease tactile feedback because sensation to the hand must first be transmitted along the instrument length.

These three unique aspects of laparoscopy (i.e., lack of depth perception, the fulcrum effect, and decreased haptic feedback) make the surgeon and FA more dependent on visual rather than tactile input during a procedure. In addition, unique psychomotor skills are required to manipulate instruments accurately and efficiently. Fortunately, validated drills (e.g., the Fundamentals of Laparoscopic Surgery [FLS]) are available to develop laparoscopic skills using box trainers (see information on the FLS program in Chapter 13, Resources). The FA should avail him/herself of these tools to hone laparoscopic skills before assisting in these procedures. Use of simulation and simulators permits ongoing feedback during skill and competency assessment in a safe, controlled setting (Rodriguez-Paz et al., 2009).

In laparoscopy, patient positioning and preparation require giving additional consideration to the placement of monitors and personnel (**Figure 3-14**). In general, monitors should be placed in such a way that surgeon and FA can view them easily and in similar alignment to the region of interest. For example, a laparoscopic cholecystectomy typically has two monitors located at the shoulder level of the

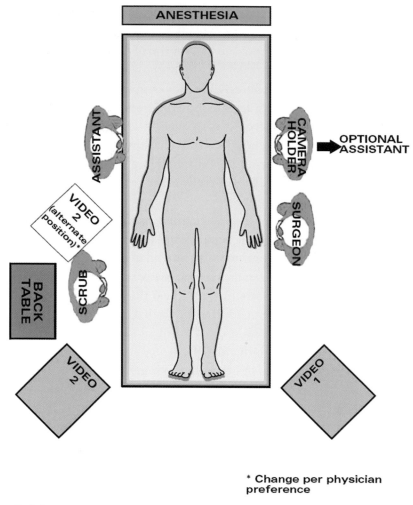

ANESTHESIA

ASSISTANT

CAMERA HOLDER

OPTIONAL ASSISTANT

SURGEON

VIDEO 2 (alternate position)*

SCRUB

BACK TABLE

VIDEO 2

VIDEO 1

* Change per physician preference

Figure 3-14

Position for laparoscopic appendectomy and herniorrhaphy.

Source: Provided courtesy of Tighe, S.M. (2007). *Instrumentation for the operating room: A photographic manual* (7th ed., Fig. 10-10, p. 52). St. Louis: Mosby. Reprinted by permission.

patient, opposite both surgeon and FA. In a laparoscopic inguinal herniorrhaphy, the monitor is placed at the patient's feet. The FA typically stands opposite the surgeon. Yet in certain upper abdominal procedures, the surgeon may take a position between the patient's legs, with the patient in a modified lithotomy position.

The uniqueness of laparoscopy has important implications for the common tissue handling techniques described above for open surgery. Incisions for laparoscopy tend to be smaller and in multiple locations. Thoughtful consideration about their placement becomes essential in order to maximize effective trocar and camera use during a procedure. A key concept is to place the camera and working trocars in such as way as to mimic the relationship between the eyes and hands. Such an arrangement can be accomplished through triangulation of the trocar ports. With this technique, the camera becomes the apex of a triangle in which the hand ports are placed on either side. If possible, a camera should not directly face a trocar because of the mirror image effect it produces on movement of an instrument through that trocar. When properly placed, a relatively small number of trocars can provide the necessary access for the procedure. If it becomes difficult to perform a procedure due to port position, additional sites may need to be created. Conversion to an open procedure should be undertaken if it cannot be safely performed using the laparoscopic approach. Finally, trocar incisions are typically made with a No. 11 blade because of their small size.

Laparoscopic dissection and retraction require particularly gentle tissue handling because of the decreased tactile feedback. Special care must be taken when grasping (Figure 3-15) and retracting tissue to avoid inadvertent tearing.

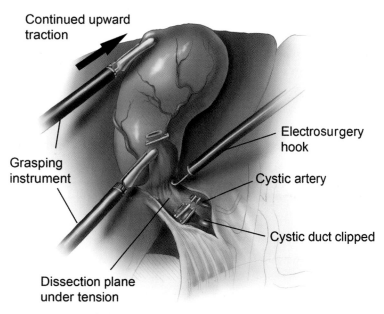

Figure 3-15

Using laparoscopic grasping instruments to provide traction and grasp the gallbladder during laparoscopic cholecystectomy.

Source: Courtesy of Phippen, M.L., Ulmer, B.C., & Wells, M.P. (2009). *Competency for safe patient care during operative and invasive procedures* (Fig. 16.7, p. 476). Denver: CCI.

Maintaining visualization of the instruments and tissues being manipulated is likewise important. In dissection, complete exposure and visualization of the structures of interest is useful. Sharp dissection with scissors is also beneficial. Heightened care using electrosurgical devices should be used to avoid unintended organ damage.

Maintaining hemostasis is particularly important in laparoscopy. Blood and clot absorb light, making visualization with the camera more difficult. In addition, light absorption can obscure planes and tissues. Spurting blood can also cover the camera, making visualization impossible. Because of the camera magnification, a comparatively small amount of bleeding can appear quite significant. Temporary hemostasis is best obtained by grasping the bleeding vessel, as direct pressure can be difficult to attain with a long instrument. Clips, staplers, and electrocoagulation are effective and definitive hemostatic measures. Ultrasonic coagulation devices can also be used to achieve hemostasis of larger vessels. Suturing also can be effective, although it is more challenging. If hemorrhage cannot be controlled, immediate conversion to an open procedure should promptly begin.

Suturing in laparoscopy also requires a skill set different from open surgery. Knots can be tied via either an intracorporeal or extracorporeal technique. Familiarity with both techniques is a necessity. The FLS drills include both techniques and allow for practice outside the operating room. Staplers specially designed to deploy in laparoscopy are often used to create anastomoses and to transect structures. Some of these devices can be articulated for highly versatile use.

The FA will often be asked to "drive" the camera during a laparoscopic procedure. In doing so, the FA becomes the eyes of the surgeon. When operating the camera, the FA should keep the instruments of the surgeon in the center of the monitor screen. When responding to a request to move the camera in a certain direction, the FA should move it based on the monitor orientation. Thus, a request to move the camera to the left should correspond with a leftward movement of the field on the monitor. Finally, the FA should also become proficient with the use of cameras with angled views in order to maximize visualization. A talented camera operator can increase the efficiency of the procedure and thereby decrease operative time.

CONCLUSION

The surgical assistant is an integral member of the operative team. As such, the FA must work diligently to facilitate effectively the work of the surgeon. By adhering to established surgical principles and using sound tissue handling techniques, the FA will contribute to the safe, efficient delivery of care to the surgical patient.

GLOSSARY

Anastomosis: a surgical joining of two anatomical structures. These may be blood vessels, as in a vascular anastomosis; ducts; tubular structures, such as parts of the bowel, or other anatomical structures. Anastomoses are performed to create an opening and consequent flow (such as the flow of blood in a vascular anastomosis) from one part to the other.

Articulated: joint that allows movement in several different directions.

Dehiscence: a separation: commonly describes a complication of wound healing in which the surgical incision opens prematurely or ruptures, especially the abdominal fascia.

Desiccation: drying out. In this chapter, it is used with reference to electrocoagulation or "drying out" of tissue.

Epithelialization: In wound healing, epithelialization refers to the process by which epithelial cells migrate across the wound bed to cover it.

Exudate: the discharge of fluids, cells, pus, or other substances from cells or blood vessels.

Granulation: tissue that forms in wounds that do not heal by first intention. Capillaries and fibrous collagen project into the wound during the healing process, filling the wound as it heals.

Haptics: the science that studies the sense of touch. Haptic technology is technology that interfaces with the user through the sense of touch. Haptic perception is the process of recognizing objects through touch.

Intra/extracorporeal: within (intracorporeal) or outside of (extracorporeal) the body.

Phagocytosis: the process by which certain cells engulf and destroy microorganisms as well as cellular debris. The prefix *phago* means to "eat" or "digest." Examples of phagocytes are macrophages and neutrophils.

Viscera: internal organs enclosed within a body cavity, such as the abdomen, thorax, or pelvis.

Viscus: singular form of viscera, meaning internal organ.

REFERENCES

1. Burt, B.M., Tavakkolizadeh, A., & Ferzoco, S.J. (2007). Incisions, closures, and management of the abdominal wound. In M.J. Zinner & S.W. Ashley (Eds.), *Maingot's abdominal operations* (11th ed.). New York: McGraw-Hill.

2. Cox, P.J., Ausobsky, J.R., Ellis, H., & Pollock, A.V. (1986). Towards no

incisional hernias: lateral paramedian versus midline incisions. *Journal of the Royal Society of Medicine, 79*(12), 711–2.

3. Dunscombe, A.R. (2007). Sutures, needles, and instruments. In J.C. Rothrock (Ed.), *Alexander's care of the patient in surgery* (13th ed.). St. Louis: Mosby Elsevier.

4. Ejlersen, E., Steven, K., & Løkkegaard, H. (1990). Paramedian versus midline incision for the insertion of permanent peritoneal dialysis catheters: A randomized clinical trial. *Scandinavian Journal of Urology and Nephrology, 24*(2), 151–4.

5. Ethicon Wound Closure Manual (2008). www.jnjgateway.com

6. Halverson, A.L., Anderson, J.L., Anderson, K., Lombardo, J., Park, C.S., Rademaker, A.W., & Moorman, D.W. (2009). Surgical team training. *Archives of Surgery, 144*(2), 107–112.

7. Haynes, A.B., Weiser, T.G., Berry, W.R., Lipsitz, S.R., Breizat, A-H.S., Dellinger, E.P., Herbosa, T., Joseph, S., Kibatala, P.L., Lapitan, M.C.M., Merry, A.F., Moorthy, K., Reznick, R.K., Taylor, B., & Gawande, A.A. (2009). A surgical safety checklist to reduce morbidity and mortality in a global population. *New England Journal of Medicine, 360*(5), 491–499.

8. Hunt, T.K. (2006). Wound healing. In G.M. Doherty & G.M. Way (Eds.), *Current surgical diagnosis and treatment* (12th ed.). New York: McGraw-Hill.

9. Kearns, S.R., Connolly, E.M., McNally, S., McNamara, D.A., & Deasy, J. (2001). Randomized clinical trial of diathermy versus scalpel incision in elective midline laparotomy. *British Journal of Surgery, 88*(1), 41–4.

10. National Quality Forum (NQF). (2009). *Safe practices for better healthcare—2009 update: A consensus report.* Washington, DC: NQF.

11. Paige, J.T., Aaron, D.L., Yang, T., Howell, D.S., Hilton, C.W., Cohn, I., & Chauvin, S.W. (2008). Implementation of a preoperative briefing protocol improves accuracy of teamwork assessment in the operating room. *The American Surgeon, 74*(9), 817–823.

12. Price, B. (2008). Medicare announces pay-for-performance rules. *The Surgical Technologist, 40*(9), 394–395.

13. Retzlaff, K. (2009). Getting on track, Tracking technologies are improving supply chain efficiency and patient safety in the operating room. *AORN Connections 7*(1), 1, 8.

14. Rodriguez-Paz, J.M., Kennedy, M., Salas, E., Wu, W.W., Sexton, J.B., Hunt, E.A., & Provonost, P.J. (2009). Beyond "See one, do one, teach one": Toward a different training paradigm. *Quality and Safety in Health Care, 18*, 63–68.

15. van Winterswijk, P. J., & Nout, E. (2007). Tissue engineering and wound healing: An overview of the past, present, and future. *Wounds, 19*(10), 277–284.

16. Vernon, A.H., & Hunter, J.G. (2007). Fundamentals of laparoscopic surgery. In M.J. Zinner & S.W. Ashley (Eds.), *Maingot's abdominal operations* (11th ed.). New York: McGraw-Hill.

17. Whitman, G., Cowell, V., Parris, K., McCullough, P., Howard, T., Gaughan, J., Karavite, D., Kennedy, M., McInerney, J., & Rose, C. (2008). Prophylactic antibiotic use: Hardwiring of physician behavior, not education, leads to compliance. *Journal of the American College of Surgeons, 207*, 88–94.

18. Zollinger, R.M. Jr., & Zollinger, R.M. Sr. (2003). *Zollinger's atlas of surgical operations* (8th ed.). New York: McGraw-Hill.

4 Providing Exposure: Retractors and Retraction

Nancy B. Davis

A major function of the surgical first assistant (FA) is to expose the operative site. Exposure is necessary to visualize organs and tissues that are being inspected, dissected, repaired, or sutured. Exposure is also necessary to prevent injury to tissues and other structures that are adjacent to the operative area. When there is bleeding, exposure is critical to identifying the site of the bleeding and controlling it.

Providing exposure is usually the first function the FA performs. An experienced FA makes this activity appear easy. However, the FA must be knowledgeable about the operative procedure, anatomy of related structures, and the potential for injury to tissues and their underlying and surrounding structures. Proper selection and utilization of exposure methods are essential. As the FA becomes more skilled at providing exposure, the surgeon can provide less direction.

Unfortunately, the act of providing exposure sometimes appears to be a simple task, merely requiring "an extra pair of hands" that are positioned by the surgeon. Some institutions may even permit the use of unlicensed assistive personnel to act as "retractor holders." As the shortage of surgeons in the United States increases and surgical residents' duty hours are limited (Iglehart, 2008), such "retractor holders" may become the norm as fewer trained staff are available to provide exposure. However, institutions cannot ignore their corporate responsibility, part of which is to ensure that there are adequate numbers of qualified perioperative personnel, appropriately educated and trained to carry out the tasks to which they are assigned (Box 4-1).

Box 4-1	Legal Brief: What Are the Consequences if a Surgeon "Drafts" a Hospital Orderly to Hold Retractors?

Assume first that the patient suffers serious injury as a result of improper retraction, for example, a sciatic nerve impingement causes serious injury. The patient will likely initiate a lawsuit as a result. Let's review the potential consequences for each of the possible parties in our hypothetical lawsuit.

The "drafted" orderly, a hospital employee, is probably uninsured and judgment proof. Therefore although, he or she may be named as a defendant, the orderly will probably obtain defense counsel and indemnity from the hospital's insurance carrier. The orderly would not need to worry much.

Likewise, our surgeon—a deep pockets target and insured—will bear direct liability for all untoward consequences to his patient, including those suffered at the hands of the orderly—controlled in all ways—by the drafting surgeon. The orderly's lack of training will prove of no benefit to the surgeon. It will be assumed by the court and jury that orderlies normally are wholly untrained in the many arts and sciences represented by health care practitioners in the OR.

As for the hospital itself, depending on the jurisdiction, the days when there was any judicial reluctance to impose liability on charitable institutions are gone. The scope of potential hospital liability appears very near boundless. Some questions about the injury would no doubt be painful for our hospital to answer.

Did the hospital's OR director, for example, know or have reason to know that this defendant surgeon was liable to draft this orderly (and had he or she done so previously, using this orderly or others)? Was the use of the orderly seen as a cost-saving measure that enjoyed the unspoken blessing of the hospital administration? Did the surgeon or his practice enjoy any economic benefit as a result of keeping hospital *per diem* costs minimized?

Those kinds of questions, if answered "yes," bode ill for the hospital, given the developing thrust of the doctrine of hospital corporate liability. By it, a hospital can be deemed *directly* responsible for what happens in the OR if it bills itself to the public as *a best provider of quality surgery and hospital care* within its community. When it does so, some courts have become quite willing to hold a hospital liable for what happens within the walls of its OR. *See, e.g., Thomson v. Nason Hospital*, 527 Pa. 330, 591 A.2d 703 (1991).

The Pennsylvania Supreme Court in *Welsh v. Bulger*, 548 Pa. 504, 698 A.2d 581 (1997), quoted approvingly from *Thomson, supra*, to expound on what is an adequate *prima facie* or "first glance" case of a hospital's direct corporate liability, needed to move a lawsuit further toward trial and a jury:

Corporate negligence is a doctrine under which the hospital is liable if it fails to uphold the proper standard of care owed the patient, which is to ensure the patient's safety and well-being while at the hospital. This theory of liability creates a nondelegable duty which the hospital owes directly to a patient. *Thompson*, 527 Pa. at 339, 591 A.2d at 707. Under *Thompson*, a hospital has the following duties:

"(1) a duty to use reasonable care in the maintenance of safe and adequate facilities and equipment; (2) a duty to select and retain only competent physicians; (3) a duty to oversee all persons who practice medicine within its walls as to patient care; and

(4) a duty to formulate, adopt and enforce adequate rules and policies to ensure quality care for the patients. Id. at 339–40, 591 A.2d at 707 (citations omitted).

'Because the duty to uphold the proper standard of care runs directly from the hospital to the patient, an injured party need not rely on the negligence of a third-party, such as a doctor or nurse, to establish a cause of action in corporate negligence.' *Moser v. Heistand*, 545 Pa. 554, 558, 681 A.2d 1322, 1325 (1996). Instead, corporate negligence is based on the negligent acts of the institution. *Moser. A cause of action for corporate negligence arises from the policies, actions or inaction of the institution itself rather than the specific acts of individual hospital employees. Id.* Thus, under this theory, a corporation is held directly liable, as opposed to vicariously liable, for its own negligent acts."
Welsh v. Bulger, supra, 548 Pa. at 512–513, 698 A.2d at 585 (emphasis added).

See and compare, Healthtrust v. Cantrell, 689 S.2d 822 (1997) (evidence sufficient to justify $800,000 Alabama award where hospital's failure to train retractor technician adequately in pediatric hip surgery caused child's sciatic nerve injury). *Also see* Blumenreich, G., "Legal Briefs: The Doctrine of Corporate Liability," *AANA Journal*, Vol. 73, No. 4, August 2005, pp. 253–257.

Compensatory damages for direct corporate liability of the hospital arise from its own negligence, *i.e.,* in our hypothetical case, knowingly allowing the surgeon to draft an orderly to perform retraction negligently. That is not, however, the end of potential consequences for the hospital or surgeon. While more difficult to prove, *punitive or exemplary damages* may also be sought and awarded. In these cases, the plaintiff needs to show either malice or, as here, gross negligence. Gross negligence is the kind of negligence that suggests to judge and jury actual or constructive knowledge of a danger of injury to a patient. Yet action was taken in the face of that danger anyway. *See, e.g.,* Thornton, R., "Malice/Gross Negligence," Baylor University Medical Proceedings, October 2006, Vol. 19, No. 4, pp. 417–418, accessed February 6, 2009, at http://www.pubmedcentral.nih.gov/articlerender.fcgi?artid=1618741

In sum, hospitals need to ensure that they as institutions know what goes on in the OR as close to "at all times" as possible. It they fail to do so, they and their insurers face major risks and potentially catastrophic damage awards.

Source: P. Alan Zulick, attorney and member, Pennsylvania and Montgomery Bar Associations; Trial and Administrative Disciplinary Law, Media, Pennsylvania

METHODS OF PROVIDING EXPOSURE

The most common method of exposure is to use retraction instruments ("retractors"). Other methods include using grasping instruments, sponges, sutures, tapes, Penrose drains, vessel loops, suctioning, plastic bags, and even the simple, but very effective, use of the assistant's hands.

When choosing how to provide exposure, the FA must consider several factors. These factors include the operative procedure and the stage of the operation. Physical characteristics of the patient should also be considered, including the patient's age, height, weight, body build, and any physical deformities or limitations. The type of tissue, the location of vascular or nerve structures, and the presence of associated organs must also be evaluated when choosing the exposure method.

Traction on tissues is the mechanism that provides exposure. If traction is inadequate, then the operative site will be poorly exposed, impeding the surgeon's work and the progress of the surgical procedure. Excessive traction may result in injuries from lacerations or pressure. Knowledge of how to provide the correct amount of traction is acquired through an understanding of surgical anatomy. An appreciation of the fragility of related tissue structures is also needed.

Retractors

Retractors are instruments designed specifically for holding tissues or organs out of the surgeon's working field during the operative procedure. Many retractors are intended only for selected operative procedures. Other retractors are more versatile and can be used for many different procedures. Selection of a retractor is based on several factors, including the:

- Operative procedure
- Stage of the operative procedure
- Tissues or organs being retracted
- Complexity of the operative procedure
- Length and depth of the wound
- Time necessary to perform the procedure
- Amount of force (effort) needed to provide exposure

Retractors are of two basic types: hand-held and self-retaining. Retractors come in several designs, and may be sharp or blunt; large or small; flat, round, or curved; wide or narrow; short or long; malleable, hinged, or fixed; straight or angled. They may be composed of one solid piece or several parts. The FA must know the types of available retractors, the names of the retractors and how to use each retractor safely and effectively.

Hand-Held Retractors   As the name implies, hand-held retractors are held continuously by the FA during use. This is the major disadvantage of this type of retractor, because the assistant's hand or hands are not available to provide other assistance during the operation. In certain operations this may not be a problem because the surgeon may only need minimal assistance during the procedure. However, if the FA is holding a retractor during more complex operations, more than one assistant may be needed for safe and efficient execution of the surgical procedure.

Box 4-2	Design, Attributes, and Use of Hand-Held Retractors

- The purpose of some retractors can be understood by their name, as in skin hooks, vein retractors, or nerve root retractors.
- The handle (or shaft) fits in the hand rather than on the fingers, as when using a clamp designed to grasp tissue.
- The handle is designed to be as comfortable as possible to permit efficient retraction for long periods; retractors with flat handles are often more difficult to hold for long periods of time.
- The handle of the retractor should not be gripped any harder than necessary.
- The blade (or endpiece) is designed to retract the tissues without damaging them; in some instances, moistened sponges are inserted between the blade and the tissue to prevent tissue injury and tissue desiccation.
- The blade may be wide or narrow, shallow or deep, or have a longer blade on one end and a shorter blade on the other.
- Blades may be sharp or dull; precautions should be used when the blades are sharp, as with sharp-toothed rake retractors.
- Although most hand-held retractors are stiff, some are flexible and malleable.
- If the assistant experiences muscle fatigue from holding the retractor, the surgeon must first be alerted before the assistant relaxes the muscles of the arm and hand.
- To prevent tissue injury, the assistant should use only as much force on the retractor as necessary.
- Do not lean or rest the arm on the patient when retracting.
- An alert assistant will vary the position of the retractor blade or its pull to adjust for requirements in exposure.
- The pull of the hand-held retractor may be sideways or upward, depending on the type of exposure required.
- Once the hand-held retractor is positioned to pull or lift upwards, it is held in that exact position without additional pull.
- The handle may be grasped with an overhand (the hand and thumb on top while the fingers curl under the retractor handle), underhand (the wrist is turned such that the majority of the hand is underneath the handle of the retractor) or dagger grip (the wrist is cocked while the handle of the retractor is grasped in the palm of the hand). The grasping technique may be determined by comfort by the assistant while still ensuring the correct amount of pull.
- Ergonomics of retraction suggest that retraction should be performed at an optimal working height (within the area between the chest and the waist height of the operative field).The retractor should be as close to the body as possible to maintain good body alignment (Applegeet, 2007) and to assist with stability when holding the retractor.

Nevertheless, the hand-held retractor has several advantages (Box 4-2). It can be put into position more quickly than a self-retaining retractor requiring adjustments, repositioned, and removed. It allows the alert FA to vary retractor position nearly instantaneously to provide exposure and to let up on pressure when tension

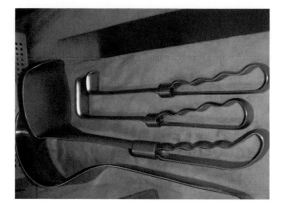

Figure 4-1

Hand-held retractors. *Top to bottom:* Malleable retractor; small Richardson retractor; medium Richardson retractor; large Richardson retractor; and Deaver retractor.

Source: Photo courtesy of Winchester Hospital, Winchester, MA.

is no longer necessary. The amount of traction placed on tissues can thus be altered as necessary. This allows the capillary network in the tissue beneath the retractor to obtain needed oxygen and nutrients. For very fragile tissue, the hand-held retractor may be essential to prevent injury. If access to the tissue needing retraction is difficult, a hand-held retractor may be the method of choice.

Hand-held retractors are designed with or without handles. The handle is designed to provide the FA with a firmer grip, but many are not designed for the handler's comfort. The handle may be round or flat and may have finger notches, rings, or curves (Figure 4-1). A flat handle is hard to hold for long periods. Retractors without handles usually have straight shafts that may have a different retracting surface on each end (Figure 4-2). Malleable retractors (see Figure 4-1), also referred to as "ribbon retractors," are flexible and may be bent into various angles. They are available in different lengths and widths. These are versatile retractors because, if a unique angle is needed, they can help hold in and protect viscera during abdominal wound closure.

Retractors with prongs are more often used for retraction of shallow tissues, such as the skin or subcutaneous tissue. The prongs may be sharp or dull, and there may be one prong or several (Figure 4-3). Sharp prongs can cause more tissue damage but are less likely to slip. The FA must be careful when using the sharp-pronged retractor because it can easily puncture gloves or tissues such as the bowel or blood vessels. Sharp-pronged retractors should be used following established safety protocols such as the hands-free technique (Allen, 2008). A neutral zone is created by the scrub person and agreed on with the surgeon and FA. Sharp-pronged instruments are placed in this neutral zone. The exchange of

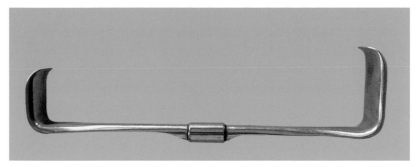

Figure 4-2

Hand-held retractor with different retracting surfaces at each end.

Source: Provided courtesy of Tighe, S.M. (2007). *Instrumentation for the operating room: A photographic manual* (7th ed., Fig. 1-3, p. 16). St. Louis: Mosby. Reprinted by permission.

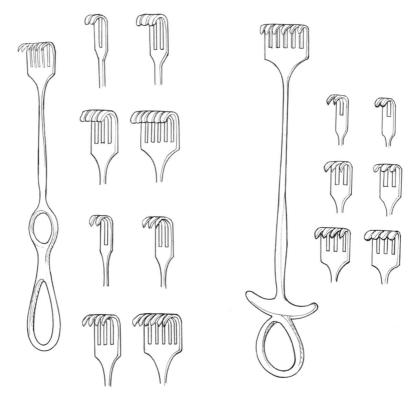

Figure 4-3

Rake retractors.

Source: Adapted by M. Borman from Rothrock, J.C. (Ed.). (1999). *The RN First Assistant: An expanded perioperative nursing role* (3rd ed., Fig. 9-4, p. 206). Philadelphia: Lippincott.

the sharp-pronged retractor may be announced with words such as "sharp rake back." To reduce risk exposure, blunt prongs are preferred when possible.

When placing the retractor, the FA must take care not to injure nerves, organs, or vascular structures. Circulation to tissues should not be compromised. Inordinate compression of tissues or organs can occur if the retractor is placed improperly. Underlying structures should be protected from excessive pressure or tension that could result in tissue damage.

The FA should hold the retractor in a position that causes the least discomfort, strain, or fatigue. FAs may wish to engage in physical conditioning exercises to develop upper body and extremity strength and endurance. Such exercises help the FA perform retraction with less risk for upper body injury (**Box 4-3**).

Box 4-3	**Physical Conditioning and Training for Upper Body and Extremity Strength**

Retracting during surgery requires upper body strength and endurance. Below is a list of assorted exercises which can be used to train the upper body and extremities. The exercises are not described or illustrated. FAs should consult a physical trainer for details on recommended exercises.

Grip strength: for use in retraction and fine manipulation; finger flexion and extension.
Exercise options: grip and spread, ball squeeze, hand gripper, towel gather, wrist roller

Forearm/wrist strength: for use in retraction, holding; wrist flexors/extensors, supination/pronation.
Exercise options: ball squeeze, wrist rolls, resistive flexion/extension and supination/pronation, towel twist, Indian club

Biceps/triceps strength: for use in lifting, holding; biceps flexion, triceps extension
Exercise options: curls, chin-ups, kick-backs, push-ups, dips

Shoulders: for use in multidirectional retracting; flexion, extension, adduction, abduction, internal and external rotation
Exercise options: Anterior deltoid: flexion, Salt & Pepper, Theraband, upright rows
Middle deltoid: scarecrow to 90°, Theraband, shoulder abduction, low/high diagonal pattern
Posterior deltoid: extension, Theraband, kick-backs, dips/reverse dips, Military press
Latissimus dorsi/shoulder adduction: lat pulls, chin-ups, high/low diagonal pattern
Internal/external rotation: resistive exercise with Theraband, weights in neutral and abducted position
Upper trapezius: shoulder shrugs, shoulder rolls, neck isometrics
Rhomboids: scapular retraction with seated rolls, bent rolls, prone fly's

Note: News, conference summaries, articles, MEDLINE abstracts, links to government and professional organizations, practice guidelines, and practical clinical tools that the FA may find useful include:

Medscape's Sport's Medicine Resource Center: www.medscape.com/resource/sportsmed

Source: Contributed by Michael Duffey, MEd., LATC, CST.

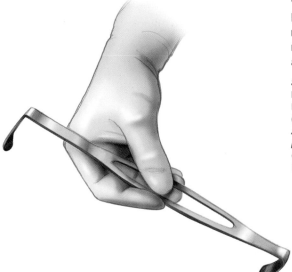

Figure 4-4

Position for holding retractor when retracting laterally or away from self.

Source: Adapted by M. Borman from Rothrock, J.C. (Ed.). (1999). *The RN First Assistant: An expanded perioperative nursing role* (3rd ed., Fig. 9-5, p. 207). Philadelphia: Lippincott.

If the assistant is retracting laterally or away from self, the retractor should rest comfortably in the hand with the palm supine and the arm flexed at the elbow (Figure 4-4). When retracting toward self, the FA will be more comfortable holding the retractor with the palm in the prone position or toward self (Figure 4-5). The retractor should not be gripped more tightly than necessary because this increases

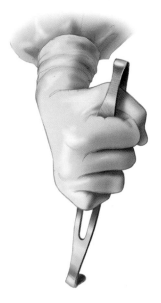

Figure 4-5

Position for holding retractor when retracting toward self.

Source: Adapted by M. Borman from Rothrock, J.C. (Ed.). (1999). *The RN First Assistant: An expanded perioperative nursing role* (3rd ed., Fig. 9-6, p. 206). Philadelphia: Lippincott.

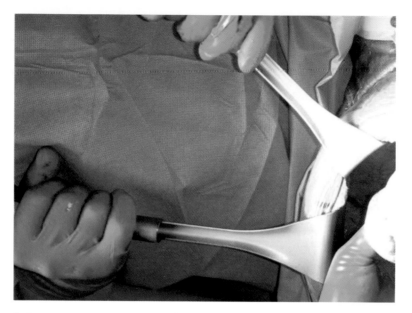

Figure 4-6

Handheld retractors. Here, the FA is using a sideways pull with an overhand grip to hold the abdominal cavity open. Once exposure is adequate, the retractors are held in a fixed position to maintain the exposure.

Source: Photo courtesy of Winchester Hospital, Winchester, MA.

arm fatigue. Also, it is important not to lean or rest the arm on the patient, as this can result in a pressure injury to soft tissues or nerves or even interfere with respiration and circulation. The FAs hand must not obstruct the surgeon's view of the operative site.

The pull on the retractor should provide adequate exposure of the operative field without distorting tissues that are being dissected or sutured by the surgeon (Figure 4-6). Excessive pull on the retractor may result in tissue laceration or slippage of the retractor from the incision. Conversely, inadequate pull may result in poor exposure and allow retracted tissues to slip into the field, obstructing the surgeon's view. The FA must observe the effect of the retraction and alert the surgeon if the retractor or tissues are slipping. Then, the retractor may be readjusted. The FA may tire with long or difficult retracting and must advise the surgeon when he or she is seriously fatigued.

Self-Retaining Retractors   The self-retaining retractor provides continuous and consistent retraction of tissues (Box 4-4). Once placed, this retractor does not need

Box 4-4	Considerations, Attributes, and Use of Self-Retaining Retractors

- They replace the assistant's muscles, relieving fatigue for the assistant by substituting for a pair of hand-held retractors.
- They must be placed and adjusted carefully as the blades are inserted and opened.
- When they are placed, excessive stretching of the tissues must be avoided.
- The handles are connected with a joint, and the two blades oppose one another.
- There is some form of ratchet or other device to keep the blades apart. The ratchet lock mechanism should be tested prior to use to validate that it locks firmly.
- Some have blades attached to a ring. If the blades are removable, they are considered part of the instrument count. The device that holds the removable blade in place [such as a wing nut] must also be accounted for to prevent it coming loose and being inadvertently retained in the patient.
- Some forms of self-retaining retractors are attached to the OR bed.

to be held, thereby freeing the FAs hands for other activities (Figure 4-7 depicts the Omni retractor, also referred to as the "Iron Intern"). Various self-retaining retractors are available, and the assistant needs to be familiar with the commonly used ones. Some are versatile and can be used for a variety of surgeries, whereas others are designed for specific operative procedures. Self-retaining retractors are

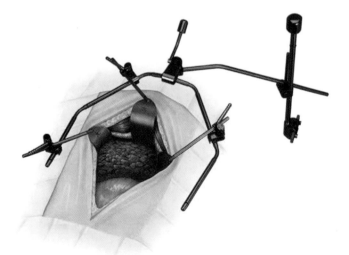

Figure 4-7

Omni retractor.

Source: Courtesy of Omni-Tract® Surgical. Reprinted by permission.

especially useful for longer procedures and are essential when concerted force is needed to provide retraction (e.g., during a thoracotomy).

Self-retaining retractors are more complex than hand-held retractors. Such retractors may be designed as a frame with fixed blades or prongs, or the retracting surfaces may be detachable, with several variations. The retracting blades or prongs may vary in width, depth, and angulation. The mechanical components of the retractor may include ratchets, springs, cranks, or nuts that open the retractor and hold it in the desired position (Figure 4-8). Any removable parts must be accounted for and included in the formal instrument count (AORN, 2009).

There are numerous self-retaining retractors designed for use in both general and specialty surgeries. For example, a self-retaining retractor with great versatility is the Bookwalter (Figure 4-9). During anterior exposure of the thoracic spine, the Book-walter may be used to provide retraction of the chest wall, lung, and diaphragm. A moist laparotomy pad and the wide malleable blades of the retractor provide excellent lung and peritoneal retraction. The two shallow bladder blades maintain

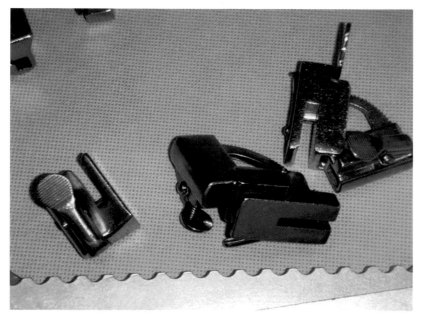

Figure 4-8

Bookwalter ratchets. Mechanical components have removable parts which must be accounted for in self-retaining retractors.

Source: Photo courtesy of Winchester Hospital, Winchester, MA.

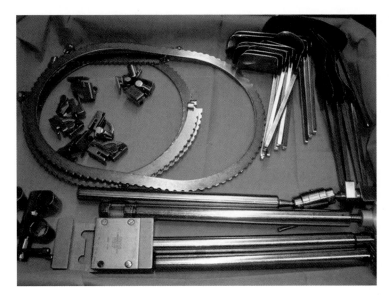

Figure 4-9A

Bookwalter retractor.

Source: Photo courtesy of Winchester Hospital, Winchester, MA.

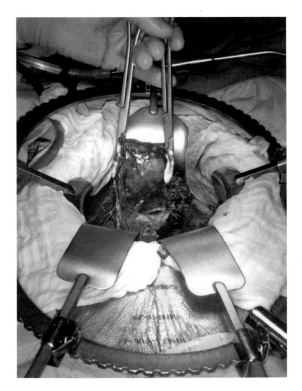

Figure 4-9B

Bookwalter being used during surgery.

Source: Photo courtesy of Winchester Hospital, Winchester, MA.

adequate chest wall separation. The deep, straight blades are effective in maintaining downward traction on the ipsilateral diaphragm (Pettiford et al., 2008).

The self-retaining Goligher retractor may be used during retroperitoneal lymph node dissection (RPLND). After the colon and small bowel are mobilized, two wide Deaver-type blades are attached to the retractor to retract the small and large bowel. Care must be taken to prevent undue traction to the pancreas and undersurface of the duodenum as well as injury to the superior mesenteric artery (Zivanovic et al., 2008).

Unlike other self-retaining retractors, the Mobius retractor consists of an elastic tube with a ring on each end. With this self-retaining abdominal elastic retractor, the larger ring is introduced in the abdominopelvic cavity while the other smaller ring remains on the skin margins of the surgical incision. The length of the elastic tube is adjusted by giving turns to the external ring, thus creating a circular area of retraction (Alcalde et al., 2007).

The selected self-retaining retractor should be opened carefully and under direct visualization. Again, care must be taken not to injure nerves, vascular structures, organs, or tissues by accidentally pinching them in or under the retracting surfaces or mechanisms within the retractor components. It may be necessary to hold the wound edges in the retractor blades while opening the retractor to prevent slipping. With self-retaining abdominal wall retractors, the assistant should keep a hand over each blade to avoid trapping viscera between the blade and the abdominal wall as the retractor is opened.

In operative procedures that require increased force for retraction, the retractor should be opened slowly and, when possible, in stages. The retractor should not be overexpanded, as this will cause excessive pulling on tissues and may cause tearing lacerations. As previously noted, it is often necessary to protect the wound edges from the retractor blades by padding with a sponge (Figure 4-10). Moistening the sponge with warm saline solution can prevent drying of the tissues, tissue friction, and abrasion. The FA should keep in mind that the greater the exposure and the longer the procedure, the more fluid loss and tissue desiccation occur. The need to use and replace warm, moist pads is determined by the length of the surgery and the exposure during the procedure. The assistant should also note the use of the sponge under a retractor blade and must remember that it has been so placed. Accounting for the sponge's location is important during a count and final retrieval to avoid inadvertent retention. To avoid relying solely on memory, which has been shown to be a root cause of retained items (Minnesota's Retained Object Protocol, 2008), the FA should also announce to the scrub person and/or circulating nurse that sponges have been placed under retractor blades.

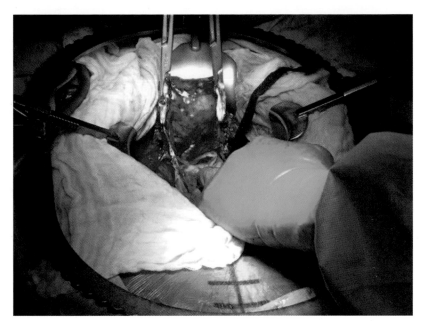

Figure 4-10

Wound edges protected from retractor blades by padding with sponges.

Source: Photo courtesy of Winchester Hospital, Winchester, MA.

For extremely long procedures, the self-retaining retractor should be removed and repositioned periodically to prevent ischemic injury to the wound edges.

Grasping Instruments

Several types of grasping instruments may be used to provide a secure hold on tissues so that traction can be more easily applied, and exposure can be achieved. Grasping instruments cause varying degrees of tissue damage, depending on the type of tissue grasped, the instrument being used, how the instrument is applied to the tissue, and the amount of traction applied to the tissue. Judgments made by the FA when using grasping instruments are based on knowledge and experience.

Tissue Forceps Tissue forceps (also referred to as "pickups") are grasping and pinching instruments that provide an extension of the thumb and fingers. Forceps are some of the most commonly used surgical instruments, and the FA must be skilled in using them with either hand. With practice, they are quick and easy to use. Forceps are held like a pencil (Figure 4-11), and the tips are forced together by applying pressure with the thumb and fingers. Grasping pressure must be sufficient

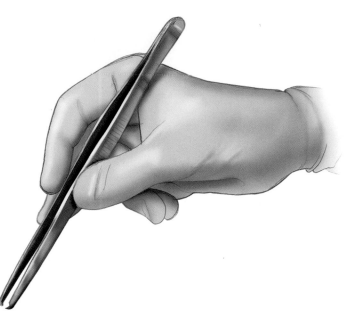

Figure 4-11

Position for holding tissue forceps.

Source: Adapted by M. Borman from Rothrock, J.C. (Ed.). (1999). *The RN First Assistant: An expanded perioperative nursing role* (3rd ed., Fig. 9-9, p. 210). Philadelphia: Lippincott.

to provide a secure hold with minimal damage to the tissues. With tissue forceps, pressure can be altered easily and more precisely than with a clamping instrument. The most commonly used tissue forceps are straight, but they vary in length, width, and tip design. Some forceps are very delicate, while others are bulky. Each forceps is designed for use on specific types of tissues.

Toothed forceps may have one tooth or several teeth. The teeth may be fine or heavy (Figure 4-12). Forceps without teeth, called "smooth forceps," are used to grasp tissues that might be easily perforated or torn, such as bowel tissue. *Smooth forceps* are also useful for holding gauze sponges because the gauze material will not become caught in the tips.

Clamps   Several types of clamps are used to grasp tissue. These clamps are available in various lengths and may be straight, curved, or angled. They have ringed handles and ratcheted boxlocks to secure their grasp. Clamp structures range from delicate to heavy, and the jaws may be smooth or serrated. The tip of the clamps may be fine, pointed, rounded, blunt, or triangular, or it may have interlocking teeth.

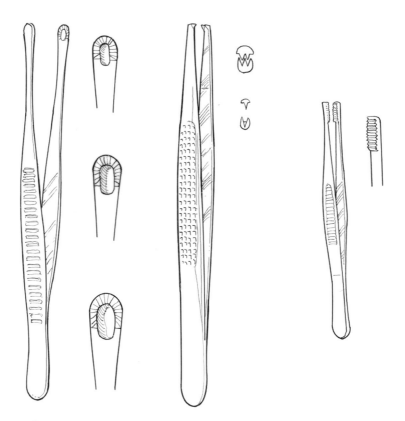

Figure 4-12

Examples of toothed forceps. Left, Russian; center, Bonney; right, Brown.

Source: Adapted by M. Borman from Rothrock, J.C. (Ed.). (1999). *The RN First Assistant: An expanded perioperative nursing role* (3rd ed., Fig. 9-11, p. 211). Philadelphia: Lippincott.

Delicate clamps cause less trauma to tissues and are therefore used on soft or fragile tissue, such as those of the lung or bowel. The Babcock clamp is an example of a clamp with a tip without teeth; it is useful for grasping structures such as the bowel, ureter, or fallopian tube without damaging the structure being grasped. Delicate clamps must not be used to grasp heavier tissues because the clamp may slip when traction is applied. Also, the clamp will be damaged if forced to clamp heavy or bulky tissue.

Clamps with teeth are used only on tissues that will not be seriously injured by tooth perforation. The teeth increase the clamp's grasping power, so that greater amounts of traction can be applied (Figure 4-13). The tips may be very sharp, and the FA must be careful not to perforate gloves or delicate structures such as bowel or blood vessels.

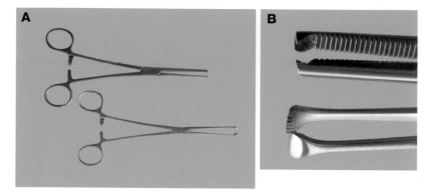

Figure 4-13

Oschner (Kocher) clamp and tip and Allis clamp and tip. A. *Top*, Oschner clamp; *bottom*, Allis clamp B. *Top*, Oschner teeth; *bottom*, Allis teeth

Source: Provided courtesy of Tighe, S.M. (2007). *Instrumentation for the operating room: A photographic manual* (7th ed., Fig. 1-6, p. 18). St. Louis: Mosby. Reprinted by permission.

Heavy clamps can cause crushing injury to tissues and must therefore be used appropriately. Frequently, just the clamp's tip is used to grasp tissue and apply traction. Excessive traction, however, will cause the clamp to slip or the tissue to tear and must be avoided.

The FA may need to simultaneously hold several clamps that provide traction at different points on a structure. When multiple clamps are attached to tissue, they should be held by the shaft rather than by the ring handles because there is less chance of accidentally unlocking the clamps (**Figure 4-14**).

Sponges

Sponges are used in different ways to provide exposure. Several types and sizes of sponges are used in the operating room. Laparotomy sponges, gauze sponges (4 $\times$ 4 $\times$ 8 inches), cottonoid pledgets, and gauze dissectors (variously referred to as "pills," "kitners," "pushers," "cherry dissectors," and "peanuts") are the most frequently used. Any sponge used during surgery must be radiopaque so that it can be visualized on x-ray if there is a count discrepancy. In addition to using x-ray-detectable sponges, approaches such as radiofrequency identification (RFID) tagging and bar coding are useful ways to prevent unintended retention of a foreign object such as a surgical sponge.

The most common use of the sponge is to absorb fluid or blood that accumulates in the operative site and obstructs the surgeon's field of vision. Sponges are designed to soak up blood and should be used to blot tissues. Rubbing tissue with the sponge, however, is abrasive and can remove clots, increase bleeding, and cause tissue damage.

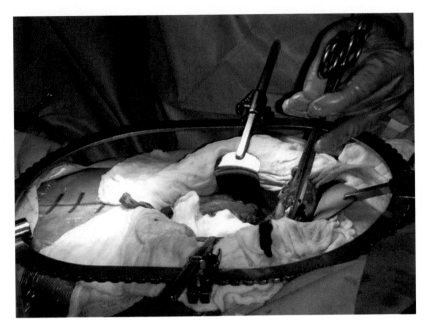

Figure 4-14

Assistant holding clamp by shaft.

Source: Photo courtesy of Winchester Hospital, Winchester, MA.

Sponges may be used with an instrument to remove blood and fluids or as dissectors or retractors to gently push (i.e., blunt dissection) or pull tissues from the operative area. A heavier clamp, such as a peon, should be used to hold a gauze dissector to prevent springing the box lock. A gauze pad can be folded and clamped into a sponge stick, often referred to as a "sponge on a stick" (Figure 4-15). It is important that sponges extend beyond the end of the clamp to protect tissue from injury by the clamp tips. The FA must be careful not to use excessive pressure with this type of sponge, or tissue may be perforated or torn. Likewise, the blood supply may be compromised if pressure is applied too firmly or in the incorrect area.

Using a sponge (gauze or laparotomy sponge) under the fingers to retract the skin edges may also reduce the likelihood of contaminating internal tissues with skin bacteria. During the procedure, slippery structures (e.g., bowel, omentum, or lung) can be held more securely by using a sponge under the fingers (Figure 4-16). The sponge's coarse fibers will increase friction and improve traction. Dry sponges provide a better grip than wet ones but also cause more tissue friction and abrasion. This tissue trauma can result in adhesion formation, which can cause postoperative complications, especially with abdominal surgeries.

Figure 4-15

Sponge stick holding folded gauze sponge.

Source: Adapted by M. Borman from Rothrock, J.C. (Ed.). (1999). *The RN First Assistant: An expanded perioperative nursing role* (3rd ed., Fig. 9-17, p. 214). Philadelphia: Lippincott.

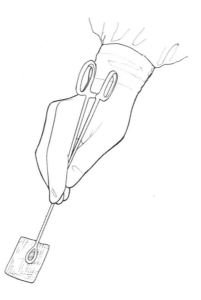

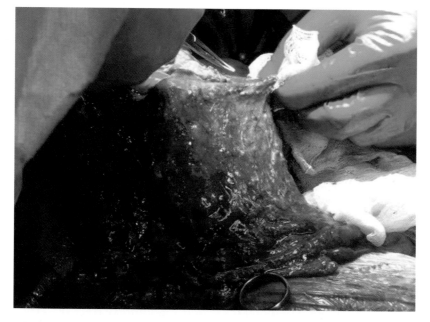

Figure 4-16

Using a sponge under fingers to more securely grip slippery tissue.

Source: Photo courtesy of Winchester Hospital, Winchester, MA.

Sponges can also be used to stabilize tissues. Loose structures such as the bowel can be more effectively retracted if they are wrapped with moistened laparotomy sponges. Organs or tissues that otherwise would fall into the operative field and obstruct the surgeon's vision can be packed out of the way with sponges. Sponges used for packing should be noted as they are placed, and removed and accounted for prior to wound closure. If the surgical procedure is lengthy, of an emergent nature, or performed on a patient with a high body-mass index, it is possible that, in addition to manual counts of sponges, confirmatory x-rays may be recommended in a particular institution where the FA works (Cima et al., 2008; Dossett et al., 2008; Egorova et al., 2008; Greenberg et al., 2008; Teixeira et al., 2008). During counts, teamwork and communication are essential, and distractions during the count must be avoided (Catchpole et al., 2007; Greenberg et al., 2007; Williams et al., 2007). This requires active participation and close attention from the assistant.

Sutures

Sutures are frequently used to provide exposure. They are particularly helpful in everting or fixing small mobile structures, such as the inner surface of the eyelid. They also can be used to stabilize or hold tissues. Skin, pleura, pericardium, dura, peritoneum, and certain other tissue edges are commonly retracted with sutures (**Figure 4-17**). Suturing is frequently considered a retraction method when delicate structures require intermittent release and retraction over an extended period.

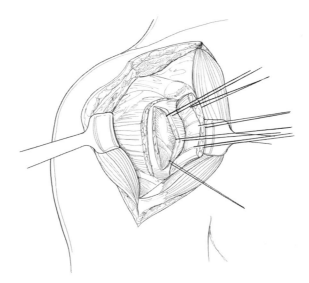

Figure 4-17

Use of sutures to retract tissue edges.

Source: Adapted by M. Borman from Rothrock, J.C. (Ed.). (1999). *The RN First Assistant: An expanded perioperative nursing role* (3rd ed., Fig. 9-18, p. 216). Philadelphia: Lippincott.

Figure 4-18

A Teflon felt pledget can be used with a suture for retracting delicate tissues

Source: Adapted by M. Borman from Rothrock, J.C. (Ed.). (1999). *The RN First Assistant: An expanded perioperative nursing role* (3rd ed., Fig. 9-19, p. 216). Philadelphia: Lippincott.

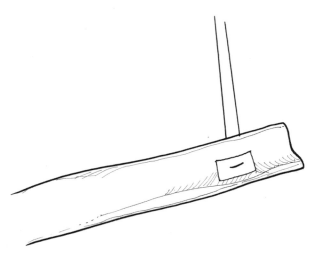

The amount of tension or pull that can be exerted on the suture depends on the tissue's fragility and the suture's tensile strength. Sutures must be placed securely in the tissue. Traction on the sutures is applied by the assistant's hand or by clamping or suturing the stitch to the drapes, wound towels, or wound edges. The jaws of the clamp might need to be shod to keep the suture from being cut. Various pre-packaged, sterile shods are available; these are surgical items that must be counted when the clamp is removed from the suture strand.

When clamps are placed on the end of a retraction suture, the clamp should not be left unattended. Holding it or fixing it to a drape minimizes the risk that someone will mistakenly pick it up without realizing that its jaws are clamped to a suture. When the sutures are stitched to drapes or to other structures, tension must be appropriate for the tissue and the sutures, knots must be tied securely, and the sutures must be cut close to the knot to prevent other sutures from catching on the knots. Once a suture is placed through a drape or wound towel, it should be considered contaminated and it cannot be removed or repositioned.

For very fragile tissues, the surgeon may use a pledget of Teflon felt (**Figure 4-18**). The felt keeps the suture from cutting into the tissue.

Sutures provide good retraction without the bulk of instruments or retractors. If fastened correctly, they will hold tissue in a continuous position.

Umbilical Tapes, Penrose Drains, and Vessel Loops

These items are often used to retract blood vessels, nerves, and gastrointestinal structures, which are fragile and slippery and difficult to hold. These tissues are also easily traumatized. Trauma to these tissues can result in serious consequences.

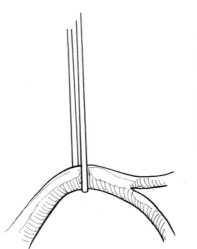

Figure 4-19

Vascular structure being retracted with a vessel loop.

Source: Adapted by M. Borman from Rothrock, J.C. (Ed.). (1999). *The RN First Assistant: An expanded perioperative nursing role* (3rd ed., Fig. 9-20, p. 217). Philadelphia: Lippincott.

Once the structure needing retraction is dissected free from surrounding tissues, an angled clamp is used to go under the structure. This clamp must be long enough and have a wide enough angle to slip around the structure easily. Various clamps are available. Those used most commonly include kidney pedicle clamps, Semb ligature carriers, Rumel thoracic right-angle forceps, and Lower gallbladder forceps.

Once the clamp is passed under the structure, it is opened, and the moistened tape, drain, or loop is inserted into the open jaw. The clamp is then closed and pulled back under the structure (Figure 4-19). This must be done carefully and gently so that the structure or surrounding tissues are not injured by the clamp or the tape, drain, or loop. The tape, drain, or loop is moistened with warm saline solution to decrease friction on surrounding tissues. The assistant usually uses two hands when placing a tape. One hand is used for the clamp or forceps which holds the end of the tape while the other holds the tape taut. To prevent excessive drag through the tissue, the FA should place just enough tape to be grasped securely into the tip of the clamp's jaws.

Once the tape encircles the structure, it is clamped with a hemostat. The FA can provide traction by pulling on the hemostat or clamping the hemostat to the wound drapes, taking care not to injure the structure by using too much tension.

Suctioning Devices

Suctioning devices remove blood or fluids from the operative area, which is essential for adequate visualization. Suction tips come in various shapes and sizes (Figure 4-20).

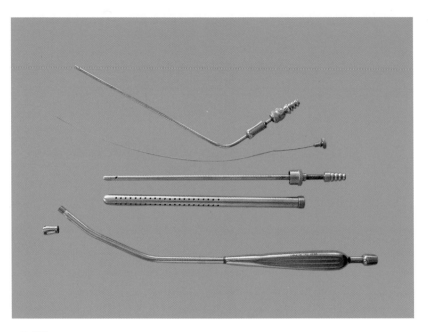

Figure 4-20

Suction tips. *Top to bottom*: Frazier suction tip with stylet below; Poole abdominal suction tip with shield protector below; and Yankauer suction tip with tip off.

Source: Provided courtesy of Tighe, S.M. (2007). *Instrumentation for the operating room: A photographic manual* (7th ed., Fig. 1-8, p. 19). St. Louis: Mosby. Reprinted by permission.

The Frazier suction tip is small and has an opening on the end (or tip). It is very useful for small incision sites with little blood loss. For operative procedures with more blood or fluid loss, a Yankauer tonsil suction tip or an abdominal suction tip may be used. The Yankauer suction tip's configuration makes it useful for retracting tissue as well as for suctioning blood or fluids. Some suction tips have a finger hole. Covering the hole increases the force of the suction. The suction tip is used to remove blood or fluids in the area where the surgeon is working. Its use must never obstruct the surgeon's or the FAs vision. The FA may need to suction frequently and briefly in coordination with the surgeon's activities, observing the operative site continuously to anticipate the need and timing of suctioning.

Aspiration tissue injury can occur with suction tips that have a single end opening. This can be avoided by protecting the tissue with a sponge so that the suction tip is not applied directly to the tissue. Should tissue be aspirated, the suction tip should not be pulled away forcibly. Instead, the suction must first be broken by bending the suction tubing and then gently removing the tissue.

In cases involving trauma or anastomosis of a structure such as bowel, the FA should ensure no cross-contamination occurs via the suction tip. Once the contaminated area is closed, the contaminated suction tip is replaced with a new one.

The FA also must be alert to the potential for losing removable parts of the suction tip. For example, the off/on controls may be held in place with a screw that can back out and drop into the wound. Occasionally, the surgeon may find it necessary to unscrew the end of the suction tip, which is then given to the scrub person for safekeeping until needed again. It is important to have a method to account for these parts (Perioperative Grand Rounds, 2008).

Retracting with Hands

The ideal retractor to provide exposure is frequently the assistant's hands (**Figure 4-21**). The hand is naturally padded, soft, and, through tactile sense, is responsive to the texture of tissue being retracted. Fingers and hands can be repositioned or removed more easily and quickly than instruments from the operative area. The amount of pressure or traction exerted on tissue can be instantly adjusted.

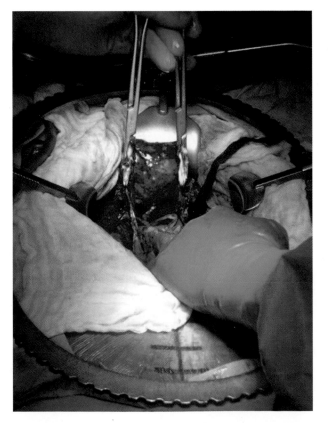

Figure 4-21

Using hands to retract. The assistant's hands are often an ideal retractor.

Source: Photo courtesy of Winchester Hospital, Winchester, MA.

After the initial incision, the assistant uses fingers to retract the skin edge while the subcutaneous layers are being cut. Fingers are usually used for retracting while the retractor is positioned. By spreading the fingers, a broad area can be retracted with one hand. In this technique, the fingers hold back the tissues while the wrist does the pulling. The FA flattens the hand as much as possible; this technique causes less obstruction to the operative area and allows better visualization for the surgeon. It also decreases the chance of a sharps injury to the FAs hand.

By placing a moistened sponge under the fingers, the FA can grip the tissue more securely; the sponge increases the friction and lessens the risk of inadvertent slippage if tissue is slick (see **Figure 4-16**). However, with prolonged retracting, the fingers and hand may become fatigued. The FA is duty bound to inform the surgeon when such fatigue begins to occur to avoid untimely slippage of the retracted tissues. A brief rest or repositioning the hand will usually relieve the fatigue.

Plastic Bags

Sterile plastic bags have been designed for retracting the small intestine during extensive abdominal operations. The bowel should be wrapped carefully in warm saline-soaked laparotomy sponges and gently placed in the bag in an anatomically correct position. Once the FA is sure the bowel is not accidentally twisted, it is secured properly within the bag to prevent it from inadvertently slipping out into the operative area.

Retraction During Laparoscopic Robotic Assisted Surgery

There are a variety of instruments which can be used during laparoscopic robotic assisted surgery to provide optimal surgical field exposure. Examples of laparoscopic instruments used for retraction are graspers, needle holders, paddle or fan-like retractors, and suction tips. Other nonlaparoscopic retraction instrument examples are Penrose drains, sutures, and sponges.

It is essential to use laparoscopic instruments with additional length during robotic surgery that involves the deep pelvis. Gastric bypass instruments are manufactured with a longer length of 42 cm compared to the 34 cm of standard laparoscopic instrument length. This longer length is highly recommended. The assistant's ports are placed in the upper portion of the abdomen away from the robotic instrument arm ports. The added length is needed to ensure that the FA can reach with laparoscopic instruments into the deep pelvis to facilitate retraction. Added instrument length also helps to reduce the possibility of instrument collision in the assistant's port and robotic arm ports. It is essential to have optimal freedom of movement in all trocar ports to facilitate safe progression of the surgical procedure.

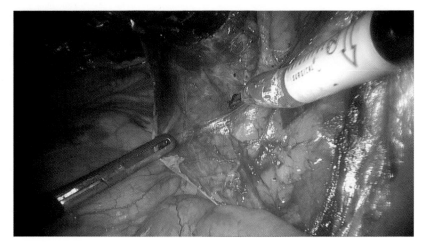

Figure 4-22

The FA grasps the peritoneum during PLND. This allows the surgeon to utilize both hands for dissection and provides safety to underlying structures.

Source: Photo courtesy of Winchester Hospital, Winchester, MA.

In a procedure such as a pelvic lymph node dissection (PLND), sponges and laparoscopic graspers can be used to retract the retroperitoneum (Figure 4-22). Sponges also act as absorbent material to clear the field of any blood and irrigation fluid.

Laparoscopic paddles (also referred to as "fans") have multiple applications in laparoscopic retraction. They can be used to retract the bowel when it falls into the surgical field during dissection. An example of this can be demonstrated by retracting the sigmoid colon from the posterior uterus during a laparoscopic hysterectomy. Retraction is performed to create the posterior peritoneal flap in order to expose the uterine vessels safely in preparation for coagulation and dissection.

The laparoscopic paddle can expand in size as it gently retracts the bowel. It can be manipulated to provide a narrow (small) or wide expansion for retraction depending on what is needed. For example, if retraction is needed in the cul-de-sac, the paddle is narrowly expanded to accommodate the smaller space (Figure 4-23). When working in the abdomen, the paddle can be fully expanded to retract a larger surface area (Figure 4-24). Paddles can also be used on the liver. Some laparoscopic paddles are constructed of a cloth-like material, which is delicate yet strong enough to retract an organ such as the liver without trauma. Paddles and fans are also useful for retraction in bariatric procedures. The FA needs to verify that any instruments chosen will fit into the port being used (e.g., a 12-mm paddle requires a 12-mm trocar port).

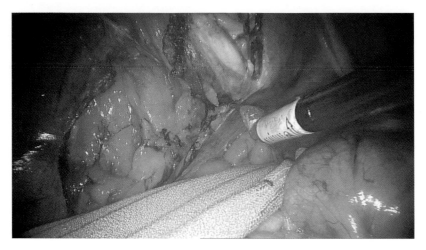

Figure 4-23

Paddle in closed position. The FA inserts the laparoscopic fan or paddle into the pelvic cavity in the closed position. While it remains in the closed position, the FA inserts it into the cul-de-sac.

Source: Photo courtesy of Winchester Hospital, Winchester, MA.

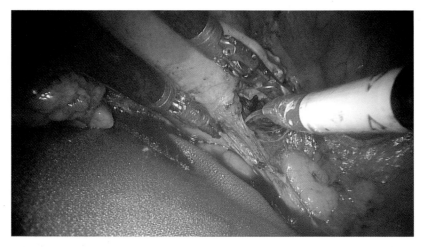

Figure 4-24

The laparoscopic fan or paddle is then opened slowly as the FA manipulates it until the bowel is safely tucked behind it. This photo demonstrates how the laparoscopic fan or paddle protects the bowel during posterior peritoneal flap exposure and dissection of uterine vessels during a Laparoscopic Robot-Assisted TAH BSO procedure.

Source: Photo courtesy of Winchester Hospital, Winchester, MA.

Sutures are another traction alternative which are sometimes used, such as during para-aortic lymph node dissection. The colon may protrude into or limit the field of view. The FA may find it beneficial to place several sutures through the tinea of the colon and temporarily attach them to the inner upper lateral abdominal wall. This allows the colon to be safely removed from the field of vision. After the para-aortic lymph node dissection is complete, the sutures are then removed, allowing the colon to fall naturally back into place within the abdominal cavity.

Laparoscopic needleholders are used to retract the running suture of the vaginal cuff anastomosis during hysterectomy procedures or during the urethral anastomosis in prostate surgery. Other laparoscopic graspers have the potential to fray the running suture if grasped too tightly. This can ultimately weaken the suture material and thus jeopardizes the integrity of the anastomosis.

Suction tips are often used in laparoscopic robotic surgery to provide both suction of fluids and retraction of anatomical structures. Suctioning clears the field of blood while the FA simultaneously provides retraction, thus optimizing the use of the instrument.

CONCLUSION

The FA's clinical acumen in retracting or providing exposure is quickly apparent during the operative procedure. If exposure is poor, the FA must find the first practical moment and method to improve it. By close observation, the FA determines the effectiveness of his or her actions. It is not uncommon for the surgeon to situate retractors or to determine the method of providing exposure. In some situations, the surgeon determines what is retracted and how retraction will be done. The FA contributes significantly to the effectiveness, efficiency, and safety of the operative procedure by providing good exposure of the operative site for the surgeon at all times. Tissue injury resulting from carelessness while providing exposure will usually be apparent at the time of the surgical procedure. However, some injuries, for example nerve injuries, may not be noticed until the postoperative period. A baseline preoperative assessment, in addition to a postoperative evaluation of the patient's status, provides the FA with information that will be helpful in determining whether any injury related to providing exposure has occurred intraoperatively. Throughout the surgical procedure, the assistant should actively participate in collaborative team communications about any difficulties encountered (or anticipated) in providing safe and effective surgical site exposure (Lingard et al., 2008).

REFERENCES

1. Alcalde, J.L., Guiloff, E., Ricci, P., Solà, V., & Pardo, J. (2007). Minilaparotomy hysterectomy assisted by self-retaining elastic abdominal retractor. *Journal of Minimally Invasive Gynecology, 14*(1), 108–112.
2. Allen, G. (2008). Evidence for practice; increasing the use of hands-free passing in surgery. *AORN Journal, 88*(3), 463, 465.
3. Applegeet, C.D. (2007). Perioperative ergonomics. *Perioperative Nursing Clinics, 2*, 345–351.
4. Association of periOperative Registered Nurses (AORN). (2009). Recommended practices for sponge, sharp, and instrument counts. *2009 Perioperative standards and recommended practices* (pp. 405–414). Denver, CO: AORN.
5. Catchpole, K.R., Giddings, S.E.B., Wilkinson, M., Hirst, G., Dale, T., & de Leval, M.R. (2007). Improving patient safety by identifying latent failures in successful operations. *Surgery, 142*, 102–110.
6. Cima, R.R., Kollengode, A., Garnatz, J., Storsveen, A., Weisbrod, C., & Deschamps, C. (2008). Incidence and characteristics of potential and actual retained foreign object events in surgical patients. *Journal of American College of Surgeons, 20*, 80–87.
7. Dossett, L.A., Dittus, R.S., Speroff, T., May, A.K., & Cotton, B.A. (2008). Cost-effectiveness of routine radiographs after emergent open cavity operations. *Surgery, 144*, 317–321.
8. Egorova, N.N., Moskowitz, A., Gelijns, A., Weinberg, A., Curty, J., Rabin-Fastman, B., et al. (2008). Managing the prevention of retained surgical instruments: What is the value of counting? *Annals of Surgery, 247*, 13–18.
9. Greenberg, C.C., Regenbogen, S.E, Lipsitz, S.R., Diaz-Flores, R., & Gawande, A.A. (2008). The frequency and significance of discrepancies in the surgical count. *Annals of Surgery, 248*, 337–341.
10. Greenberg, C.C. Regenbogen, S.E., Studdert, D.M., Lipsitz, S.R., Rogers, S.P., Zinner, M.J., et al. (2007). Patterns of communication breakdowns resulting in injury to surgical patients. *Journal of American College of Surgeons, 204*, 533–540.
11. Iglehart, J.K. (2008). Revisiting duty-hour limits: IOM recommendations for patient safety and resident education. *New England Journal of Medicine, 359*, 2633–2635.
12. Lingard, L., Regehr, G., Orser, B., Reznick, R., Baker, G.R., Doran, D., et al. (2008). Evaluation of a preoperative checklist and team briefing among surgeons, nurses, and anesthesiologists to reduce failures in communication. *Archives of Surgery, 143*: 12–17.
13. Minnesota's retained object protocol. (2008). *OR Manager, 24*(12), 14, 16.
14. Pettiford, B.L., Schuchert, M.J., Jeyabalan, G., Landreneau, J.R., Kilic, A., Landreneau, J.P., et al. (2008). Technical challenges and utility of anterior exposure for thoracic spine pathology. *The Annals of Thoracic Surgery, 86*(1), 1762–1768.
15. Perioperative Grand Rounds: Where is the suction tip? (2008). *AORN Journal, 88*(5), 876.
16. Teixeira, P.G.R., Inaba, K., Salim, A., Brow, C., Rhee, P., Browder, T., et al. (2007). Retained foreign bodies after emergent trauma surgery: Incidence after 2,526 cavitary explorations. *The American Surgeon, 73*, 1031–1034.
17. Williams, R.G., Silverman, R., Schwind, C., Fortune, J.B., Sutyak, J., Horvath, K.D., et al. (2007). Surgeon information transfer and communication: Factors affecting quality and efficiency of inpatient care. *Annals of Surgery, 245*, 159–169.
18. Zivanovic, O., Sheinfeld, J., & Abu-Rustum, N.R. (2008). Retroperitoneal lymph node dissection (RPLND). *Gynecologic Oncology, 111*(2), Supplement 1, S66–S69.

5

Methods for Assuring Surgical Hemostasis

James R. McCarthy

Hemostasis is the process of controlling or stopping the flow of blood from a vessel or organ. The control of such bleeding is necessary to preserve physiologic function for the patient and to provide clear visualization of anatomic structures for the surgeon and the surgical first assistant (FA) (Villanueva, 2008). The alleviation of vulnerabilities, like bleeding, is considered a part of patient-centered care (PCC) (Hobbs, 2009). Alleviating vulnerability such as bleeding by achieving hemostasis is essential to the role of the FA. Effective hemostasis not only provides a clear surgical field, but also results in fewer transfusions, reduced surgical time, and decreased morbidity and mortality (Samudrala, 2008).

During surgery, the patient's usual clotting mechanisms are often insufficient to provide adequate hemostasis, necessitating the use of surgical hemostatic techniques. A primary expectation and responsibility of the FA is to provide and assure hemostasis. Thus, the FA must not only be technically skilled, but must have a functional understanding of the physiologic and mechanical aspects of coagulation, bleeding, and methods to achieve hemostasis. Application of the appropriate method depends on the type of bleeding, its location, and the structures involved.

Physiologic, or "natural," processes may be used to achieve hemostasis. Natural physiologic responses may be inhibited by preexisting medical conditions. Thus, an artificial process may be used, employing mechanical strategies such as sutures, ties, pressure, instruments, surgical staples, ligating clips, or bonewax; chemical hemostatic adjuncts; tourniquets; electrosurgical devices; ultrasonic energy devices; argon beam-enhanced electrosurgery; or any combination of the above. The physiologic response to bleeding is a series of interactions represented by the coagulation cascade (Figure 5-1). Bleeding during or after a surgical intervention

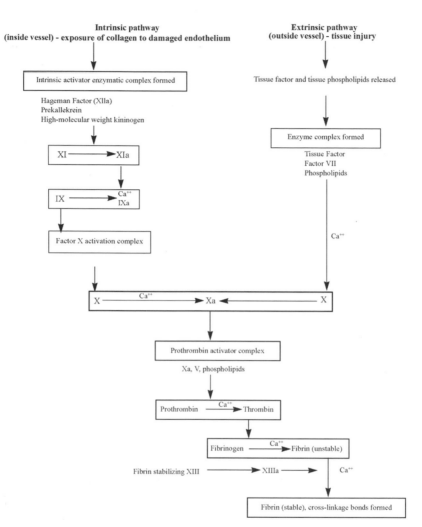

Intrinsic pathway
(inside vessel) – exposure of collagen to damaged endothelium

Extrinsic pathway
(outside vessel) – tissue injury

Intrinsic activator enzymatic complex formed

Tissue factor and tissue phospholipids released

Hageman Factor (XIIa)
Prekallekrein
High-molecular weight kininogen

Enzyme complex formed

Tissue Factor
Factor VII
Phospholipids

$XI \longrightarrow XIa$

$IX \longrightarrow \overset{Ca^{++}}{IXa}$

Factor X activation complex

Ca^{++}

$X \overset{Ca^{++}}{\longrightarrow} Xa \longleftarrow X$

Prothrombin activator complex

Xa, V, phospholipids

Prothrombin $\overset{Ca^{++}}{\longrightarrow}$ Thrombin

Fibrinogen $\overset{Ca^{++}}{\longrightarrow}$ Fibrin (unstable)

Fibrin stabilizing XIII $\longrightarrow$ XIIIa $\longrightarrow$ Ca^{++}

Fibrin (stable), cross-linkage bonds formed

Figure 5-1

In the coagulation sequence, the intrinsic pathway is initiated by surface contact, whereas the extrinsic pathway is initiated by the release of tissue factor from injured tissues. The pathways are interrelated and operate in tandem to achieve hemostasis.

Source: Adapted from Rothrock, J.C. (Ed.). (1999). *The RN First Assistant: An expanded perioperative nursing role* (3rd ed., Fig. 13-1, p. 298). Philadelphia: Lippincott.

is influenced by multiple factors, including the type of procedure, anatomy, certain medications, coagulopathies, fibrinolytic activity, patient position, and the patient's medical condition and nutritional status, all of which can have a profound impact on expected outcomes.

NORMAL CLOTTING MECHANISMS

Coagulation is a process that changes compounds circulating in the blood into an insoluble gel that is able to plug leaks in blood vessels and stop the loss of blood. Injury to a blood vessel causes the recruitment and activation of platelets, which adhere to each other at the site of injury. This leads to the initial formation of a platelet plug and the eventual formation of a fibrin clot. This intricate process requires three elements: coagulation factors, calcium, and phospholipids. Coagulation factors are produced by the liver, calcium is recruited from intracellular sources in the blood, and phospholipids are components of platelets. Platelets are essential in the process because their aggregation is vital to the initial formation of the platelet plug (Spry, 2009).

Coagulation occurs through either an intrinsic or extrinsic pathway. The intrinsic pathway is initiated from within the blood vessel, and the extrinsic pathway is initiated by events such as the severing of a vessel during surgery. When either pathway is initiated, platelets are exposed to collagen, which activates them to form the initial platelet plug within seconds. The "clotting cascade" starts sooner when the extrinsic pathway is initiated, because some of the steps required for the intrinsic pathway are bypassed. Both pathways complete the coagulation process through a common pathway that involves the activation of factors X, V, II, XIII, and I. Deficiencies or abnormalities in any one factor (**Box 5-1**) can slow the overall process and increase the risk of hemorrhage.

In both pathways, thrombin plays an essential role in the eventual formation of the hemostatic plug. Thrombin generation is induced by blood vessel injury. Injury results in exposure of tissue factor, which is then able to interact with activated factor VII to generate thrombin. Thrombin carries out several actions, including conversion of fibrinogen to fibrin and activation of factors V, VIII, XI, which stimulate the production of additional thrombin molecules (DiNisio et al., 2005). This additional thrombin enhances cross-linkage of fibrin strands and formation of the hemostatic plug.

Conditions Associated with Impairments in Normal Coagulation

Significant physiologic conditions that affect clotting include platelet deficiencies and coagulation factor deficiencies. The most common congenital platelet deficiency, Von Willebrand disease, is an inherited platelet membrane receptor defect in which von Willebrand factor (vWF) is missing. Von Willebrand factor is necessary for the platelets' adherence to collagen. Most other clotting deficiencies are the result of coagulation factor defects, of which hemophilia is an example. Hemophilia presents in two forms: hemophilia A (classical hemophilia) is a Factor VIII deficiency, and

Box 5-1	Factors in the Clotting Cascade

Each step of the coagulation cascade is initiated and completed by a series of coagulation factor reactions that involve multiple coagulation factors. As shown in the list below, the number associated with the factor does not represent the order in which the factor is involved in the coagulation cascade:

- Factor I (fibrinogen) is converted to fibrin by thrombin.
- Factor II (prothrombin) is converted to thrombin by factor X. After activation, thrombin converts fibrinogen (factor I) to fibrin. Its synthesis is vitamin K-dependent.
- Factor III (tissue factor or tissue thromboplastin) interacts with factor VII, which is the primary reaction that initiates the extrinsic cascade.
- Factor IV (calcium) and factors VII, IX, X and XIII, which require calcium to be activated, enhance platelet aggregation and red cell clumping.
- Factor V Leiden (proaccelerin, accelerator globulin, labile factor) is essential for converting prothrombin to thrombin.
- Factor VI (accelerin) is a subset of factor V and is also known as factor Va; there is no actual factor VI in blood coagulation.
- Factor VII (proconvertin, cothromboplastin, serum prothrombin conversion accelerator) binds to factor III (tissue factor), then activates factors IX and X. It is essential for conversion of prothrombin to thrombin, and its synthesis is vitamin K-dependent.
- Factor VIII (antihemophilic globulin) is a substance similar to factor V that activates other parts of the coagulation process. Lack of this factor is the cause of hemophilia A.
- Factor IX (Christmas factor) reacts with other factors to activate factor X. It is essential in the common pathway between intrinsic and extrinsic pathways. Lack of this factor causes hemophilia B.
- Factor X (Stuart-Prower factor) reacts with other factors to activate conversion of prothrombin to thrombin.
- Factor XI (plasma thromboplastin antecedent, Fletcher factor [or prekallikrein] and high-molecular-weight kininogen) is part of a complex chain reaction that catalyzes other parts of the coagulation process (activation of factor IX). Patients deficient in factor XI often have mild bleeding problems postoperatively.
- Factor XII (Hageman factor or contact factor) is a substance that reacts with other factors to activate factor XI in the intrinsic pathway.
- Factor XIII (fibrin-stabilizing factor and protein C) assists in forming cross-links among fibrin threads to form fibrin clot.

hemophilia B (also known as Christmas Disease) is a factor IX deficiency. Hemophilia is treated by replacement therapy, and dosing is often dependent upon the classification of surgery as major or minor. Other rare deficiencies, including factors XI and XIII, and inherited fibrinogen abnormalities can be treated by transfusion of fresh frozen plasma (FFP) and cryoprecipitate.

Thrombocytopenia is probably the most common hemostatic deficiency occurring as a result of surgery. Thrombocytopenia may occur as result of massive blood loss and replacement in trauma or by the administration of heparin, which is commonly referred to as heparin-induced thrombocytopenia (HIT). The effects of thrombocytopenia may include hemorrhage or thrombotic events. Direct thrombin inhibitors (DTIs) are a newer class of anticoagulants primarily used in the treatment of HIT (DiNisio et al., 2005). Trauma is a severe physiologic insult that can also impair normal coagulation by affecting clotting from multiple directions. Massive blood loss and temperature loss may profoundly increase bleeding, as well as hemodilution caused by volume replacement to treat shock. Hemorrhage control and product replacement are essential to prevent hypovolemic shock after trauma (**Box 5-2**).

Box 5-2	**Hypovolemic Shock**

Depletion of vascular volume caused by hemorrhage during surgery can limit heart filling, thereby decreasing cardiac output. After about 10% loss of total blood volume, cardiac output and central pressure fall. The following compensatory mechanisms then occur:

- Peripheral vasoconstriction
- Improved cardiac output
- Improved pulmonary gas exchange
- Diaphoresis
- Glucogenolysis
- Reduced glomerular filtration rate
- Further vasoconstriction

These changes can lead to "compensated shock," so termed because the body is able to compensate for volume loss. If blood loss is not corrected, compensatory mechanisms fail and the following sequence of events occurs:

- Vasoconstriction further depletes peripheral cells of oxygen
- Peripheral cells function in an anaerobic state
- Metabolic waste products overtake the cell
- The cell dies, releasing inflammatory mediators
- Inflammatory mediators cause capillary permeability and vasodilatation
- Blood pressure falls

Classification of hypovolemic shock

- Mild: loss of 20% or less of circulating blood volume
- Moderate: loss of 20% to 40% of circulating blood volume
- Severe: loss of 40% or more of circulating blood volume

(continued)

Box 5-2	Hypovolemic Shock (*Continued*)

Fluid resuscitation
   Three main fluids are considered: crystalloid solution, colloid solutions, or blood and blood products.

Crystalloid solutions:
Isotonic electrolyte solutions such as normal saline, lactated Ringer's, Plasma-Lyte

Colloid solutions:
   Albumin

   Dextran

   Hetastarch

Blood and blood products:
   Packed red blood cells (PRBC)

   Blood components containing clotting factors (platelets, fresh frozen plasma, cryoprecipitate)

Source: Adapted from Hoogerwerf, B.J. (2009). Provide hemostasis. In M.L. Phippen, B.C. Ulmer, & M.P. Wells (Eds.), *Competency for safe patient care during operative and invasive procedures.* Denver: Competency & Credentialing Institute; Solheim, J. (2008). Hypovolemic shock. *Nursing Spectrum, 17*(23), 20–25.

Core temperature loss can result from massive blood loss in trauma surgery or during prolonged surgical procedures. Temperature loss has a direct affect on clotting; when the core temperature approaches 34 °C, the platelets' ability to aggregate is significantly diminished (i.e., hypothermic coagulopathy). Preoperatively, skin surface may be warmed with forced-air devices (forced-air blanket or gowns) or circulating fluid garments (Paulikas, 2008). In the operating room (OR), the patient is kept warm to prevent inadvertent hypothermia. The head and feet should be covered. Core temperature in trauma and major surgery should be routinely monitored, and application of warming devices (such as forced-air warming systems) (Constantine & Payne, 2009), warmed irrigation solutions, and elevated ambient temperature should be employed. Similarly, the postoperative hypothermic patient should be actively rewarmed.

Disseminated intravascular coagulation (DIC), a complex, life-threatening condition, is another devastating sequela of massive trauma and transfusion. This hypercoagulative state inappropriately activates the coagulation cascade. Tissue factor (TF) release initiates the cascade, causing an excess of thrombin to be released. With the unregulated release of thrombin, plasminogen is converted to plasmin, inducing fibrinolysis. Fibrinolysis, in turn, results in an excess of fibrin degradation products (FDPs), thereby promoting excessive bleeding (McGraw & Lyon, 2008). When the coagulation system is initiated in DIC, the activated fibrinolytic pathway (see Figure 5-1) results in the deposition of fibrin and contributes to multiple organ dysfunction syndrome (MODS) (Owings, Utter, & Gosselion, 2007).

Another physiologic factor that should not be overlooked or minimized is steroid dependence. Any patient with a medical condition requiring chronic steroid treatment should be considered a higher risk for coagulation complications.

Increased risk for bleeding may also be affected by anatomic anomalies because an incidental injury to major vessels may occur. Arterial venous malformations (AVM), for example, may occur in any location and can present technical challenges to maintaining vascular control and planned surgical outcomes. Accessory vascular structures, whether known or unknown, may also present a surgical challenge.

Cardiac surgery typically requires the use of extracorporeal circulation and oxygenation. The blood circuit exerts physiologic and mechanical effects on clotting. Because the blood circuit is synthetic, it can stimulate the body's inflammatory response to a foreign substance. In addition, blood products are absorbed and injured by the tubing, filters, and membranes necessary to oxygenate and cleanse blood before reinfusing. Large doses of heparin are required to enable blood to flow through the circuit and oxygen membrane without clotting, which encourages bleeding during the procedure and may require blood and volume replacement. Core temperature is also reduced to 34 °C and occasionally as low as 18 °C to reduce oxygen demand and the risk for cell death. This induced hypothermia interrupts the coagulation cascade by significantly impairing platelet adhesion. As previously described, large doses of heparin, platelet loss, hemodilution, and hypothermia all have profound effects on the coagulation cascade; thus, continuous monitoring by the surgical team is required as well as an established plan for replacement therapies.

PREOPERATIVE ASSESSMENT

Adequate hemostatic control during surgery begins with the preoperative assessment and review of the patient's history (see Chapter 7 for a thorough discussion of patient assessment). The preoperative assessment will alert the surgical team to any cardiovascular comorbidity that predisposes the patient to intraoperative problems. Collaboration with the surgeon, as well as coordination with nursing staff and the anesthesia provider for any additional supplies, equipment, fluids and/or blood products will improve chances for achieving an optimal outcome.

The history and physical examination (H&P) provide information about the patient's present condition, past history, and medication use. The H&P is performed no more than 30 days prior to any procedure requiring anesthesia (Further changes, 2009). After reviewing the H&P, the FA focuses on preoperative considerations relating to potential problems with hemostasis during the planned procedure (**Box 5-3**). Sepsis, deficiencies in blood clotting mechanisms, anticoagulant

---

Box 5-3	**Preoperative Considerations**

- Is the patient on anticoagulants?
- Is the patient taking antiplatelet drugs?
- Does the patient take aspirin-containing medication (prescription or over-the-counter [OTC]) or other nonsteroidal anti-inflammatory drugs (NSAIDS)?
- Does the patient take vitamin supplements (E) or herbs which may contribute to increased bleeding times (bilberry, gingko biloba, garlic, cayenne, ginger, ginseng, feverfew, bromelain, dong quoi, fish or flaxseed oil, chamomile, grape seed extract, dandelion root, horse chestnut, saw palmetto, or quinine)?
- Does the patient have a personal or family history of bleeding disorders, such as hemophilia or sickle cell disease?
- Does the patient acknowledge easy bruising, bleeding gums, easy superficial bleeding after things such as razor nicks, or severe nosebleeds?
- Is the patient anemic?
- Does the patient have renal or hepatic disease?
- What are the results of the patient's coagulation profile?
- Has the patient been typed and cross-matched?
- Has consent been signed for administration of blood or blood products?
- Are there restrictions to consent for blood products, such as transfusion of own (autologous) blood, use of cell recovery system (blood salvage/autotransfusion), or directions regarding which blood components are acceptable?
- Has preoperative autologous blood been donated?
- Have plans been made for perioperative blood salvage and autotransfusion?
- Does the patient have signed refusal for transfusion of blood products?
- Have bloodless surgery alternatives been discussed with the patient?
- Are there cultural, religious or ethnic beliefs that affect the administration of blood or blood products?

Sources: ASA practice guidelines for perioperative blood transfusion and adjuvant therapies. (2006). *Anesthesiology,* 105, 198–208; Backman, S.B., Bondy, R.M., Deschamps, A., et al. (2007). Perioperative considerations for anesthesia. In W.W. Souba (Ed.), *ACS surgery: Principles & practice* (6th ed., p. 49). New York, NY: WebMD; Black, J.M., & Hawks, J.H. (2005). *Medical-surgical nursing,* 263–312. St. Louis, MO: Elsevier; Fox, J., Brown, S., & Vigil, R. (2008). Bloodless surgery and patient safety issues. *Perioperative Nursing Clinics, 3*(4), 345–354; Hulisz, D.T. (2008). Top herbal products efficacy and safety concerns. Medscape general surgery. Retrieved February 22, 2009 from www.medscape.com/viewarticle/568235; *Nursing 2008 drug handbook.* Philadelphia: Lippincott Williams & Wilkins; Valentine, W., & Craig, S. (2007). Integrated health practices: Complementary and alternative therapies. In J.C. Rockrock (Ed.), *Alexander's care of the patient in surgery* (13th ed., pp. 1211–1214). St. Louis MO: Mosby.

drugs, allergies, or diseases such as leukemia, thrombocytopenia, lymphoma, or multiple myeloma increase a patient's risk of bleeding. Ask the patient about hemostatic responses to previous surgical interventions, easy bruising, epistaxis, gingival bleeding, menorrhagia, and consumption of alcoholic beverages. Patients with a history of excessive alcohol intake are at risk due to altered nutritional status and possible liver damage. Medication history should be reviewed for such drugs as anticoagulants, aspirin (and aspirin-containing drugs), or other nonsteroidal anti-inflammatory medications, including over-the-counter medications. The use of dietary supplements or herbs should be raised because many interact directly with medications, affect platelet function, or increase bleeding time.

During this part of the patient interview, questions should be very direct and specific. Use queries such as "Do you take over-the-counter drugs?" "What are they?" "Do you use cold medicines?" and "Which cold medicines do you use?" because patients need to be specifically asked about such use. If one simply asks the patient what medications they take, they are likely to list only prescription medications, and the FA may lose potentially critical parts of the history.

The presence of anemia in surgical patients should be carefully considered, because a study by Campbell et al. (2008) suggested that absence of anemia (along with shorter operative times and fewer blood transfusions) was associated with lower incidences of surgical site infection (SSI). A review of laboratory results identifying clotting characteristics should include results of the hemoglobin and hematocrit (H&H) tests. Other laboratory studies are requested for patients with a history suggestive of a bleeding disorder or if major bleeding is anticipated due to the nature of the surgical procedure (Merrick et al., 2006). Activated partial thromboplastin time (APTT), prothrombin time (PT), international normalized ratio (INR), bleeding time, and a platelet count are common laboratory tests performed to assess risk of bleeding. Activated coagulation time (ACT) is used as a trend indicator and requires a baseline reading. The ACT is most often used for open heart and major vascular surgeries. See Appendix I for a complete review of laboratory studies and normal values.

The OR Briefing

The type and extent of the planned surgical procedure are important to consider when determining the risk of bleeding. Although all procedures require a thorough preparation, some procedures clearly present a significantly higher risk for hemorrhage. OR briefings enhance team communication and increase patient safety (Paige et al., 2008). Although it often lasts only a few minutes, the briefing should include the critical steps of the planned procedure and any potential problems. Any potential problems with coagulation should be addressed at this time so that the entire team is prepared to mitigate potential coagulation issues (Nundy et al., 2008). During the briefing, procedures posing exceptional hematological risks such as abdominal organ removal, tumor resection, major vessel resection, or extracorporeal blood circulation should be discussed. Patients who have had previous surgery may have adhesions, which can increase bleeding. Difficult or prolonged surgery requiring extensive exposure causes core temperature to drop, which in turn increases the risk for excessive bleeding. Measures to address these and other potential coagulation or hemostasis issues should be discussed during the briefing. The World Health Organization's Safe Surgery Saves Lives campaign has developed a surgical safety checklist and tested it in eight countries worldwide. Research on the use of the checklist concluded that implementation of the checklist during major operations was associated with a significant reduction in complications and mortality. This checklist recommends that during the time out, the surgeon reviews critical events anticipated in the surgery, the anticipated duration of the procedure, and the anticipated blood loss (Haynes et al., 2009).

FLUID REPLACEMENT THERAPIES

An essential part of the surgical plan includes proper planning for fluid balance and replacement therapies. Identifying fluid imbalances and clotting deficiencies during the preoperative assessment helps the surgical team avoid or treat potential hemostatic risks. Decisions about transfusing blood products depend on the patient's need for additional oxygen-carrying capacity. When significant hypovolemia or active bleeding is present, transfusion is initiated to increase intravascular volume and to prevent deficits in additional oxygen-carrying capacity.

Packed red blood cells (PRBCs) are administered to improve oxygen delivery when blood is lost during surgery. PRBCs contain hemoglobin, which transports oxygen through the bloodstream to the body's tissues. The hematocrit and hemoglobin tests monitor red blood cell volume. The transfusion of one unit of PRBCs (or whole blood) increases the hematocrit by approximately 3% and the hemoglobin by about 1 g/dL. The American Society of Anesthesiologists (ASA) guidelines state that transfusion is rarely recommended when the hemoglobin value is greater than 10 g/dL and is almost always indicated when less than 6 g/dL. (ASA Practice Guidelines, 2006). Intermediate hemoglobin values require an assessment of the patient's risk for developing complications of inadequate oxygenation that would necessitate PRBC transfusion. The administration of PRBCs requires ABO and Rh cross-matching.

Whole blood is rarely administered during surgery. However, massive blood loss may necessitate immediate replacement of RBCs and volume expansion with the colloid plasma proteins that whole blood contains. Whole blood must be ABO identical and Rh compatible.

Platelets are concentrates from whole blood. Administration of platelets, according to the ASA guidelines (ASA Practice Guidelines, 2006), is usually indicated in patients with microvascular bleeding if the platelet count is less than 50×10^9/L. Intermediate platelet counts require a determination of the patient's risk for developing more significant bleeding. Patients with an apparently adequate platelet count may still require a platelet transfusion if there are known platelet dysfunction and microvascular bleeding. Platelets do not require ABO or Rh crossmatching.

Plasma component therapy (fresh frozen plasma, "FFP") may be necessary for patients at risk of adverse effects from inadequate coagulation factors. FFP contains normal components of blood plasma, including fibrinogen, and is commonly administered to surgical patients undergoing procedures in which bleeding is anticipated (Bielefeldt and DeWitt, 2009). Plasma component therapy requires ABO crossmatching. FFP may be administered to reverse the effects of warfarin therapy, to correct known coagulation factor deficiencies when the specific concentrate is unavailable, or when there is microvascular bleeding secondary to coagulation deficiency in transfused patients. The ASA guidelines (ASA Practice Guidelines, 2006) recommend administering FFP in doses calculated to achieve a minimum of 30% plasma factor concentration; this is usually achieved with 10 to 15 mL/kg of FFP.

For patients with inherited or acquired coagulopathies, cryoprecipitate, which contains factors VIII and XIII, fibrinogen, fibronectin, and von Willebrand's factor, is used. Cryoprecipitate may also be indicated to correct microvascular bleeding in massively transfused patients. The ASA recommends that fibrinogen concentrations lower than 80 to 100 mg/dL be used as an indication for component therapy (ASA Practice Guidelines, 2006).

Transfusion-Free Surgery

Given the risks associated with blood transfusions, as well as religious beliefs that forbid transfusions, the surgical community has developed interventions that reduce or eliminate the need for blood transfusion in the surgical patient. Referred to as "bloodless" or transfusion-free surgery, perioperative strategies may employ a variety of medications, blood conservation, and surgical techniques to achieve transfusion-free surgery. Bloodless techniques vary from hospital to hospital.

Preoperatively, medicinal and nutritional approaches may be used to increase the patient's blood count before surgery. Efforts are made to guard against unnecessary

Box 5-4	Hematopoietic Agents to Stimulate Blood Cell Growth and Development

Recombinant Erythropoietin (rHu-EPO) (epoetin, Epogen®, Eprex®, Procrit®, Recormon®)
Use: stimulates red blood cell production.
Recombinant Granulocyte Colony-Stimulating Factor (rHu-G-CSF)
Use: stimulates production of neutrophils.
Recombinant Interleukin-11 (rHu-IL-11)
Use: stimulates platelet production.

Sources: Alternatives to transfusion. *The University Center for bloodless surgery and medicine at University Hospital in Newark, NJ.* Retrieved February 22, 2009 from www.theuniversityhospital.com/bloodless/html/bloodlessterms/ alternatives.htm; Skidmore–Roth, L. (2008). *Mosby's nursing drug reference.* St. Louis, MO: Mosby.

blood loss from lab tests, and microanalyzers may be used to assess smaller blood samples. Hematopoietic agents can be specifically selected to stimulate blood cell growth and development (**Box 5-4**), and medications such as Aprotinin, vitamin K, or Desmopressin may be prescribed (Alternatives to transfusion, 2009). The anesthesia provider may select hypotensive anesthesia or hemodilution.

Intraoperatively, blood loss can be minimized when the FA uses immediate and deliberate hemostatic techniques, such as immediate clamping or coagulation of bleeding vessels. Other techniques include the use of nontraditional cutting scalpels which minimize blood loss, such as argon beam coagulators, the ultrasonic cutting and coagulation surgical device, surgical lasers, or the cyber-knife, which facilitates image-guided radiosurgery. The use of a cell-saver, when appropriate, can minimize blood loss during surgery. In a process referred to as "blood salvage," blood lost during certain surgical procedures is collected, filtered and continuously reinfused when a cell-saver is used.

Acellular blood substitutes are currently undergoing clinical trials for use during surgery. They possess a number of beneficial attributes (Owings et al., 2007) including increased shelf life, increased availability not tied to donor supply, reduced risk of viral transmission, and reduced risk of incompatibility.

MECHANICAL HEMOSTATIC TECHNIQUES

Surgery is a profound insult to the human body, which in turn exhibits systemic responses. The amount and severity of tissue and organ manipulation have direct effects on bleeding and healing. One of the primary tasks of the FA during a surgical procedure is to provide surgical exposure (see Chapter 4 for a full discussion of surgical exposure). Understanding that tissue manipulation and injury impact hemostasis, the FA must provide adequate exposure for the surgeon to perform the surgical task safely while simultaneously ensuring limited tissue injury. Proper use of surgical instruments reduces tissue damage and thus the incidence of bleeding.

Direct Pressure

The first type of mechanical hemostatic control is direct pressure. When exposure is limited, particularly in peripheral vascular surgery, the standard surgical technique is to achieve proximal and distal control of the objective vessels with instruments or vascular tourniquets. This is not always easily performed or achieved. If injury occurs prior to adequate control, direct pressure at the source of bleeding usually prevents major blood loss. Applying direct pressure for 7 to 10 minutes will resolve most minor bleeding, but when injury to a significant vascular structure occurs, pressure is used until proximal and distal control is achieved.

Arterial bleeding lends itself to direct pressure more readily than venous bleeding because the arterial vessel is muscular and the flow is pulsatile. Venous bleeding may not be readily controlled with direct pressure in the same manner, and in some situations the application of direct pressure may increase the severity of the vascular injury. Packing the area of venous bleeding with surgical sponges can reduce blood loss when direct pressure control cannot be achieved or generalized bleeding is present as a result of a coagulopathy. Systemic coagulopathy may occur as a result of trauma, infection, massive blood loss, or platelet dysfunction.

When sponges are used to control bleeding, it is useful for the FA who places them to announce the number of sponges that have been packed in the cavity. This helps to ensure the retrieval of all the sponges at the time of reexploration. Foreign objects unintentionally left in patients (often referred to as a "retained foreign object" or RFO) are a significant surgical safety issue and are considered a "never event" by the Centers for Medicare and Medicaid Services (CMS) (Retzlaff, 2009). In a study by Cima and colleagues (2008), retained surgical sponges accounted for 68% of the inadvertently retained items in RFO patients. Approaches such as radiofrequency identification (RFID) tagging are gaining attention as methods to mitigate against unintended retention of a foreign object such as a surgical sponge (Figure 5-2). The risk for RFOs is higher in a patient undergoing an emergency procedure, unplanned changes in a procedure, or possessing a higher body-mass index (Gawande et al., 2003). As noted by Catalano (2008), communication, team awareness and effort, and collaboration help reduce the likelihood of a safety-compromising event. The FA has a primary accountability for engaging in productive and useful communication. If sponges are used to pack a bleeding site and intentionally left in the patient, the FA should communicate to the circulating nurse the number and types of sponges in the patient leaving the OR. The

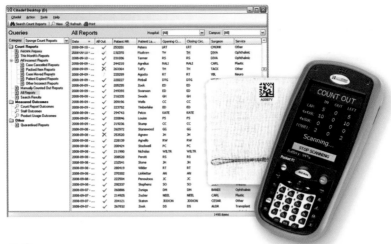

Figure 5-2

The SurgiCount Safety-Sponge™ system—comprised of uniquely identifiable surgical sponges, the SurgiCounter handheld scanning device, and customized software—allows the surgical team to precisely account for each sponge used in a procedure and documents the successful result in a database or patient record formats.

Source: Courtesy of SurgiCount Medical. Reprinted by permission.

circulating nurse will then document that information, along with the reason for the intended variation in the count (that is, the count is not correct in this situation, but the sponges are accounted for). When the patient later returns to surgery, the surgical team will reconcile the number and types of sponges it removes with the record from the previous surgery (AORN Recommended practices for sponge, sharp and instrument counts, 2009).

On occasion, moistened sterile towels may be requested by the surgeon for packing a surgical site in an obese patient. The FA should verify that the towels have radiopaque markers. The towels should be included in the surgical count as "miscellaneous items" (Downing, 2008). As in using sponges to pack a cavity, the FA who places the sterile towels should announce the number of towels in the cavity. This helps to ensure their retrieval when the count is done.

Hemostats

Hemostats (also referred to as "snaps") are the surgical instruments most commonly used to clamp vessels (**Figures 5-3** and **5-4**) and tissue to control or stop bleeding. Hemostats are designed with many shapes and sizes for a wide variety of applications.

Curved hemostats (see **Figure 5-3**, top) may be preferred because the FA can apply them while maintaining visualization of the clamp tip. This reduces the risk of inadvertently applying the clamp on unintended tissue. On the other hand,

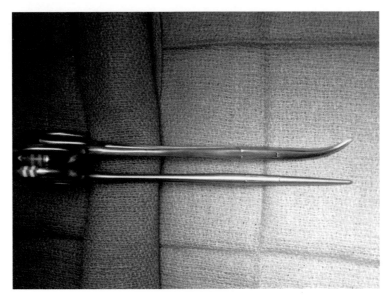

Figure 5-3

Hemostats. Curved (top) and straight (bottom).

Source: Photo courtesy of Winchester Hospital, Winchester, MA.

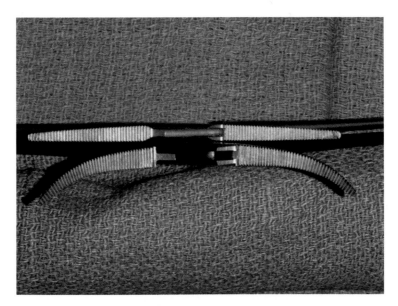

Figure 5-4

Hemostat jaws are serrated along their entire length to secure a vessel or tissue during temporary hemostasis.

Source: Photo courtesy of Winchester Hospital, Winchester, MA.

some prefer the straight hemostat (see Figure 5-3, bottom), believing that it is easier to show the clamp tip by simply elevating it when the first throw of a tie is being placed. The FA, through acquisition of surgical skill, will develop a technique that is effective but does not compromise surrounding tissue or twist the vessel to expose the hemostat tip when placing a tie.

To apply a hemostat, the open end of the bleeding vessel is grasped in the tip of the clamp (known as the "tip" technique; Figure 5-5). Only the minimum amount of the vessel should be clamped. If the open end of the vessel cannot be held securely with the tip of the hemostat, it should be cross-clamped with the hemostat jaws (known as the "jaw" technique; Figure 5-6).

To decrease blood loss, blood vessels are clamped before being cut whenever possible. As noted above, either the tips or the jaws may be used, depending on the vessel size and location and the content of surrounding tissues. The vessel is usually clamped with two hemostats, with space left between the clamps for cutting the vessel. The amount of vessel left between the clamps must be sufficient to prevent the clamps from slipping off the vessel once it is severed. When placing a

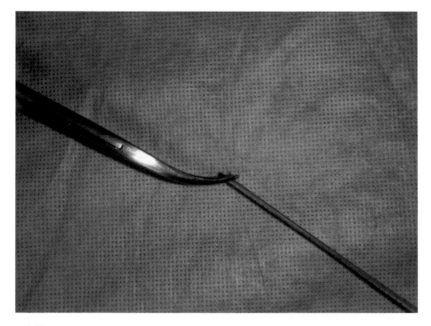

Figure 5-5

Method of the tip technique when clamping a blood vessel (represented by rubber tubing) with a curved hemostat.

Source: Photo courtesy of Winchester Hospital, Winchester, MA.

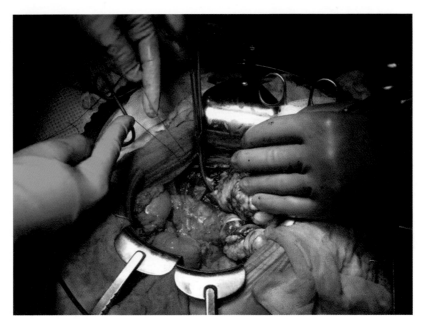

Figure 5-6

If the open end of the vessel cannot be held securely with the tip of the hemostat, it should be cross-clamped with the hemostat jaws as shown here.

Source: Photo courtesy of Winchester Hospital, Winchester, MA.

hemostat on a branch of a blood vessel, the FA should allow space on the branch between the clamp and the major vessel; this allows placement of a ligature around the cut branch and prevents fracturing (or injuring) the major vessel (**Figure 5-7**). If curved hemostats are used, the tips of the two clamps should point toward each other. This facilitates cutting between the clamps and the subsequent placement of ligatures.

Removing a hemostat during vessel ligation requires coordination between the person holding the clamp and the person tying the ligature. The hemostat handle is lifted so that the ligature can be placed behind the clamp. This must be done carefully, so that the hemostat is not pulled off the vessel. The hemostat is then lowered or flattened to hold the ligature behind the clamp and elevate the point (tip) of the hemostat. The ligature is then brought around the tip of the hemostat, encircling the vessel to be ligated. As the first throw of the ligature knot is being tightened, the hemostat is slowly and carefully opened, thereby releasing the end of the vessel. The hemostat should be removed in a direction that will not interfere with the placement of the ligature or obstruct the vision of the person doing the tying. The

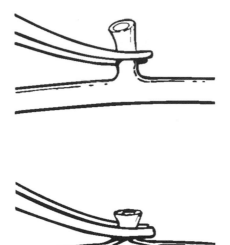

Figure 5-7

Application of clamp. *Top*: Proper application of clamp to branch of blood vessel allows room for ligating without injuring vessel. *Bottom*: Improper placement of clamp on branch of blood vessel. Note injury to vessel.

Source: Adapted from Rothrock, J.C. (Ed.), (1999). *The RN First Assistant: An expanded perioperative nursing role* (3rd ed., Fig. 13-5, p. 305). Philadelphia: Lippincott.

hemostat can be opened and removed with precise control by placing the third finger and thumb into the ring handles. In many instances the hemostat can be removed with the use of leverage on the handle. This method is acceptable when ligature placement and tying are easy, although the release of the hemostat is not as precise. The leverage method becomes quicker and easier as the skill is developed.

There are three basic techniques for clamping and ligating blood vessels deep within a wound. The method used is usually related to the accessibility, size, and fragility of the vessel or surrounding tissue structures. In one technique, the vessel is clamped with longer, fine hemostats and then divided with a scissor or knife. The ligature is held at one end with a tissue forceps or a tonsil hemostat, and the free end of the ligature is passed around the handle of the clamp and held taut with the free hand. The clamped end of the ligature is then placed under the tip of the hemostat. The FA, holding the hemostat, then tilts the hemostat tip downward and holds the ligature.

The hemostat's position must be changed very cautiously to prevent it from slipping off the end of the vessel. After the ligature is passed under the tip of the hemostat holding the vessel, the ligature is pulled until enough length is available for easy tying. The ligature is released from the clamp or tissue forceps, and the first throw of the knot is slipped down behind or to the side of the hemostat clamped to the vessel as the hemostat is slowly removed by the FA.

In another method, the blood vessel is clamped and cut in the same manner. However, instead of using a free ligature, the surgeon uses a ligature on a needle (stick tie). The surgeon holds the hemostat clamped to the vessel as the suture needle is placed through the blood vessel behind the hemostat. The ligature is pulled through the vessel, leaving enough length on the free end for easy tying. The ligature is then tied behind and around the vessel as the FA slowly removes the hemostat.

In the third technique, the ligatures are placed before the vessel is cut. The vessel is dissected free of surrounding tissue so that it can be visualized. An angled clamp of the appropriate length is used. The tip of the clamp is placed under the vessel and opened. The assistant then passes the ligature into the open tip of the angled clamp. It will be necessary for the FA to hold the ligature with both hands: one hand to keep the ligature taut and the other hand to hold the end of the ligature that will be placed in the angled clamp. In deep wounds, a tonsil hemostat or tissue forceps can be used to hold the end of the ligature to be placed in the open clamp tip. The angled clamp is closed so that the ligature is gripped securely between its jaws as the FA releases the ligature. Care must be taken not to close surrounding tissue in the clamp jaws. The angled clamp is then withdrawn and the ligature passed under the vessel. Sufficient ligature is pulled under the vessel to allow easy tying. The ligature is released from the angled clamp and tied securely around the vessel. The procedure is then repeated. The second ligature is positioned on the vessel to allow space between the two ligatures. The vessel is then cut between the two ligatures. The amount of vessel between the cut ends and the ligatures must be long enough to prevent the tie from slipping off. It is easier to cut the vessel if both ligatures are held taut, thereby pulling on the vessel.

Right angled clamps (Figure 5-8) are often used for exposure of vessels to pass suture and tapes or to clamp larger vessels and tissue pedicles containing vessels. The goal is to apply the clamp before incising or transecting the vessel. This is accomplished by applying the ends of the clamp across the vessel with only minimal segments extending beyond the clamp. Having applied the clamp, the vessel is transected, and a surgical tie or suture ligature is passed around the base of the clamp and tied. When a vessel is unexpectedly injured, a clamp applied grossly to the vessel or tissue ensures complete and immediate occlusion of the vessel. This technique is modified when the source of bleeding is a vessel that cannot be ligated without risking damage to the organ, such as a vital organ artery. In this situation, an atraumatic vascular clamp is applied to allow temporary control while performing a vascular repair.

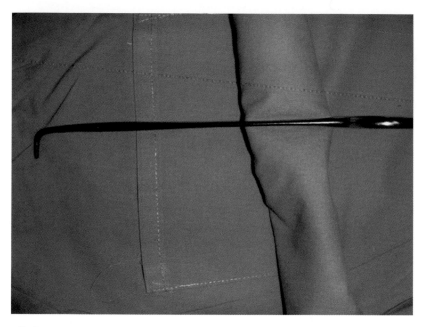

Figure 5-8

Right angled clamps are often used to expose vessels in order to pass suture and tapes or to clamp larger vessels and tissue pedicles.

Source: Photo courtesy of Winchester Hospital, Winchester, MA.

Vascular Clamps

When performing a vascular procedure, it is standard practice to gain control of the intended vessel by isolating the vessel proximal and distal to the intended surgical location. The vascular clamp is an atraumatic clamp that is used to occlude a blood vessel temporarily (Figure 5-9). Such clamps come in many shapes (Figure 5-10) and are designed to provide complete or partial occlusion of the vessel. Pioneers in cardiovascular surgery such as Cooley, DeBakey, Statinsky, and Derra have designed clamps that still bear their names today. Some of these clamps have been modified to accept an insert, known as a Fogarty™ insert, that is soft and malleable on one side of the clamp jaw. This insert is preferred in many situations because the soft insert accommodates occlusion with minimal trauma.

Vascular clamps are designed with tiny non-opposing teeth that provide firm, partial, or complete compression of the vessel without injuring the vessel lining (intima). Partial occlusion is used, for example, when suturing the vein to the aorta during a coronary artery bypass. In this situation, applying a partial occlusion clamp permits creation of an aortotomy without blood flow in the operative portion of

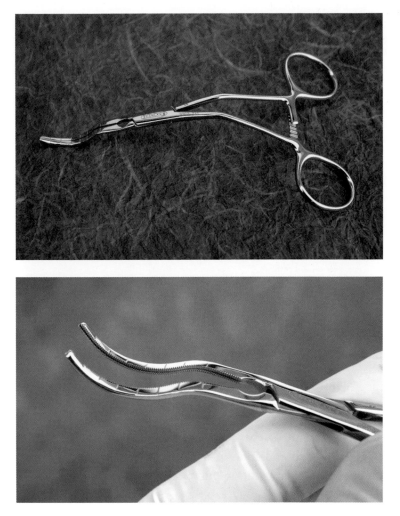

Figure 5-9A and Figure 5-9B

Vascular clamps, like the one shown (A, full clamp), may have very fine atraumatic teeth to secure vascular occlusion (B, clamp jaws). They are available in various sizes, angles, and lengths.

Source: Photographs courtesy of Scanlan International, Inc. Reprinted by permission.

the aorta. An example of the use of complete occlusion is during a femoro-popliteal bypass. When performing this procedure, the femoral artery does not have sufficient diameter for placement of a partial occlusion clamp to perform an arterial anastomosis safely. Instead, the artery is occluded (commonly referred to as "crossclamped") proximal and distal to the arteriotomy site to provide a bloodless

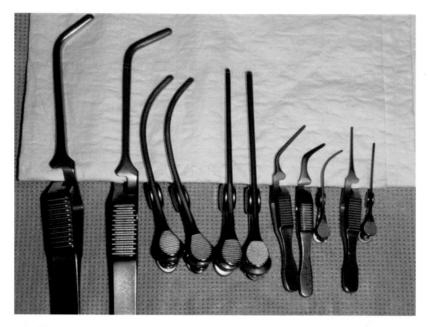

Figure 5-10

Vascular clamps come in many different shapes. Shown here are bulldog clamps, which occlude an artery or vein with correct tension to avoid vessel trauma. Their jaws vary in length and they may be straight or curved.

Source: Photo courtesy of Winchester Hospital, Winchester, MA.

operative field. Crossclamp times are recorded by the circulating nurse and anesthesia provider; the FA should announce when the vessel is clamped and when the clamp is removed for documentation purposes.

Should the FA be in the position to apply or remove a vascular clamp, it must be understood that although the clamp is atraumatic, its application or removal is not risk-free. The action of applying or removing a vascular clamp must be performed in a deliberate and controlled fashion. Undue hesitation or abrupt movement can have severe and devastating consequences.

Tourniquets

Another method to control blood flow is the application of a tourniquet. Tourniquets may be used directly on the vascular structure (referred to as a "vascular tourniquet") or by applying the tourniquet to a limb. The vascular tourniquet, usually a commercially prepared item such as a vessel loop (Figure 5-11) (moistened umbilical tape is also used), is applied directly to the vascular structure and pulled through a semi-rigid tube like a red rubber catheter

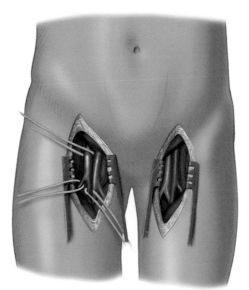

Figure 5-11

Vessel loops applied to the femoral artery.

Source: Courtesy of Phippen, M.L., Ulmer, B.C., & Wells, M.P. (2009). *Competency for safe patient care during operative and invasive procedures* (Fig. 16.3, p. 472). Denver: CCI.

cut to length, pulled tight, and clamped with a hemostat. Commercially prepared vascular tourniquets such as vessel loops are preferred when the vascular structure is to be preserved.

Limb tourniquets control blood flow by application of a pneumatic device, are set to specific pressures, and are closely time-monitored (Box 5-5). In orthopedic procedures, this method provides a bloodless field and expedites the surgery. When occluding a limb, ischemia and permanent nerve and/or tissue damage are significant risks; prolonged surgeries may require deflating the pneumatic tourniquet to reestablish tissue perfusion. During this period, direct pressure achieves hemostasis until the pneumatic tourniquet is reinflated.

Hemostatic Clips

Ligating hemostatic clips (also referred to as "hemoclips") are quickly and easily applied. The clips may be manually loaded in a reusable applier. The scrub person loads and then passes the clip positioned in the applier. Clip appliers come in a variety of sizes with straight or angled jaws. The finger ring of the applier is often color-coded to match the clip cartridge. Before application, blot the bleeding area with a sponge. If necessary, apply direct pressure to the bleeding area with the sponge. Then, roll the sponge off the bleeding vessel, and grasp it with forceps or hemostat. Place the clip across the vessel, squeeze the applier handles together, and then release them. Apply additional clips as necessary. Clips may also be used in lieu of ties to achieve distal and proximal control of a vessel prior to its transection (Figure 5-12).

Box 5-5	Safety Measures When Using the Pneumatic Tourniquet

- Be familiar with the risks and benefits of tourniquet use. Tourniquet use is contraindicated in neonates and in patients with peripheral vascular disease, thrombosis, embolism, crushing injuries, open fractures, infection, or presence of a shunt or vascular access device in the extremity being operated on.
- If the FA has not used the pneumatic tourniquet previously, manufacturer's written instructions should be reviewed. Automated tourniquet systems may recommend a limb occlusion pressure (LOP) and contain audible indicators for cuff status, pressure changes, and time limits. The FA must be familiar with the specific tourniquet system being used and the unique instructions for its use.
- Select an appropriate size cuff. The cuff should be:

  ■ Wider than half the diameter of the patient's limb
  ■ Long enough to overlap and fully fasten; too much overlap can cause increased pressure in the area of the overlap
  ■ Contoured, if necessary, for a tapered (conical) limb

- Place a soft, lint-free padding with interlocking fibers that will not come apart (e.g., stockinette) or a limb protection device around the limb prior to cuff placement.
- Verify that the selected tourniquet cuff is clean (single-use cuffs are also available).
- Verify the correct surgical site/side prior to placing the cuff on the extremity.
- Choose an appropriate site for tourniquet application. These vary according to surgical site (upper arm, thigh, forearm, calf, or ankle).
- Use care when applying the cuff on an obese patient's extremity. The circulating nurse or another surgical team member should apply traction to the excess skin until the tourniquet cuff is applied. This prevents possible shearing injury.
- When applying the cuff, avoid crinkling, folding, or bending the cuff. To prevent damage to the underlying skin and soft tissue, the cuff should be applied smoothly, with no wrinkles or tunneling effect. There should be sufficient room to insert two fingers under the proximal edge of the cuff.
- Place the cuff such that the tubing connection is close to the lateral aspect of the extremity.
- When using a limb-positioning device, avoid compressing the tourniquet cuff against the device during patient positioning.
- Use caution when prepping so that fluids do not pool under the cuff.
- When using perforating towel clips for draping, place them to avoid damaging or puncturing the cuff (the cuff contains the inflated bladder).
- Verify with the anesthesia provider that antibiotics or other medications have been administered and sufficient time has elapsed to ensure appropriate tissue concentrations prior to extremity exsanguination and cuff inflation.
- When the extremity is exsanguinated prior to inflation, it should be:

  ■ Elevated to promote the exit of venous blood
  ■ Compressed with an elastic wrap unless that is contraindicated by malignancy, fracture, infection, or other conditions as determined by the surgeon

- Follow recommended guidelines for inflation pressure and inflation times. Confirm these with the surgeon.

- Note when the audible activation indicator or alarm sounds to alert the FA to a change in pressure or to alert the FA that the designated inflation time has been reached.
- If the designated inflation time has been reached and continued tourniquet time is necessary, the limb should be reperfused. This should be coordinated with the anesthesia provider, surgeon, and circulating nurse.
- At the conclusion of tourniquet use, deflation should proceed according to manufacturer's recommendations.
- After deflation, look for and control any bleeding at the surgical site.
- Collaborate with the circulating nurse in monitoring the patient following tourniquet deflation.

Sources: AORN. (2009). Recommended practices for the use of the pneumatic tourniquet in the perioperative practice setting. *Perioperative standards and recommended practices* (pp. 373–385). Denver: AORN; FDA medical device safety. Retrieved December 29, 2008 from www.fda.gov/cdhr/medicaldevicesafety/tipsarticles/tourniquet.html; Spry, C. (2009). *Essentials of Perioperative Nursing* (pp. 203–206). Sudbury, MA: Jones and Bartlett Publishers; Retrieved December 29, 2008 from www.tourniquets.org

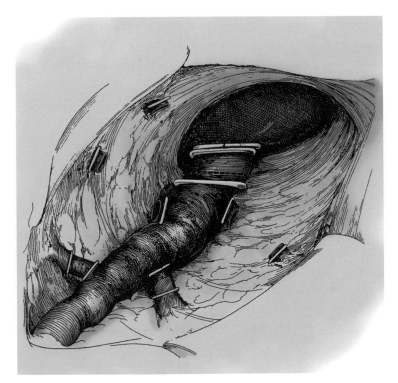

Figure 5-12

Distal and proximal application of hemostatic clips to the saphenous vein.

Source: Courtesy of Phippen, M.L., Ulmer, B.C., & Wells, M.P. (2009). *Competency for safe patient care during operative and invasive procedures* (Fig. 17.2, p. 511). Denver: CCI.

Disposable appliers are often used. They are preloaded with ligating clips and are available in a variety of applier lengths and clip sizes. The clips are constructed from stainless steel, titanium, or an absorbable material.

Surgical Staplers

Sterile, disposable staplers with removable cartridge inserts or preloaded with a set number of staples come in a variety of sizes for use in either open or endoscopic procedures (see Chapter 3, Figure 3-13). They are generally used for resection of the bowel or lung, but they are also available for vascular control, particularly in thoracic surgery, and for closing skin (see Chapter 6). These staplers offer a safe, efficient method to achieve hemostasis in many surgical procedures.

Tying Sutures

As a surgical assistant, the FA must possess the vital skill of "tying" ligatures and sutures. The FA may find herself/himself in the position of having to tie a critical suture. Surgeons train for many years to meet the requirements of surgery and to make decisions that determine the course of surgery. The FA's role imposes similar burdens, which cannot be minimized. As a collaborating surgical professional, the FA should practice tying skills more than any other skill and must be equally proficient with all tying techniques.

Sutures are categorized as absorbable or nonabsorbable as well as multifilament or monofilament. These characteristics are additional factors in determining the type of knot used. Monofilament nonabsorbable suture is preferred for vascular repairs, and braided suture is most often preferred when strength and ease of tying are deemed important. Chapter 6 provides a full discussion of sutures and suturing techniques.

Surgical knots can be tied by using one-handed (Figure 5-13), or two-handed techniques (Figure 5-14), or with an instrument (Figure 5-15). The two-handed technique is the mainstay for tying, and the FA must have proficiency in this method before all others. Surgical knots have different applications that must be well understood. The granny or slipknot allows the FA to cinch the knot on the second or third throw, ensuring hemostasis with minimal risk of injury to the vessel.

The basic knots are the square knot (Figure 5-16), the surgeon's knot, and the granny or slipknot. The square knot is used most frequently and is the most secure. The surgeon's knot is helpful when tying under a moderate amount of tension. If the first throw is doubled, the suture will not slip while the second knot is being placed (Figure 5-17). The granny knot, or slip knot, is especially useful in wounds that provide limited access. It is made by placing two identical throws of the suture, allowing the FA to cinch the knot on the second or third throw, thus ensuring hemostasis with minimal risk of injury to the vessel. A square knot is tied on the granny knot to keep it from slipping.

Figure 5-13

One-handed tie. Step-by-step instructions for one method of completing the one-handed tie with a square knot.

Source: Photos courtesy of Winchester Hospital, Winchester, MA.

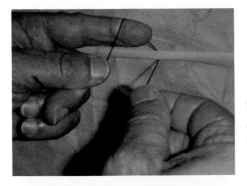

Figure 5-13A

Grasp the outer strand of the ligature material and loop it over the left index finger. Hold the other end of the strand with the right thumb and index finger.

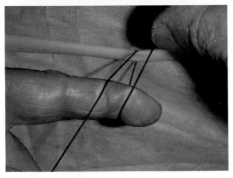

Figure 5-13B

Loop the strand in right hand over the extended left index finger. Slightly close the left index finger to secure the strand.

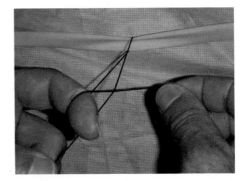

Figure 5-13C

Bring the left index finger over the strand held by the left hand, pulling toward the left hand.

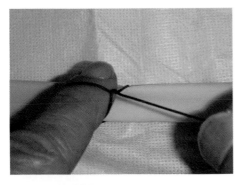

Figure 5-13D

Pull loop through.

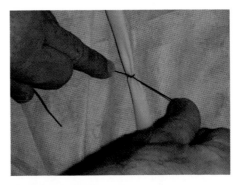

Figure 5-13E

Use the left index or middle finger to push the knot down flat and securely.

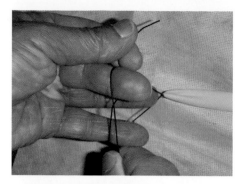

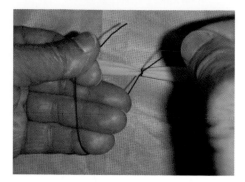

Figure 5-13F

Grasp the strand in the left hand, turn hand toward yourself to loop strand around the three fingers of the left hand. Hold the end of the strand between the left thumb and index finger while holding the other end between right thumb and index finger.

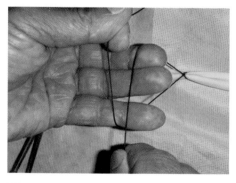

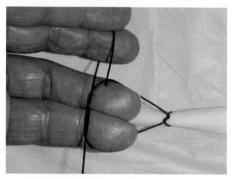

Figure 5-13G

Take the strand in the right hand and loop it around the same three fingers, starting from the middle finger ending over the small finger of the right hand.

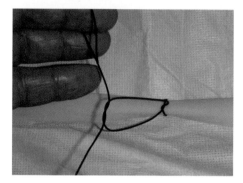

Figure 5-13H

Top to bottom: Flex the left middle finger slightly toward the palm. Bring the middle finger with the strand beneath and over the strand in the left fingers. Extend the left middle finger and pull the strand held by the left thumb and index finger, completing the knot.

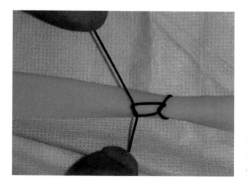

Figure 5-13I

Using the right index finger, push the knot down flat and securely to complete the square knot.

Figure 5-14

Two-handed tie. Step-by-step instructions for one method of completing the two-handed tie with a square knot.

Source: Photos courtesy of Winchester Hospital, Winchester, MA.

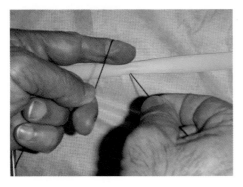

Figure 5-14A

Place the strand of ligature material over extended left index finger, holding the end of that strand in palm of left hand. Hold other end of strand with right thumb and index finger.

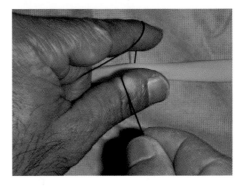

Figure 5-14B

Place the shorter strand (held between right thumb and index finger) over the inner portion of left thumb.

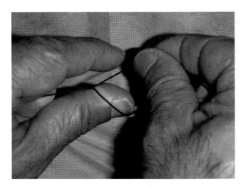

Figure 5-14C

Take the short strand (held between right thumb and index finger) and cross it over the other (longer) strand. Grasp crossed strand with left thumb and index finger.

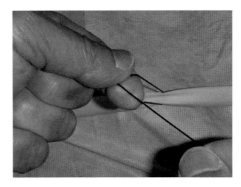

Figure 5-14D

Rotate the left index finger, switching knot through loop from left thumb to left index finger. Grasp end of strand with right thumb and index finger to pull through loop.

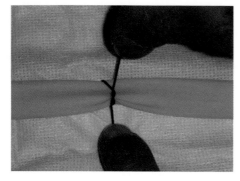

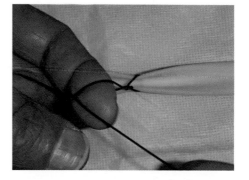

Figure 5-14E

Release knot and use left index finger to push knot flat and securely down. Secure the shorter end with the right thumb and index finger. Pull strands in separate directions, applying even tension.

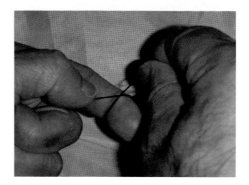

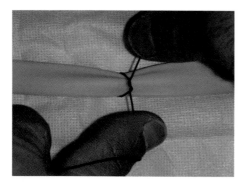

Figure 5-14H

Top to bottom: Rotate the left thumb and index finger so the strand sits on left index finger. Then, bring short strand in the right thumb and index finger towards the end of the left thumb and index finger.

Figure 5-14F

Place the thumb under and over the strand held by left hand. Note that strand is over outer portion of the left thumb.

Figure 5-14G

Use the right index finger and thumb to pull the short strand over the left thumb.

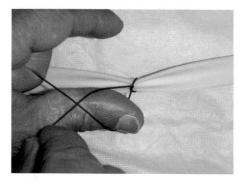

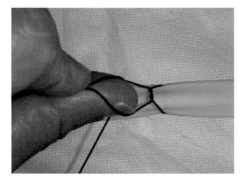

Figure 5-14I

Grasp the short strand in the left thumb and index finger (the longer strand remains on the left palm, not pictured). Then, rotate the left thumb so the knot is on top of the left thumb. Now, grasp the end of the short strand in the loop with the right thumb and index finger.

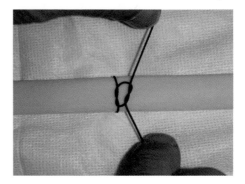

Figure 5-14J

Pull the strands in separate directions, applying equal tension. Use the right index finger to push knot down squarely to complete the square knot.

Figure 5-15

Step-by-step instructions for one method of completing an instrument tie.

Source: Photos courtesy of Winchester Hospital, Winchester, MA.

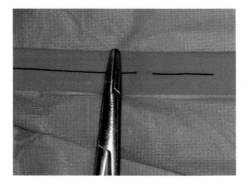

Figure 5-15A

Instrument tie #1: After the suture is placed through the tissue (represented here by rubber tubing), pull the suture and leave a short end. Place the needleholder against the suture.

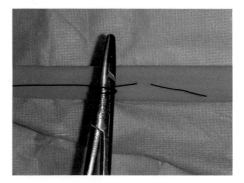

Figure 5-15B

Instrument tie #2: Wrap the suture around the needleholder (once or twice).

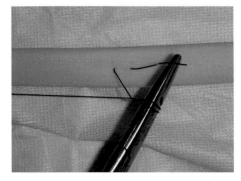

Figure 5-15C

Instrument tie #3: Grasp the short end of the suture with the needleholder and pull it through the suture wrapped around the needleholder.

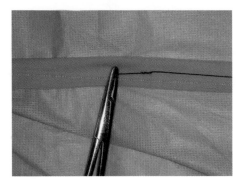

Figure 5-15D

Instrument tie #4: Secure the knot.

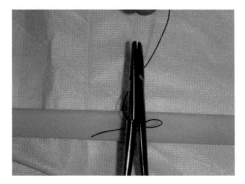

Figure 5-15E

Instrument tie #5: Wrap the suture over the needleholder in the direction opposite that of the initial loop.

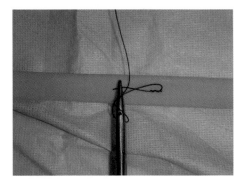

Figure 5-15F

Instrument tie #6: Grasp the short end of the suture with the needleholder and pull it through the suture wrapped around the needleholder.

Figure 5-15G

Instrument tie #7: Secure the second half of the knot.

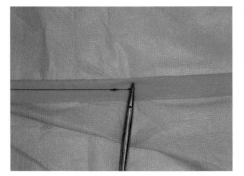

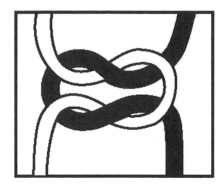

Figure 5-16

Square knot.

Source: Adapted from *Knot Tying Manual.* (1983). Somerville, N.J.: ETHICON, Inc., a Johnson and Johnson Company. In J.C. Rothrock (Ed.), (1999). *The RN First Assistant: An expanded perioperative nursing role* (3rd ed., Fig. 13-16, p. 313). Philadelphia: Lipincott.

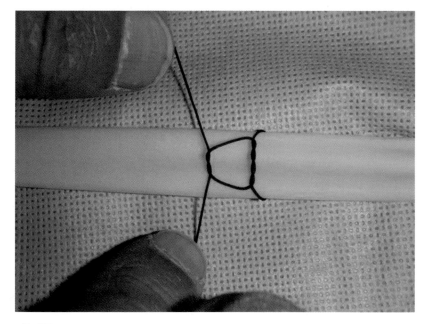

Figure 5-17

The surgeon's knot.

Source: Photo courtesy of Winchester Hospital, Winchester, MA.

A ligature may also be deployed as a suture ligature (or "stick tie") attached to a needle. This is performed with the ligature on a needle holder and passed through the vascular structure or tissue that has been clamped. The suture is then passed around the clamp, and the knot is tied and cinched down while the clamp is slowly released. This prevents the vessel from retracting before the tie is completed. Forceps are required when placing suture ligatures. When not in active use, the forceps may be palmed and supported by extending the ring and little finger (**Figure 5-18**). The unflexed middle finger remains free for use. Palming, while alternately grasping with forceps when placing suture ligatures, can save time.

Regardless of the technique used, some basic principles guide knot tying. The free end of the suture must be of sufficient length to allow easy grasping; excessive length, however, is clumsy and interfering. The amount of tension exerted on the suture while the knot is being secured depends on the suture type and size. The knot should be tied tightly enough that it holds securely without cutting through the tissue or breaking the suture. The knot is usually secured with three throws if the vessels are small or the tissues are not under tension. Four throws are advised for larger vessels or tissues under tension. Monofilament (e.g., nylon) or coated sutures may require five or more throws for security.

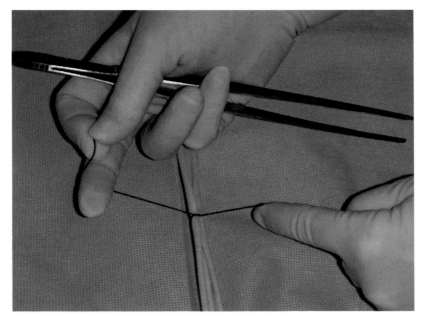

Figure 5-18

When not in active use while performing a suture ligature, the forceps may be palmed and supported by extending the ring and little finger, as shown here. The unflexed middle finger is then available for use in tying the knot. Palming while alternately grasping with forceps when placing suture ligatures can save time.

Source: Photo courtesy of Winchester Hospital, Winchester, MA.

THERMAL HEMOSTASIS

Heat generated from electrical current, lasers and ultrasonic devices are thermal means to control bleeding. When any "energy-based" hemostatic adjunct is used, appropriate safety precautions must be initiated by the FA and the other members of the surgical team.

Electrosurgery Unit (ESU)

The electrosurgical unit (ESU) has been the device of choice for dissection and hemostasis since the 1920s. However, today's ESUs are solid state, isolated units that do not recognize alternate grounds and function with return electrode monitoring (REM). These features make modern ESUs much safer than their predecessors. "Electrocautery" and "electrosurgery," are not the same, although the terms are used synonymously. The ESU uses alternating current to produce different types of current, or waveforms, often referred to as the "mode." The coagulation mode produces an interrupted waveform that produces spikes that create heat, thereby coagulating the cell. This is sometimes referred to as "fulguration" (Figure 5-19). The ESU's cutting mode is a continuous current at lower energy, which produces a cutting effect to vaporize tissue with little or no hemostasis. Use of the blend mode simultaneously cuts tissue and coagulates bleeding (Figure 5-20). Desiccation is

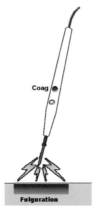

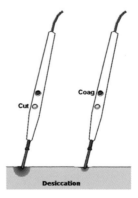

Figure 5-19

Fulgeration of tissue using the coagulation waveform.

Source: Courtesy of Phippen, M.L., Ulmer, B.C., & Wells, M.P. (2009). *Competency for safe patient care during operative and invasive procedures* (Fig. 17.4, p. 514). Denver: CCI.

Figure 5-20

Desiccation of tissue using the cut and coagulation waveforms.

Source: Courtesy of Phippen, M.L., Ulmer, B.C., & Wells, M.P. (2009). *Competency for safe patient care during operative and invasive procedures* (Fig. 17.7, p. 515). Denver: CCI.

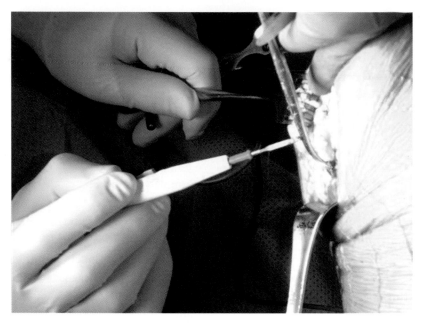

Figure 5-21

When current is applied to a surgical instrument such as a forceps or hemostat, it is sometimes referred to as "buzzing the hemostat." The vessel is grasped with the instrument and the activated electrode touched to the instrument for only as long as it takes to blanch the tissue.

Source: Photo courtesy of Winchester Hospital, Winchester, MA.

produced by all three modes and is accomplished through direct contact of the electrode tip. The pencil handpiece can deliver current directly to the tissue or to an instrument (sometimes referred to as "buzzing the instrument") (Figure 5-21). The energy is delivered through the pencil and returned to the unit through a special dispersive pad that is placed on the patient over a large muscle mass (Figure 5-22).

Electrosurgical principles

By understanding the basics of electricity and electrosurgery, clinical applications, and available technologies, the FA can collaborate in preventing patient injury and maximizing the capabilities of the ESU.

Basics of Electricity Electricity arises from the existence of positively and negatively charged particles. As particles move, like charges repel each other and unlike charges attract each other. *Electricity* is the movement of electrons. Two

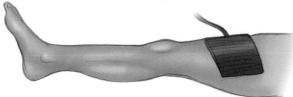

Figure 5-22

The ESU dispersive pad (also called the "patient return electrode" and "grounding pad") is placed after the patient is positioned on the OR bed. It is placed on a clean, dry skin surface over a well-vascularized, large muscle mass. Placement as shown in this example avoids risk areas such as bony prominences, pressure points, metal prostheses, and adipose tissue.

Source: Courtesy of Phippen, M.L., Ulmer, B.C., & Wells, M.P. (2009). *Competency for safe patient care during operative and invasive procedures* (Fig. 11.10, p. 311). Denver: CCI.

properties of electricity affect patient care in surgical and other invasive procedures. As electricity moves at nearly the speed of light, it always follows the path of least resistance and always seeks to return to ground. Electron movement through a conductor to ground is known as the *electrical circuit.* The variables associated with the electrical circuit must be considered when using electricity for patient care. Two types of current are used in the operating room, *direct current* (DC) and *alternating current* (AC). Direct current follows a simple circuit as the electricity flows in one direction. For example, batteries contain a simple circuit. Energy flows from one terminal on the battery and must return to the other terminal to complete the circuit.

Alternating currents switch, or alternate, direction of electron flow. The frequency of these alterations is measured in cycles per second, or Hertz (Hz), with 1 Hz being equal to 1 cycle per second. Household current alternates at 60 cycles per second, as does much of the equipment in the operating room. Alternating current at 60 Hz can cause tissue reaction and damage. Neuromuscular stimulation ceases at about 100,000 Hz, as the alternating currents move into the radiofrequency (RF) range. Electron flow is measured in *amperes,* or amps.

Resistance (or impedance) is the opposition to the flow of current; it is measured in ohms. In the OR, one source of resistance or impedance is the patient. A push is needed to overcome this resistance, and that push is *voltage.* Voltage is the force that will cause 1 amp to flow through 1 ohm of resistance. It is measured in volts and provides the electromotive force that pushes electrons through the circuit in an ESU generator. *Power,* measured in watts, is the energy that is produced. The power setting used by the FA or surgeon is either printed on an LED screen in watts, or a percentage of the wattage is demonstrated on a numerical dial setting.

Modes of Electrosurgical Current   There are different modes (cut, fulgeration, and desiccation) of producing electrosurgical current from generators, and each has a distinct effect on tissues. The cutting current from an electrosurgical generator is a continuous waveform. Since the delivery of current is continuous, much lower voltages are required to achieve the desired effect, which is tissue vaporization. To achieve the cutting effect, the FA should hold the active electrode (ESU pencil tip) just above the target tissue to let the spark divide tissue by vaporization, creating a clean tissue cut.

Tissue *fulgeration* is achieved using the *coagulation mode* on the ESU generator. The coagulation mode produces an interrupted or dampened waveform with a duty cycle that is activated approximately 5% to 6% of the time, producing spikes of current. The tissue is heated as the wave spikes and cools down during the off cycle, thereby coagulating the cell. To achieve tissue fulgeration when using the coagulation mode, the FA should hold the active electrode (ESU pencil tip) slightly above the target tissue. Like electrosurgical cutting, electrocoagulation is a non-contact use of the active electrode (ESU pencil tip).

The *blended mode* on an ESU generator is a function of cut. Blended currents produce voltage higher than that of the pure cut mode. The current is modified to a dampened waveform that produces some hemostasis during cutting. Several blend settings provide different ratios of coagulation with the cutting current. Because these vary among manufacturers, the FA must be familiar with the specific manufacturer's information regarding cut and coagulation ratios when using the blended mode.

Tissue Sensing Energy ESU Generators

Referred to as "hemostasis with division," these generators provide a high level of coagulation and are capable of dissecting a larger array of tissue types. They must be used with a specific ESU device (active electrode) (Figure 5-23). Hoogerwerf (2009) notes the following benefits when using tissue sensing energy ESU generators:

- Tissue division is more efficient while maintaining hemostasis.
- Thermal injury to surrounding tissue is minimized.
- ESU current is precisely controlled.
- ESU energy is precisely dosed according to tissue needs.

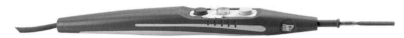

Figure 5-23

The Force TriVerse™ Electrosurgical Device used for hemostasis with division. The device has three buttons: cut and blend (yellow), dissection with hemostasis (clear), and blue (coagulation).

Source: Courtesy of Phippen, M.L., Ulmer, B.C., & Wells, M.P. (2009). *Competency for safe patient care during operative and invasive procedures* (Fig. 17.6, p. 515). Denver: CCI.

Other Variables Influencing Tissue Effect

There are also additional variables that can alter the outcome of electrosurgical tissue effect:

- Time—the length of time the active electrode is on determines the extent of tissue effect. Activating the electrode too long produces wider and deeper tissue damage. However, an activation that is too short will not produce the desired tissue effect.
- Power—the power setting alters the tissue effect. The FA should always use the lowest setting that is capable of achieving the desired tissue effect.
- Electrode—the size of the active electrode (pencil tip) influences the tissue effect. A large electrode requires a higher power setting than a smaller one. The FA should also remember that a clean electrode will conduct current more effectively than a dirty one; using a clean electrode requires lower power settings.
- Tissue—patient tissue can determine the effectiveness of the generator. A lean, muscular patient will conduct the electrical current better than an obese or emaciated patient. The physical condition of the patient determines the amount of impedance encountered as the current attempts to return to the generator to complete the circuit.

Safety Considerations When Using the ESU

It is not uncommon for FAs or surgeons to report receiving a shock during ESU use. Holes in gloves have been implicated as the cause; holes may be present as a manufacturing defect or may occur during the surgical procedure. To avoid being shocked by the ESU (Table 5-1), the FA should not lean on the patient because this includes the FA in the electrosurgical circuit. When preparing to "buzz" a hemostat that is attached to target tissue, hold it with a full grip; this disperses the current over a wider surface area. Touch the clamp before activating the ESU pencil. Open-circuit activation of the ESU pencil causes the current to jump the air gap to reach conductive

TABLE 5-1   Techniques for Avoiding Hemostat Burns

- Know and follow the manufacturer's recommendations.
- Use the lowest power setting possible.
- Use cut mode (low voltage).
- Avoid touching the patient.
- Hold the hemostat (or other instrument, like forceps) with a full grip.
- Touch the active electrode tip to the instrument before activating the electrode.
- Activate the electrode by depressing, then releasing, the appropriate switches on the handpiece (**Figure 5-24**).
- Remember that surgical gloves do not insulate against radio-frequency current.

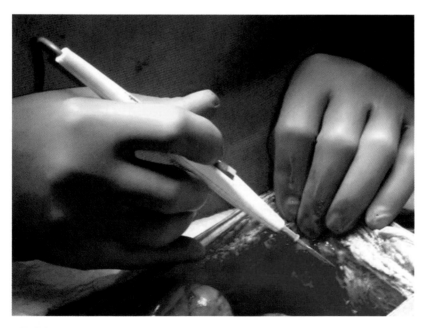

Figure 5-24

When using the ESU, touch the tissue with the activated electrode for as long as it takes to blanch the tissue. The electrode is activated by depressing and then releasing the appropriate switch.

Source: Photo courtesy of Winchester Hospital, Winchester, MA.

metal. Current demodulation can then occur and shock the person holding the clamp and blow a hole in the glove. The cut waveform should be used because the voltage is much lower. Use brief, intermittent activations and avoid overheating the target tissue. As tissue becomes charred, the ESU current may seek a more conductive path back to the dispersive pad. That path can be the clamp and the hand of the FA (or other operator), creating a shock and subsequent hole in the glove. When not in use, place the active electrode in a safety holster—do not leave it lying on the surgical field. When using the ESU, the FA must rigorously adhere to fire-prevention safety measures (Box 5-6) and recommendations for surgical smoke evacuation.

Box 5-6	Safety Measures When Using the Electrosurgery Unit (ESU)

- Participate in any communication that takes place regarding the safe use of heat sources (this may be part of a preop briefing, part of a fire risk assessment, or part of the time-out).
- Verify that skin prep solutions have dried and vapors have dissipated before applying the surgical drapes and activating the ESU.
- Use a water-based jelly to coat the patient's body hair that is close to an active electrode.
- In an oxygen-enriched atmosphere, arrange the surgical drapes so that anesthetic gases flow to the floor. Consider creating a seal between drapes and skin edges with an incise drape to decrease venting to the surgical site. Communicate with the anesthesia provider prior to activating the ESU.
- Inspect the active electrode at the surgical field before use. Of particular importance is impaired insulation; this may allow an alternate current path and result in electrical shock.
- Holster the active electrode to prevent accidental activation.
- Do not allow another person to activate the active electrode; only the person using it should activate it.
- Ensure that the circulating nurse confirms the power settings with you before activation of the ESU.
- Activate the active electrode only under direct vision, when it is in contact or ready to be used with the tissue or appropriate instrument.
- Use settings consistent with the intended application and the manufacturer's written instructions for patient size and active electrode type. Use cut or blend mode whenever possible.
- Keep the ESU active electrode clean of char build-up, which can impede the current flow and serve as a fuel source in a fire. Visually inspect the tip for damage caused by repeated cleaning with an abrasive pad. Preferred methods of cleaning the ESU tip include moistened sponges or instrument wipes for nonstick coated tips, or abrasive electrode cleaning pads for noncoated electrodes.
- At the end of the procedure, do not disconnect the cord of the active electrode while the ESU is still on. Cord should be disconnected and disposed of as a single unit with other hazardous waste.
- Know fire suppression strategies, fire containment techniques, and the evacuation plan for the OR. Be prepared to assist the surgical team in patting out or smothering small fires, or removing burning material from patient (rip burning material off patient).

(continued)

Box 5-6	Safety Measures When Using the Electrosurgery Unit (ESU) *(Continued)*

- If possible, prepare the patient by controlling the bleeding and covering the surgical site with sterile drapes before moving the patient in a fire evacuation.

Sources: AORN. (2009). *AORN guidance statement: Fire prevention in the operating room* (pp. 187–201). Denver, CO: AORN; Everson, C.R. (2008). Fire prevention in the perioperative setting: Perioperative fires can occur anywhere. *Perioperative Nursing Clinics, 3*(4), 333–343; Guidance article: Surgical fires: A patient safety perspective. (2006). *Health Devices, 35*(2), 45–48; James, E. (2008). Breaking the fire triangle. *Advance for Nurses, 10*(2), 27–28; Williams, S. (2008). Fire in the OR! *Nursing Spectrum, 17*(2), 22–25.

Surgical Smoke

Exposure to surgical smoke (also referred to as "plume") presents health concerns for patients and members of the surgical team. Surgical smoke and bio-aerosols are produced by surgical devices such as lasers, ESUs, radiofrequency devices, ultrasonic devices, and power tools. Measures to reduce exposure to surgical smoke are presented in **Box 5-7**. Smoke evacuation systems are designed to filter airborne

Box 5-7	Measures to Reduce Exposure to Surgical Smoke

- Air exchanges in operating rooms/procedure rooms should be at least 15 exchanges per hour.
- Rooms in which procedures are performed should be maintained at positive pressure; keeping the door to the room closed assists with maintaining positive pressure.
- Filters in general ventilation systems should be changed according to manufacturer's recommendations.
- High-filtration surgical masks should fit snugly around all facial contours and should be changed after each surgical procedure (or if they become wet).
- In procedures that generate a small amount of surgical smoke, the wall suction unit with an in-line filter can be used.
- Portable or central smoke evacuation systems are more effective for surgical smoke.
- Laparoscopic evacuation/filtration systems should be used in those surgical procedures.
- The capture device (e.g., suction wand, ESU active electrode with smoke evacuation attachment) should be held within 2 cm of the point of smoke origin.
- Single-use supplies such as electrosurgery handpiece, suction tubing, prefilter (if used), and high efficiency filters should be disposed of appropriately as contaminated waste.

Sources: Modified from AORN. (2008). *AORN Position statement on surgical smoke and bio-aerosols.* Anaheim, CA: AORN; AORN (2009). Recommended practices for safe environment of care. *Perioperative standards and recommended practices* (pp. 415–437). Denver, CO: AORN; CCI. Sample policy: Smoke evacuation in the OR. *CCI electrosurgery competency module* (p. 30); Ulmer, B.C. (2008). The hazards of surgical smoke. *AORN Journal, 87*(4), 721–734.

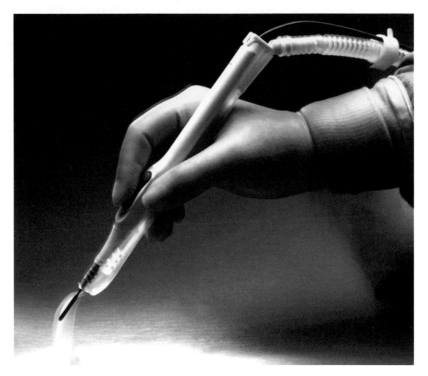

Figure 5-25

Surgical smoke plume and aerosol evacuators capture plume at the point of creation and isolate the biological particulate and harmful gaseous by-products that exist within the plume. Smoke evacuation systems must be rated to capture virus and bacteria, as well as the gaseous by-products, to ensure staff safety.

Source: Courtesy of Buffalo Filter. Reprinted by permission.

contaminants from the surgical site and the operating room itself. These systems have filters which trap very small particulates (as small as 0.12 microns). While the main purpose of surgical smoke evacuation systems is reducing a potential health hazard, they also help clear the surgical site of the smoke so the view of the surgical field is not impaired (**Figure 5-25**).

SAFE USE OF ELECTROSURGERY DURING ENDOSCOPIC PROCEDURES

The primary hazards associated with endoscopic electrosurgery are direct coupling, insulation failure, and capacitative coupling, which may result in injury outside the field of vision of the surgical team. *Direct coupling* can occur when the active electrode is activated close to another object inside the abdomen. Care must be taken to prevent activation of the active electrode when it is in contact with, or close to, other instruments in the operative area. Using lower power settings minimizes damage from direct coupling when the active electrode is activated while near another metal device inserted into an adjacent trocar port (AORN, Recommended Practice for Electrosurgery, 2009). Instrumentation in adjacent ports is often unavoidable, and the FA works assiduously to avoid instrument collisions as well as direct coupling.

Insulation failure occurs when the material used to coat the active electrode is compromised in some way. This can result from rough handling, repeated uses, or high voltages used during electrosurgery. Current can escape from the active electrode at any break in the insulation. Methods used to detect insulation failure include active electrode shielding and monitoring (continuously monitor endoscopic instruments to minimize the risks of insulation failure or capacitive coupling), active electrode indicator shafts that have two layers of insulation each a different color (a different color in the inner layer shows through the outer black layer if there is an insulation break), and active electrode insulation integrity testers that use high DC voltage to detect full thickness insulation breaks (AORN, Recommended Practice for Electrosurgery, 2009). In the last method, the electrode is either tested before the procedure or tested during the procedure with the sterilizable probes.

Keep in mind that using the coagulation mode instead of the cut mode results in the use of higher voltages, which is undesirable. Consider checking with the manufacturer of active electrodes purchased by the surgery department to verify that they meet the standards for electrosurgical devices set by the Association for the Advancement of Medical Instrumentation (AAMI) or the American National Standards Institute (ANSI).

Capacitative coupling may be the least understood of the hazards that can occur endoscopically. A capacitor consists of two conductors separated by an insulator. Inserting an active electrode down a metal cannula creates a capacitator. Capacitatively coupled electrical current can be transferred from the active electrode, through intact insulation and into the conductive metal cannula. If the cannula then comes into contact with body structures, the energy can be discharged, damaging those structures. A metal cannula provides a pathway for any energy stored in the cannula to disperse along the patient's conductive abdominal wall. For this reason, it is unwise to use plastic anchors to secure the cannula; this isolates the current from the abdominal wall. Some institutions use plastic trocar cannula systems, believing them to be safer. However, the plastic systems can be just as hazardous because the patient's own conductive tissue in the abdomen can form the second conductor, creating a capacitator. Omentum or bowel draped over the

TABLE 5-2   Techniques for Preventing Accidental Patient Injury During Endoscopic Electrosurgery

- Always use the lowest possible power setting.
- Use the lower voltage cut waveform.
- Inspect insulation on the active electrode carefully.
- Activate the electrode only when near or in contact with target tissue; do not activate electrode if it is in contact with other metal objects in the abdomen.
- Activate the electrode only when in your field of vision.
- Use all-metal or all-plastic trocar systems; do not combine metal and plastic cannula systems (hybrid systems).

plastic cannula could discharge stored energy to adjacent body structures. Activating the electrode when it is not in close proximity to target tissue increases the risk of capacitive coupling. Methods the FA should use to prevent accidental injury during endoscopic electrosurgery are presented in Table 5-2.

Bipolar Electrosurgery

Bipolar electrical energy delivers lower peak voltages and high current concentrations. Like monopolar electrosurgery, heat is produced in the tissue as current flows through it. The circuit of current is completed through parallel electrodes in the tips of the hand piece as the electricity flows back and forth between the tines of the instrument (Figure 5-26). Because the current is so carefully controlled, it is often used in close proximity to nerve structures or in the case of an implanted electrical device, like a pacemaker. A return pad is not necessary with this type of energy delivery. Newer bipolar instruments have a mechanical cutting mechanism that enables both cutting and coagulation, which older instruments did not have. Newer generators can sense tissue impedance and decrease the current in response to increased impedance. Some models of bipolar generators will interrupt energy delivery at certain levels of impedance.

Electrocautery Unit (ECU)

An electrocautery device uses a closed circuit with direct current. A battery-powered cautery pencil is the most common form of this device. In this application, the current travels from the electrode of the battery to a wire filament (similar to a light bulb), which is heated. The current then returns to the other electrode of the battery. The heated cautery tip is used in direct contact with tissue. This type of cautery does not perform well as a dissection tool or for vessels of any significant

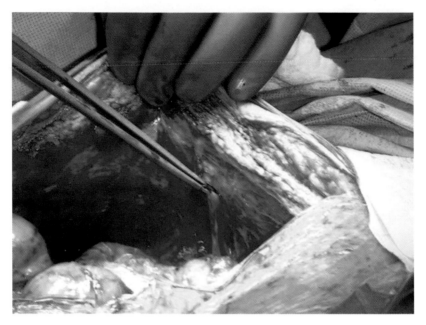

Figure 5-26

With bipolar electrical energy, the circuit of current is completed through parallel electrodes in the tips of the hand piece; the electricity flows back and forth between the tines of the instrument.

Source: Photo courtesy of Winchester Hospital, Winchester, MA.

size. The small, hand-held eye cautery is an example of this device. The battery heats a wire loop at the end of the cautery pencil; the current never leaves the device to travel through patient tissue. Thus, a patient return electrode (dispersive pad) is not required. In ophthalmic surgery and other minor procedures where minimal bleeding is encountered, an electrocautery pencil is useful. Limitations include the inability to cut tissue or coagulate large bleeders, and the tendency of target tissue to stick to the electrode.

Ultrasonic Cutting and Coagulation Surgical Device

The ultrasonic cutting and coagulation surgical device is an ultrasonic instrument that oscillates longitudinally at the point of contact. It can seal vessels up to a diameter of 5 mm. Because there is no dispersed current, the device affects only the tissue with which it is in contact, thus causing minimal thermal injury to surrounding tissues. There is no need for a dispersive pad when using the ultrasonic cutting and coagulation surgical device. Applications of the ultrasonic cutting and coagulation surgical device include sharp or blunt dissection, coagulation, or separating tissue. Some ultrasonic dissectors incorporate an aspirator to remove tissue or fluids from the surgical field. Smoke evacuation systems are required with the use of this device.

Argon-Enhanced Coagulation (AEC)

Argon-enhanced coagulation (AEC), or argon-enhanced electrosurgery, is another form of thermal hemostasis. Argon coagulation delivers current to the tissue in a directed beam of ionized argon gas. The flow of gas blows away blood and debris from the surgical field and produces a coagulated surface that is more uniform and superficial than that produced in standard electrosurgical coagulation. As a result, the FA may find that he or she is able to coagulate bleeding tissue faster, with reduced blood loss and tissue damage. Argon coagulation has also been found to produce less smoke than conventional electrosurgery (Figure 5-27). However, the same safety measures implemented with monopolar ESUs must be implemented with AEC. Additional precautions include purging air from the argon gas line and electrode by activating the system before use, after moderate delays between activations, and between uses; limiting argon gas flow to the lowest level that still provides

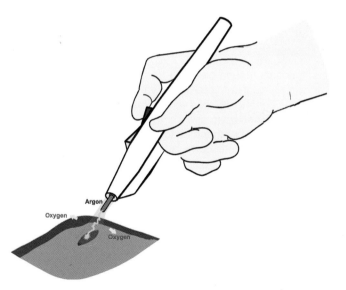

Figure 5-27

Argon-enhanced electrosurgery uses a stream of argon gas to conduct electrosurgical current. The inert and noncombustible argon gas is heaver than air, displacing oxygen and nitrogen. The ESU's current ionizes the argon gas, producing less tissue damage and a more flexible eschar.

Source: Courtesy of Phippen, M.L., Ulmer, B.C., & Wells, M.P. (2009). *Competency for safe patient care during operative and invasive procedures* (Fig. 17.10, p. 519). Denver: CCI.

the desired clinical effects; refraining from placing the active electrode in direct contact with tissue; and moving the active electrode away from the patient's tissue after each activation (AORN, Recommended Practice for Electrosurgery, 2009).

CHEMICAL HEMOSTASIS

Chemical hemostatic agents are employed when standard surgical techniques to stop blood loss are ineffective or impractical. For example, if pressure, electro-coagulation, or a suture can safely resolve bleeding, then one of these should be considered as the first choice to achieve hemostasis. If a topical agent is selected as a hemostatic adjunct, safe medication practices should be followed (Wanzer et al., 2008). The FA should verbally confirm and acknowledge the scrub person's announcement of the topical agent being provided for use. The syringe or container (if applicable) for hemostatic agent preparation must be labeled.

Topical agents are generally implied when chemical hemostatic agents are considered. These agents are readily available, well accepted, and are available in a variety of forms (Box 5-8).

Box 5-8	Topical Hemostatic Agents

Topical hemostatic agents reduce bleeding from small vessels by accelerating natural blood clotting or by forming an artificial clot. A variety of agents are available to facilitate hemostasis, and some commonly used topical hemostatic agents are presented here. When using absorbable hemostatic agents, the FA should review the agent's labeling, paying particular attention to contraindications, warnings, and precautions. In general, when these agents are used near bony or neural spaces, only the minimum amount required to achieve hemostasis should be used, and as much as possible should be removed thereafter. This will reduce the possibility of neural and other soft tissue damage from agent swelling and/or migration.

Absorbable Collagen

(Collastat®, Helistat®, Lyostypt®)

Indications:
Use as adjunct to hemostasis when control of bleeding by ligature or conventional procedures is ineffective or impractical. Collagen activates the coagulation mechanism, particularly the aggregation of platelets, thus accelerating the formation of a clot. Available in sponges or felt.

Administration Guidelines:
1. Use dry.
2. Apply directly to the bleeding surface as supplied from the sterile package with dry gloves or instruments.

3. Use only amount needed.
4. Material should not be used in skin incision closures because it will create a mechanical barrier to healing.
5. Material may reduce bond strength of methyl methacrylate adhesives.

Contraindications:
- Patients with known sensitivity to materials of bovine origin.
- Infected or contaminated areas; areas where blood or other body fluids have pooled.

Side Effects/Adverse Reactions:
Adhesion formation, allergic reaction, foreign body reaction, and hematoma.

Absorbable Gelatin

(Gelfoam®)

Indications:
Use as adjunct to hemostasis when control of bleeding by ligature or conventional procedures is ineffective or impractical. Available in powder or compressed (gelatin sponge) forms. When placed on areas of capillary bleeding, it deposits fibrin in the interstices, and then the sponge swells, forming a considerable clot. The compressed sponge is not soluble.

Administration Guidelines:
1. If material is used dry, the scrub person will provide an appropriate-sized piece. Compress with fingers. Then apply to bleeding site and gently compress with dry laparotomy pad for 10 to 15 seconds.
2. If used wet, the sponge is dipped in warm saline and then squeezed or pressed against the side of a basin by the scrub person to remove the air. The sponge may be blotted to remove dampness. Apply to bleeding site and gently compress with dry laparotomy pad or a moist cottonoid sponge for 10 to 15 seconds. Suction may be directly used on gelatin sponge to draw in blood and hasten clotting.
3. The sponge is often soaked in a thrombin or epinephrine solution. In this case, the same procedure is used, but the sponge is then placed back into the solution and allowed to absorb solution back to its original size. Use safe medication practices to verify solution (announcements, label checks).
4. The gelatin in powder form is mixed with sterile saline to make a paste for application to cancellous bone or denuded areas of skin or muscle.
5. Gelatin sponges may be left in place. They do not need to be removed prior to wound closure, but they are commonly removed to prevent compression of adjacent structures.

Contraindications:
- Patients with known sensitivity to materials of porcine origin.
- Should not be used for closure of skin incisions, as it may interfere with healing of the skin edges; should not be placed in intravascular compartments, because of the risk of embolization.

(continued)

Box 5-8	Topical Hemostatic Agents (*Continued*)

Side Effects/Adverse Reactions:
Local infection, abscess formation, foreign body reactions, encapsulation of fluid, and hematoma.

Gelatin Matrix

(FloSeal® [Baxter]; Surgiflo® [Ethicon])

Indications:
Use as adjunct to hemostasis when control of bleeding by ligature or conventional procedures is ineffective or impractical.
    FloSeal: Available as gelatin matrix granules and topical thrombin, packaged as a kit with syringes and mixing bowl.

Administration Guidelines:
1. Matrix particles form a composite clot that seals the bleeding site; thrombin component converts the fibrinogen in the patient's blood to fibrin.
2. Product achieves maximum expansion after approximately 10 minutes.
3. Excess product should be removed with gentle irrigation.
4. Do not inject or compress gelatin matrix into blood vessels or tissue.
5. Do not apply in the absence of active blood flow, (i.e., to clamped or bypassed vessels); extensive intravascular clotting and even death may result.
6. Do not use in the closure of skin incisions because mechanical interposition of gelatin may interfere with the healing of the skin edges.

Surgiflo:

1. Prefilled syringe is mixed with 3 to 5 ml of sterile saline or thrombin solution.
2. Mixing is done with five to six syringe-to-syringe transfers. Results in 9 to 11 ml of hemostatic matrix. Tip of choice is applied (or endoscopic applicator may be used), and matrix is expressed on surgical site.
3. Care should be exercised to avoid overpacking the site.
4. Matrix may swell; therefore, it should be removed from confined spaces (e.g., optic chiasm, foramina in bone, spinal cord).

Contraindications:
Patients with known allergies to materials of bovine origin.

Side Effects/Adverse Reactions:
Anemia, atrial fibrillation, infection, hemorrhage, pneumonia, urinary tract infection, rash, edema, hypotension, respiratory distress, confusion, dural tear, ventricular fibrillation, arrhythmia, right heart failure, arterial thrombosis, fever, atelectasis, and pleural effusion.

Microfibrillar Collagen

(Avitene®, Instat®)

Indications:
Use as adjunct to hemostasis when control of bleeding by ligature or conventional procedures is ineffective or impractical. Available in compacted nonwoven web or loose fibrous forms. Tissue cohesion is an inherent property of the collagen itself. It functions as a hemostatic agent only when applied directly to the bleeding source or directly to active bleeding. When in contact with bleeding surfaces, it attracts platelets that aggregate into thrombi, thus initiating the formation of a physiologic plug.

Administration Guidelines:
1. Apply dry pieces of cut collagen sponge to bleeding site. Dry, clean forceps may be used for application.
2. Compress for 2 to 5 minutes.
3. Effective application is demonstrated by a firm, adherent coagulum with no breakthrough bleeding from the surface or edges.
4. Excess material should be removed from application site before wound closure.

Contraindications:
Should not be used in the closure of skin incisions as it may interfere with the healing of the skin edges; should not be used on bone surfaces to which prosthetic materials are to be attached with methyl methacrylate adhesives, as it may significantly reduce the bond strength of methyl methacrylate adhesives by filling porosities of cancellous bone. Due to fluid absorption and expansion of sponge, not recommended for use where it may exert pressure on adjacent structures.

Cannot use blood scavenging system after use of microfibrillar collagen. FA must communicate use to circulating nurse.

Side Effects/Adverse Reactions:
Adhesion formation, allergic reaction, foreign-body reaction, inflammation, and potentiation of infection.

Oxidized Regenerated Cellulose

(Surgicel®, Surgicel Nu-Knit®)

Indications:
Use as adjunct to hemostasis. Available in a pad of oxidized regenerated cellulose in a knitted fabric strip that is either high-density (Surgicel) or low-density (Surgicel Nu-Knit). Clot forms on contact with blood; as it reacts with blood, it increases in size and forms a gel. Absorbs 7 to 10 times its own weight.

Administration Guidelines:
1. Blot area dry with laparotomy sponge or other surgical sponge. Area may also be suctioned dry prior to application.
2. Apply dry (effect is diminished when moistened) with clean forceps, using only the amount of material required.

(continued)

Box 5-8	**Topical Hemostatic Agents** (*Continued*)

3. May be sutured to, wrapped around, or held firmly against a bleeding site, or laid dry on an oozing surface until hemostasis is achieved. Then, remove from the application site when possible.

4. May be removed before wound closure or left in place if applied in small amounts. Must be removed if used around optic cord or spinal cord due to potential harm from product swelling.

Contraindications:
• Not recommended for use on bone defects (unless it is removed after hemostasis), because it may interfere with bone regeneration.
• Should not be used to control hemorrhage from large arteries; should not be used on nonhemorrhagic serous oozing surfaces because body fluids other than whole blood (e.g., serum) do not react well with oxidized regenerated cellulose; should not be used for adhesion prevention.

Side Effects/Adverse Reactions:
Encapsulation of fluid and foreign-body reaction.

Topical Thrombin

Indications:
Use as adjunct to hemostasis; works directly at the end of the blood coagulation cascade. Accelerates coagulation of blood, rapidly binding with fibrin to form a clot. For topical use only; may be used topically as a dry powder; as a solution that gelatin sponges are dipped in; mixed with a gelatin matrix; or as a spray. Should be used within 3 hours of reconstitution. If supplied as frozen solution, must thaw prior to application.

Dosing:
Available in:
5,000 I.U. per vial with 5 mL diluent
20,000 I.U. per vial with 20 mL diluent
20,000 I.U. per vial with 20 mL diluent, spray pump, and actuator
20,000 I.U. per vial with 20 mL diluent, spray tip, and syringe

Administration Guidelines:
1. Implement safe medication practices. Verify that correct concentration has been prepared verbally with scrub person and by reading solution label.

2. Flood the surface when spraying. Do not suction or sponge area overly dry; thrombin is most effective when it mixes with blood.

3. For thrombin-soaked gelatin sponges: use dry forceps to apply appropriate sized sponge piece. Hold in place with surgical sponge (gauze sponge or cottonoid) for 10 to 15 seconds.

Contraindications:
Patients known to be sensitive to any of its components and/or to material of bovine origin.

Side Effects/Adverse Reactions:
May cause fever or allergic-type reaction in persons known to be sensitive to bovine materials; inhibitory antibodies which interfere with hemostasis may develop in small percentage of patients.

Sources: Heltemes, L. (2008). Ceasing blood flow with absorbable hemostatic agents. *OR Nurse, 2*(5), 19–20; Moss, R., & Smart, T. (2008). Hemostatic agents. In *Perioperative pharmacology reference book* (pp. 63–65). Denver, CO: Competency & Credentialing Institute; Samudrala, S. (2008). Topical hemostatic agents in surgery: A surgeon's perspective. *AORN Journal, 88*(3), S2–S11; Spry, C. (2009). *Essentials of perioperative nursing* (pp. 199–224). Sudbury, MA: Jones and Bartlett Publishers; Topical Thrombin. Retreived February 12, 2009 from www.thrombin-jmi.com/thrombin-jmi-how.aspx; Vaiden, R.E. (2005). *Core curriculum for the RN First Assistant* (pp. 260–263). Denver, CO: AORN.

Thrombin

Thrombin is perhaps the most widely used topical agent for chemical hemostasis in surgery. Thrombin can be derived from human or cattle plasma ("bovine") or manufactured using recombinant DNA techniques (recombinant thrombin). The best form to use is debatable, but is generally determined by personal preference, cost, and availability. Topical thrombin is available as either a liquid or powder and must be reconstituted according to the manufacturer's recommendations. It promotes hemostasis by directly clotting the fibrinogen in the blood and is most useful in controlling bleeding or oozing from small blood vessels or capillaries. In neurosurgery, it is applied to small cottonoid sponges that are placed on brain and nerve structures for their protection.

Before applying thrombin, excess blood should be removed from the operative area by sponging or suctioning. When absorbable gelatin sponges soaked in thrombin are used, it is important to squeeze the sponge gently to remove any trapped air. The sponge is then completely saturated with thrombin and is therefore more effective in promoting hemostasis. Once the area has been treated, it should not be sponged, because the clots will be removed or dislodged.

Thrombin must never be injected into the bloodstream or allowed access to the bloodstream through open, large blood vessels (Heltemes, 2008), or extensive intravascular clotting and possible death may ensue. The use of topical hemostatic agents is also contraindicated if a blood scavenging system (cellsaver) is being used, and in a patient with an allergy to bovine products if cattle plasma-derived thrombin is used.

Gelatin Sponges

Absorbable gelatin sponges are prepared from a purified gelatin solution that has been whipped into foam, dried, and sterilized. Gelatin sponges can be applied to the bleeding surface dry or moistened with normal sterile saline. Frequently thrombin or epinephrine is added to the saline to enhance the hemostatic effect. The sponge is often cut into the desired size and, if used moist, immersed in the solution, squeezed to remove air, and then stored in the solution until used. The sponge absorbs many times its own weight in blood, which then clots within the sponge. The blood is drawn passively into the sponge by capillary action, but it can be suctioned actively into the sponge if the sponge is protected with a gauze sponge or cotton pledget.

The gelatin sponge liquefies within two to five days following its application to bleeding mucosal areas and is absorbed completely in four to six weeks. A gelatin sponge should not be used in the presence of an infection that could localize in the sponge. When used in cavities or closed tissue spaces, care must be taken not to overpack the area because swelling of the sponge can cause pressure and consequent injury to surrounding tissues, nerves, and vascular structures.

Epinephrine

Epinephrine is a hormone that causes direct vascular constriction. It also acts on cardiac function and increases heart rate. Increased epinephrine production in emergency situations (i.e., the body's fight-or-flight defense mechanism) preserves brain and organ function by increasing heart rate and cardiac output and constricting the peripheral blood supply. Epinephrine's vasoconstrictive property makes it desirable as a hemostatic agent in surgery, where it can be topically applied with a sponge or injected in combination with a local anesthetic. When added to local anesthetics, it not only reduces bleeding, but also slows the absorption of the local anesthetic, thereby prolonging its analgesic effect.

Epinephrine's vasoconstrictive action must also be recognized as a significant risk when performing procedures on fingers, toes, ears, male genitalia, and any structure with a compromised blood supply. Normally, its use in such procedures is avoided.

Microfibrillar Collagen

A hemostatic agent derived from bovine dermis, microfibrillar collagen (MC) is an effective agent in a wet surgical field with generalized bleeding ooze. MC promotes hemostasis by initiating the coagulation mechanisms that activate platelets. MC is available in a loose fibrous form and in a compacted, "nonwoven" web form. Collagen itself adheres to wet surfaces; therefore, MC is applied with dry, smooth forceps to the bleeding site. The site is compressed with a dry sponge, the MC applied, and pressure then applied with a sponge. If bleeding continues through the MC, its application can be repeated. MC should not be used in patients with an allergy to bovine products or when a blood scavenging system (cell saver) is being used. Excess amounts of loose MC should be removed, and MC should not be applied to wound edges.

Absorbable Collagen Sponges

Absorbable collagen sponges consist of collagen derived from bovine flexor tendon. The sponge can be cut to size and applied directly to the bleeding area. They will not disperse as MC does, making collagen sponges easier to handle and place. Collagen sponges are also handled with dry, smooth tissue forceps. After placement on tissue, the sponges control bleeding in two to four minutes by causing platelet aggregation and clot formation.

Oxidized Cellulose

Oxidized cellulose is available impregnated in treated gauze or cotton. Applied directly to a bleeding surface, it promotes clotting of capillaries and smaller vessels that cannot be controlled by other means. The treated gauze can be cut into strips or to the desired size, and then placed dry on the bleeding site, using a dry sponge to hold it in place. The oxidized cellulose is absorbed in two to seven days. It must not be packed tightly because it swells. In particular, it must never be left in the patient near the spinal cord, optic nerve, or any area where swelling could seriously damage surrounding tissues or nerves. Oxidized cellulose is not used as permanent packing in bone fractures or other orthopedic procedures because it interferes with bone regeneration. Finally, it should never be used with thrombin because it interferes with thrombin's hemostatic action.

Fibrin Gel

Fibrin gel, also called "fibrin glue" or "fibrin sealant," is useful to control generalized oozing of blood, but it will not control vigorous bleeding. It is a biological adhesive that recreates natural physiological coagulation. In the presence of other ingredients, fibrinogen, which has been cryoprecipitated from human plasma, and thrombin, usually of bovine origin, are applied directly to tissue. The thrombin then converts fibrinogen to fibrin, forming an effective clot.

The gel can be prepared with banked plasma or the patient's own (autologous) plasma in one syringe, and thrombin (10,000 units per ampule) mixed with 10% calcium chloride in a second syringe. Each solution is drawn into a separate syringe because combining them would rapidly form a fibrin clot. The two solutions are then sprayed (or injected) simultaneously on the bleeding site. The fibrin clot begins to form within a few seconds.

Other fibrin sealants are available in separate frozen vials. After thawing, the vials are attached to an accompanying syringe device which combines the vial contents. The tip of choice is then added to the syringe containing the preparation and the sealant is sprayed or dripped on the tissue surface.

Tissue Adhesive

A new generation of topical hemostatic agents has recently gained popularity in surgery. Polyethylene glycol polymer is a synthetic adhesive that links with tissue proteins to adhere to the area of application. Polymerization occurs very rapidly to seal the areas of bleeding. The sealant can be applied in liquid or aerosolized form. When aerosolized, it is very effective in treating diffuse surfaces such as adhesions or synthetic grafts. A pressurized spray clears the field and the adhesive adheres to the surface, providing a polymer seal. This sealant is fully absorbed in four weeks.

Microporous Polysaccharide Hemosphere

Another recently introduced hemostatic topical agent is microporous polysaccharide hemosphere (MPH). This agent is derived from vegetable starch and is available as a powder. When applied, the MPH particles interact with the blood to form a gel, enhancing the clotting cascade. MPH is easily applied to surfaces and poses little risk because it contains no human or animal components.

HANDOFF AND SIGN-OUT REPORT

The FA is responsible for clear, focused, and concise communication when writing the operative note in the medical record and sharing patient and procedure information with other caregivers. During the handoff report to the postanesthesia care unit (PACU), intensive care unit (ICU), or another discharge unit, pertinent information should be communicated including problems with hemostasis (gleaned from the patient's history and assessment or from intraoperative assessment), treatments rendered (such as the administration of blood products or volume expanders), description of drains, and any anticipated changes resulting from problems with achieving hemostasis. It is important that the FA uses the standardized handoff report tool or approach for the institution where he or she assists in surgery. During the handoff report, interruptions should be minimized and the staff in the receiving patient care unit should have the opportunity to ask questions (Chard, 2008). In addition, estimated blood loss (EBL) should be included in the handoff report. In some institutions, a surgical Apgar score is calculated at the end of the surgical procedure from the EBL, lowest mean arterial pressure (expressed in mm of Hg), and the lowest heart rate rhythm recorded on the anesthesia record during the procedure. The score may be used to identify patients with a higher likelihood of developing complications after surgery (Regenbogen et al., 2009).

If the FA follows the patient during the course of hospitalization and will be passing care responsibilities to another provider, then the sign-out to the other care provider should also include major events during surgery and information about deviations from the expected intraoperative plan to achieve hemostasis (Kemp et al., 2008).

CONCLUSION

In a study undertaken by Antonacci and others (2008), a profile of incidents affecting quality outcomes after surgery was created by developing a usable operating room and perioperative clinical incident report database. Clinical incidents associated with unplanned returns to the OR (24.3%; 1056 of 4343) were all recognized in the postoperative period and could be directly related to the original surgical procedure. Hemorrhage was one of the most common issues; there were 290 hemorrhage events, accounting for 27.8% of unplanned returns to the OR. Clearly, the critical thinking and clinical acumen demonstrated by the FA in achieving effective hemostasis is a critical factor in preventing such unplanned returns to the OR.

REFERENCES

1. Alternatives to transfusion. The University Center for Bloodless Surgery and Medicine at University Hospital in Newark, NJ. Retrieved February 22, 2009 from www.theuniversityhospital.com/bloodless/html/bloodlessterms/alternatives.htm

2. Antonacci, A.C., Lam, S., Lavarias, V., Homel, P., & Eavey R.D. (2008). Benchmarking surgical incident reports using a database and a triage system to reduce adverse outcomes. *Archives of Surgery, 143*(12), 1192–1197.

3. ASA practice guidelines for perioperative blood transfusion and adjuvant therapies. (2006). *Anesthesiology, 105*, 198–208.

4. Association of periOperative Registered Nurses (AORN). (2009). Recommended practices for electrosurgery. *Perioperative standards and recommended practices* (pp. 331–345). Denver, CO: AORN.

5. Bielefeldt, S., DeWitt, J. (2009). The rules of transfusion: Best practices for blood product administration. *American Nurse Today, 4*(2), 27–30.

6. Campbell, D.A., Henderson, W.G., Englesbe, M.J., Hall, B.L., O'Reilly, M., Bratzler, D., Dellinger, E.P., Neumayer, L., Bass, B.L., Hutter, M.M., Schwartz, J., Ko, C., Itani, K., Steinberg, S.M., Siperstein, A., Sawyer, R.G., Turner, D.J., & Khuri, S.F. (2008). Surgical site infection prevention: The importance of operative duration and blood transfusion—results of the first American College of Surgeons–national surgical quality improvement program best practices initiative. *Journal of American College of Surgeons, 207*(6), 810–820.

7. Catalano, K. (2008). Knowledge is power: Averting safety-compromising events in the OR. *AORN Journal, 88*(6), 987–995.

8. Cima, R.R., Kollengode, A., Garnatz, J., Stovrsveen, A., Weisbrod, C., & Deschamps, C. (2008). Incidence and characteristics of potential and actual retained foreign object events in surgical patients. *Journal of the American College of Surgeons, 207*(1), 80–87.

9. Chard, R. (2008). Clinical issues: Implementing a process for hand-off communications. *AORN Journal, 88*(6), 1005–1006.

10. Constantine, T., & Payne, C. (2009). Prevent the dangers of hosing. *OR Nurse, 3*(1), 56.

11. Di Nisio, M., Middeldrorp, S., Buller, H.R. (2005). Direct thrombin inhibitors. *New England Journal of Medicine, 353*, 1028–40.

12. Downing, D. (2008). Clinical issues: Counting sterile towels. *AORN Journal, 87*(4), 823–825.

13. Further changes for 2009 standards. (2009). *OR Manager, 25*(5), 10.

14. Gawande, A.A., Studdert, D.M., Orav, E.J., Brennan, T.A., & Zinner, M.J. (2003). Risk factors for retained instruments and sponges after surgery. *New England Journal of Medicine, 348*(3), 229–235.

15. Haynes, A.B., Weiser, T.G., Berry, W.R., Lipsitz, S.R., Breizat, A-H.S., Dellinger, E.P., Herbosa, T., Joseph, S., Kibatala, P.L., Lapitan, M.C.M., Merry, A.F., Moorthy, K., Reznick, R.K., Taylor, B., & Gawande, A.A. (2009). A surgical safety checklist to reduce morbidity and mortality in a global population. *New England Journal of Medicine, 360*(5), 491–499.

16. Heltemes, L. (2008). Ceasing blood flow with absorbable hemostatic agents. O*R Nurse,* (May), 19–20.

17. Hobbs, J.L. (2009). A dimensional analysis of patient-centered care. *Nursing Research, 58*(1), 52–61.

18. Hoogerwerf, B.J. (2009). Provide hemostasis. In M.L. Phippen, B.C. Ulmer, & M.P. Wells (Eds.), *Competency for safe patient care during operative and invasive procedures.* Denver: Competency & Credentialing Institute.

19. Kemp, C.D., Bath, J.M., Berger, J., Bergsman, J., Ellison, T., Emery, K., Garonzik-Wang, J., Hui-Chou, H.G., Mayo, S.C., Serrano, O.K., Shridharani, S., Zuberi, K., Lipsett, P., & Freischlag, J.A. (2008). The top 10 list for a safe and effective sign-out. *Archives of Surgery, 143*(10), 1008–1010.

20. McGraw, B., & Lyon, D.E. (2008). Diagnosing disseminated intravascular coagulopathy in acute promyelocytic leukemia. *Clinical Journal of Oncology Nursing, 12*(5), 717–720.

21. Merrick, H.W., Smith, M.R., & MacFayden, B.V. (2006). Surgical bleeding and blood replacement. In P.F. Lawrence (Ed.), *Essentials of general surgery* (4th ed.). Philadelphia: Lippincott Williams & Wilkins.

22. Nundy, S., Mukherjee, A., Sexton, B., Pronovost, P.J., Knight, A., Rowan, L.C., Duncan, M., Syin, D., & Makary, M.A. (2008). Impact of preoperative briefings on operating room delays. *Archives of Surgery, 143*(11), 1068–1072.

23. Owings, J.T., Utter, G.H., & Gosselin, R.C. (2007). Bleeding and transfusion. In Souba, Fink, Jurkovich, et al. *ACS surgery-principles & practice* (pp. 61–76). New York: WebMD Professional Publishing.

24. Paige, J.T., Aaron, D.L., Yang, T., Howell, D.S., Hilton, C.W., Cohn, I., & Chauvin, S.W. (2008). Implementation of a preoperative briefing protocol improves accuracy of teamwork assessment in the operating room. *The American Surgeon, 74*(9), 817–823.

25. Paulikas, C.A. (2008). Prevention of unplanned perioperative hypothermia. *AORN Journal, 88*(3), 358–364.

26. Recommended practices for sponge, sharp, and instrument counts. (2009). In 2009 *Perioperative standards and recommended practices* (pp. 405–414). Denver, CO: AORN.

27. Regenbogen, S.E., Ehrenfeld, J.M., Lipsitz, S.R., Greenberg, C.C., Hutter, M.M., & Gawande, A.A. (2009). Utility of the surgical Apgar score. *Archives of Surgery, 144*(1), 30–36.

28. Retzlaff, K. (2009). Getting on track. Tracking technologies are improving supply chain efficiency and patient safety in the operating room. *AORN Connections, 7*(1), 1–8.

29. Samudrala, S. (2008). Topical hemostatic agents in surgery: A surgeon's perspective. *AORN Journal, 88*(3), S2–S11.

30. Spry, C. (2009). *Essentials of perioperative nursing* (pp. 199–224). Sudbury, MA: Jones and Bartlett Publishers.

31. Tan, S.R., Tope, W.D. (2004). Effectiveness of microporous polysaccharide hemospheres for achieving hemostasis in mohs micrographic surgery. *Dermatologic Surgery, 30*(6), 908–14.

32. Ulmer, B.C. (2008). The hazards of surgical smoke. *AORN Journal, 87*(4), 721–734.

33. Villanueva, M. (2008). Introduction: Effective hemostasis in surgery. *AORN Journal, 88*(3), S1.

34. Wanzer, L.J., Hicks, R.W., Goecker, B., Cole, L. (2008). A focused review: Perioperative safe medication use. *Perioperative Nursing Clinics, 3*(4), 305–316.

6

Suturing Materials and Techniques

Nancy B. Davis

For a surgical first assistant (FA) suturing aptitude is a fundamental clinical skill during operative and other invasive procedures. As with any skill acquisition, learning and performing the techniques of suturing means graduating from basic competency to excellence in skill performance.

The FA first learns about the types of sutures and various suturing techniques in his/her basic educational program (Physician Assistant [PA], Surgical Assistant [SA], Registered Nurse First Assistant [RNFA], Certified First Assistant [CFA], medical internship, or residency). Further information is obtained by observing the surgeon, engaging in clinical discussions about suture characteristics and suturing techniques, taking professional continuing education, and reviewing manufacturer's literature. In the interest of patient safety, practice by novices should initially be done in a simulated setting. Laboratory practice is especially helpful when learning more complex suturing techniques, such as those used in microsurgery. After practice and initial skill evaluation, suturing skills are refined in the operating room under the direction and supervision of the surgeon. The application of this skill varies depending on the clinical privileges awarded by the credentialing body and is based on scope of practice, practice setting, and any legal constraints.

Although the choice of suture materials and techniques is primarily determined by the operating surgeon, many factors must be considered. The patient's condition and age, the presence of infection, and the type of tissue being sutured are some important factors. Preoperative assessment of the patient provides data that can help the assistant to identify potential complications. Suture materials are foreign substances; therefore, in selecting the type of suture and suturing techniques, the FA should consider patient risk factors and the potential for wound infection, inadequate or delayed wound healing, wound dehiscence, and excessive scarring. The goal is to leave minimal foreign material in the wound. This result is achieved, in part, by selecting the suture with the highest tensile strength, the smallest diameter (size), and one that holds knots well, requiring fewer turns and throws during tying.

USES AND SELECTION OF SUTURES

The three common uses for sutures during operative procedures are as follows:

1. Hemostasis: strands of sutures are used as ligatures to tie off blood vessels and control bleeding.
2. Wound closure: sutures are used to sew tissues together and to hold the tissues securely until healing occurs.
3. Wound exposure: sutures are used to retract tissues and expose the operative site for the surgeon, when tension is applied to the sutures.

Sutures are medical devices and must meet certain standards established by the Federal Food and Drug Administration (FDA, 2003). Government regulations have established criteria for ensuring the safety and effectiveness of sutures. Sterility, tensile strength, size, dyes, needle attachments, coating or impregnation of suture material with other substances, biocompatibility, absorption profile, packaging and labeling are some of the areas addressed in these regulations.

The three main characteristics of sutures are *physical characteristics, handling characteristics*, and *tissue-reaction characteristics. Physical characteristics* include physical configuration (single- or multistrand), capillarity, diameter (size), tensile strength, knot strength, elasticity, and memory. *Handling characteristics* include pliability, tissue drag, knot tying, and knot slippage. *Tissue-reaction characteristics* include inflammatory and fibrous cell reaction, absorption, potentiation of infection, and allergic reaction (Rothrock, 2007). Allergic reactions to sutures have been reported (Woo, 2008) in the scientific literature and must be anticipated by the surgical team. Patients with known allergies to certain suture materials should inform their health care providers and should wear a medical-alert identification bracelet with information about any allergies. The FA should always check any patient's arm for a wristband noting an allergy. In some states, wristband standardization initiatives require the use of a red-colored wristband for allergies (Texas Hospital Association, 2008). Any patient allergies should be communicated during the preop briefing or time-out, which are designed to improve teamwork and communication (Nundy et al., 2008).

The FA should consider the type of tissue when selecting a suture. The suture must be as strong as the tissue it is holding, and the strength of the suture must last until the tissue is healed. Thus, the rate of suture absorption should correspond to the rate of healing. Tissues heal at different rates, and healing can be affected by such factors as infection, obesity, the presence of malignancies or debilitating injuries, immunodeficiency, blood loss, fluid and/or electrolyte imbalances, debilitation, inadequate nutrition, chronic disease, inadequate blood supply, radiation therapy, and age. The smallest diameter of suture is used to minimize tissue reaction and injury. The suture material should be pliable, strong, and hold knots securely. Suture security depends on the suture material's intrinsic tensile strength and ability to hold a knot. Other factors to be considered include location and length of the incision, desired cosmetic results, personal experience, cost, and product availability.

CLASSIFICATION OF SUTURES

Sutures are classified according to the effects of tissue enzymes and body fluids on the material. A suture is a foreign body, and the body reacts to it by secreting substances in an attempt to dissolve or digest it. If the suture can dissolve or be digested, it is considered absorbable. Nonabsorbable sutures, in contrast, cannot be dissolved or digested; rather, they become encapsulated by body tissues or must be removed (as in skin sutures).

Sutures are also classified according to the number of strands of material used. A suture with two or more strands of suture material twisted or braided together is termed a multifilament suture. Although the multifilament suture's higher coefficient of friction helps it hold knots, the multiple strands may make it "drag" through tissue, thus increasing tissue trauma and tissue reaction. This type of suture has a capillary or wicking effect whereby body fluids can adhere to the suture strand. This capillary action can be reduced by coating the suture with silicone or paraffin. A monofilament suture consists of a single strand of suture material that has no capillary action, and consequently causes very little tissue reaction.

Absorbable Sutures

Absorbable sutures are temporary and will be digested or dissolved. Tensile strength and retention and absorption rates vary among the absorbable sutures, and these factors must be considered separately. For example, a suture may lose its strength quickly and be absorbed slowly. These sutures can be treated to delay the absorption rate or coated with agents that have antimicrobial action. Absorbable sutures vary in texture, structure, size, and color (Table 6-1).

Surgical Gut   Surgical gut (catgut) is used less frequently than synthetic absorbable sutures. Gut is made from the submucosal layer of sheep intestine or the serosal layer of beef intestine; it is a highly purified collagen. Gut is processed by electronically spinning and polishing the strands into various sizes. The suture can be left "plain"

Table 6-1 **Absorbable Sutures Commonly Used in Surgery**

Suture and Type	Frequent Uses	Tissue Reaction	Contraindications	Absorption Rate	Tensile Strength Retention *In Vivo*
Surgical gut/plain	Soft tissue approximation and/or ligation	Moderate	Should not be used where extended approximation of tissues under stress is required. Should not be used in patients with known sensitivities or allergies to collagen or chromium.	Absorbed by proteolytic enzymatic digestive process.	Individual patient characteristics can affect rate of tensile strength loss. Lost within 7–10 days.
Surgical gut/chromic	Soft tissue approximation and/or ligation	Moderate	Same as surgical gut/plain	Same as surgical gut/plain	Individual patient characteristics can affect rate of tensile strength loss. Lost within 21–28 days.
Polydioxanone monofilament	All types of soft tissue approximation, including pediatric, cardiovascular, and ophthalmic procedures	Slight	Should not be used where extended approximation of tissues under stress is required. Should not be used with prosthetic devices (heart valves or synthetic grafts), adult cardiovascular tissue, microsurgery, or neural tissue.	Minimal until about 90th day. Essentially complete within 6 months. Absorbed by slow hydrolysis.	Approximately: 70% remains at 2 weeks; 50% remains at 4 weeks; 25% remains at 6 weeks

Polyglactin braided or monofilament	Soft tissue approximation	Minimal	Should not be used where extended approximation of tissue is required. Not for use in cardiovascular and neurological tissues.	Essentially complete between 56 and 70 days. Absorbed by hydrolysis.	Approximately: After 2 weeks 75% remains. After 3 weeks 50% remains. After 4 weeks 25% remains.
Poliglecaprone 25 monofilamente	Soft tissue approximation	Minimal	Should not be used where extended approximation of tissue is required. Undyed versions not indicated for use in fascia.	Complete at 91–119 days	Approximately: After 1 week 50–60% remains. After 2 weeks 20–30% remains. After 3 weeks, it is lost.

Source: From *Wound closure manual* (pp. 20–21), by ETHICON, 2007, Somerville, NJ: Johnson and Johnson. Copyright 2007, ETHICON, Inc. Adapted with permission from ETHICON.

or may be dipped in chromium salt solution. "Chromicizing" the suture increases its resistance to the digestive action of tissue enzymes, thereby delaying absorption. This treated suture is called "chromic." Chromic sutures cause less tissue reaction than plain sutures, which may elicit a marked foreign-body response.

Surgical gut suture must be handled as infrequently as possible because handling may cause the suture to fray. The suture material loses its pliability if allowed to dry. Pliability can be restored by moistening the suture with sterile water or saline. The suture must not be soaked any longer than a few seconds because soaking decreases tensile strength and knot security. When removed from its packaging, chromic suture may retain its memory, which is not desirable for suture material. It should be straightened by holding both ends and stretching the strand taut once. Repeated pulling or running fingers down the length of the suture will weaken it.

Generally, plain surgical gut loses its tensile strength in approximately 7–10 days and is absorbed in about 70 days. Chromic suture's tensile strength lasts approximately 21 to 28 days and is absorbed in about 90 days.

Synthetic Absorbable Sutures   Polymers made from polyglycolic acid, polyglactin 910, polyglyconate, poliglecaprone 25, or polydioxanone are used to make synthetic absorbable sutures that are prepared as monofilament or multifilament sutures. Tissue reactions are mild and are decreased further when a monofilament suture is used. This type of suture is stronger than surgical gut, and the tensile strength lasts longer. After seven days, about 60% or more of the suture's tensile strength remains. Absorption occurs through hydrolysis, which accounts for the mild tissue reaction, and the suture is usually absorbed after 42 to 70 days. The polydioxanone suture is usually absorbed after 90 to 180 days.

The braided polymers handle as silk sutures, and, because of their higher coefficient of friction, knot security is good. On the other hand, the monofilament or the coated sutures are smoother and slicker, requiring additional throws for better knot security.

Poly-4-hydroxybutyrate suture (TephaFLEX) is a monofilament absorbable suture based on recombinant DNA technology and has been approved by the FDA. It is more flexible than the synthetic absorbable polymers and is very biocompatible (Clinical Rounds, 2007; Martin & Williams, 2003).

Nonabsorbable Sutures

Nonabsorbable sutures are not digested by tissue enzymes or hydrolyzed by body fluids. They are considered permanent sutures. Nonabsorbable sutures are used when the suture strength needs to be retained longer than two to three weeks (Table 6-2).

Table 6-2 Nonabsorbable Sutures Commonly Used in Surgery

Suture and Type	Frequent Uses	Tissue Reaction	Contraindications	Absorption Rate	Tensile Strength Retention *In Vivo*
Silk Braided	Soft tissue approximation and/or ligation.	Acute inflammatory reaction	Should not be used in patients with known sensitivities or allergies to silk.	Gradual encapsulation by fibrous connective tissue.	Progressive degradation of fiber may result in gradual loss of tensile strength.
Surgical Stainless Steel Suture Monofilament or Multi-filament	Abdominal or sternal wound closure, hernia repair, and orthopedic procedures.	Minimal	Should not be used in patients with known sensitivities or allergies to stainless steel or constituent metals such as chromium and nickel.	Nonabsorbable	Indefinite
Nylon Monofilament or Braided	Soft tissue approximation and/or ligation.	Minimal	Should not be used where permanent retention of tensile strength is required.	Gradual encapsulation by fibrous connective tissue.	Progressive hydrolysis may result in gradual loss of tensile strength.
Polyester Fiber Monofilament or Braided	Soft tissue approximation and/or ligation.	Minimal	None known	Gradual encapsulation by fibrous connective tissue.	No significant change known

(continued)

Table 6-2 (*Continued*)

Suture and Type	Frequent Uses	Tissue Reaction	Contraindications	Absorption Rate	Tensile Strength Retention *In Vivo*
Polypropylene Monofilament	Soft tissue approximation and/or ligation.	Minimal	None known	Nonabsorbable	Not subject to degradation or weakening from action of tissue enzymes.
Hexafluoro-propylene-VDF Monofilament	Soft tissue approximation and/or ligation.	Minimal	None known	Nonabsorbable	Not subject to degradation or weakening from action of tissue enzymes.

Source: From *Wound closure manual* (pp. 20–21), by ETHICON, 2007, Somerville, NJ: Johnson and Johnson. Copyright 2007, ETHICON, Inc. Modified with permission fom ETHICON.

With the exception of wire sutures, nonabsorbable sutures should not be used in the presence of infection. The suture itself could become the site of an infection, requiring suture removal.

The United States Pharmacopoeia (USP) classifies nonabsorbable surgical sutures as:

Class I: silk or synthetic fibers (monofilament, twisted or braided construction);

Class II: cotton or linen fibers or coated natural or synthetic fibers (coating contributes to suture thickness but not strength); and

Class III: metal wire (may be monofilament or multifilament).

(*Wound Closure Manual*, 2007, p. 21).

Surgical Silk   In the past, surgical silk was the most commonly used nonabsorbable suture material, because of its ease in handling, its tensile strength, and the security of its knots, requiring a minimal number of throws. Silk is made from the silk of silkworms. After the silk filaments are processed, the strands are braided or twisted, treated to decrease capillary action, and usually dyed black. All other sutures are compared with silk in relation to handling properties. Silk, however, causes a higher degree of tissue reaction than do the other commonly used nonabsorbable sutures. Moisture weakens the silk suture, and therefore it is used dry. Its tensile strength decreases after 90 to 120 days, and the suture is usually absorbed within two years. Thus, silk is not a true nonabsorbable suture but is classified as such because it remains in the tissues so long. Silk should not be used in an infected wound.

Surgical Stainless Steel Wire   Surgical stainless steel wire sutures are made from strong, flexible, and uniform steel alloy and can be used with stainless steel hardware or prostheses. They should not be used in the presence of another alloy because electrolytic reactions may occur. Stainless steel wire is strong, minimally tissue reactive, and one of the most secure suture materials available. The suture is prepared as a monofilament or multifilament wire. Monofilament wire kinks easily. Both types can be held securely in place by twisting or knotting the suture. The major disadvantage is related to handling the suture, as gloves can be punctured or tissue injured by the sharp ends of the wire. Wire's tensile strength is very high, and, as stated, tissue reaction is minimal. Wire cutters must be used to cut the suture, since the wire will damage suture scissors.

Nylon   Nylon is made from a synthetic polyamide polymer. Its tensile strength is high, and tissue reaction is minimal. Monofilament nylon suture is noncapillary and easy to handle. It does require additional throws for knot security. Moistening nylon suture makes it easier to handle and more pliable. Multifilament nylon is braided very tightly and treated for noncapillarity. Nylon handles like silk, but with less tissue reaction. Nylon suture loses 15 to 20% of its tensile strength per year in tissue and will not provide indefinite support.

Polyester Suture Polyesters are made from polyethylene terephthalate fibers braided together. This suture is strong and very little tissue reaction occurs as the suture is coated with polybutylate, a synthetic coating developed as a surgical suture lubricant.

Polypropylene Polypropylene suture is an isostatic, crystalline steroisomer of a linear hydrocarbon polymer that allows little or no saturation. It is a smooth monofilament suture that does not weaken in tissues, causes very little tissue reaction, is easy to handle, and hold knots securely.

Hexafluoropropylene VDH This suture is a polymer blend of vinylidene fluoride and vinylidene fluoride-cohexafluoropropylene. This monofilament suture does not adhere to tissue and resists infection.

Expanded Polytetrafluoroethylene (ePTFE) Expanded polytetrafluoroethylene is a soft, supple suture that is easy to handle, does not have memory, and causes minimal tissue irritation. This suture is known as GOR-TEX® and is used for selected vascular and cardiac procedures.

Surgical Cotton Surgical cotton is made from natural cellulose cotton fibers. This is the weakest nonabsorbable suture and is rarely used. The tensile strength increases if moistened immediately prior to use.

Linen Linen suture is made from twisted flax fibers. It is rarely used as its strength is inferior to other nonabsorbable sutures.

Quill SRS Suture Recently introduced, the Quill SRS suture is a new concept in suturing. The suture has "barbs" that grasp the tissue securely, and knots are not required (Figure 6-1). It can be used for subcuticular or multilayer closures (Figure 6-2). Tension is more evenly distributed, and knot complications are avoided. It is available in absorbable (polydioxanone) and nonabsorbable (nylon and polypropylene) types.

SURGICAL NEEDLES

The surgical needle transports the suture through the tissues during surgical operations with as little trauma to tissues as possible. High-quality steel alloy is used in manufacturing surgical needles. The different size needles are made from wire of

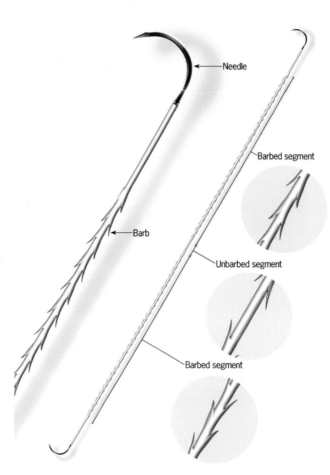

Figure 6-1

Quill SRS suture anatomy.

Note: The Quill™ is a knotless surgical wound closure system that has tiny barbs on its surface; these barbs are arrayed in opposing directions on either side of a transitional, unbarbed segment. To facilitate tissue insertion and deployment, a needle is crimped onto both ends of the suture. The barbs penetrate into the surrounding tissue and lock the suture in place.

Source: From *Quill SRS techniques and procedures: A novel approach to soft tissue approximation*, by Angiotech Pharmaceuticals, Inc.: Vancouver, B.C. Copyright 2008 by Angiotech Pharmaceuticals, Inc. Reprinted with permission.

various thicknesses. The wire is heat treated and tempered to provide the necessary strength and flexibility. A needle must be strong enough to penetrate the tissue without bending, breaking, or deforming. The needle can bend slightly without breaking because it is flexible. Bending alerts the user that the tissue may be too tough for the chosen needle.

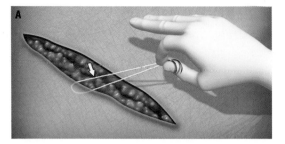

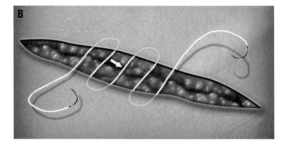

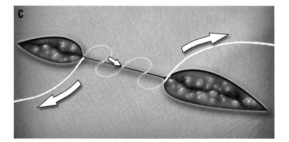

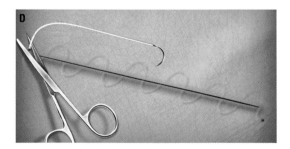

Figure 6-2A–D

Deep subcuticular closure using Quill SRS suture.

Note: Suture is started in the center.

Source: From *Quill SRS techniques and procedures: A novel approach to soft tissue approximation*, by Angiotech Pharmaceuticals, Inc.: Vancouver, B.C. Copyright 2008 by Angiotech Pharmaceuticals, Inc. Reprinted with permission.

Needles are carefully sharpened, finely polished and smoothed for easier tissue penetration. Silicone coatings are occasionally used. Blunt needles are available for use with heavier sutures. All surgical needles are noncorrosive so that flaking of foreign material from needles into the surgical wound cannot occur.

Needle Designs

Basically, needles have three components: the eye, the shaft or body, and the point (Figure 6-3).

Eye   The eye of the needle is located at the end of the needle where the suture is attached. The three types of needle eyes are closed, French eye or split, and swaged (Figure 6-4). The swaged design is most commonly used, although there are occasions when the FA may opt for an alternate needle design.

The *closed-eye needle* has a round, square or oblong hole through which the suture is threaded. The eye must be smooth to avoid cutting the suture.

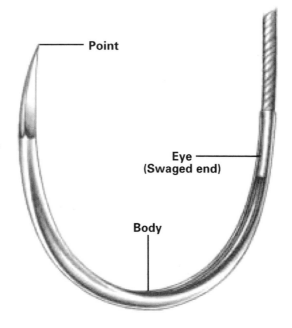

Point

**Eye
(Swaged end)**

Body

Figure 6-3

Suture needle components.

Figure 6-4

Suture needle eyes. *Top to bottom*: Closed eye, French eye, and Swaged.

Source: Wound Closure Manual (2007). (Ch. 3, Fig. 5, p. 46) by ETHICON, 2007, Somerville, NJ: Johnson and Johnson. Copyright 2007, ETHICON, Inc. Reprinted with permission.

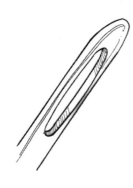

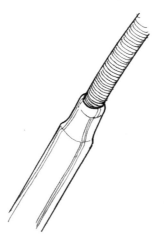

Eyed needles may be reusable or disposable. Although eyed needles may be economical, the eye must be larger than the suture. The additional bulk of a double suture can cause increased damage to the tissue when the needle is pulled through the tissue. Additional skill and speed are also required on the part of the scrub person to manually thread the needle and to have it ready for use without slowing the surgeon or FA.

The *French eye or split-eye needle* has a spring opening that allows the suture and the needle to be almost the same size, which decreases tissue trauma. The double suture still must be pulled through the tissue. Although French eye needles are quicker to thread, they are usually finer needles that have a limited use.

The *swaged or atraumatic needle* is actually an eyeless needle. The suture is attached to the end of the needle during the manufacturing process and is only as large as the needle itself. This type of needle provides the least amount of tissue trauma. Although more costly, sutures with swaged needles are easier and quicker to use, and are necessary in some situations. Fine synthetic nonabsorbable sutures, employed for delicate surgery, such as microsurgery or vascular surgery, are attached to a swaged needle because this use causes minimal tissue injury. Sharpness is ensured, because the swaged needle is used only with that one suture and then discarded.

Sutures are available with swaged needles that can be removed from the suture with a slight tug. Generically called "pop-off" or "breakaway" sutures (**Figure 6-5**), these are used for interrupted suturing techniques in which several sutures can be placed rapidly.

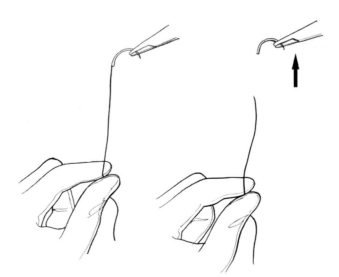

Figure 6-5

Control release suture needle.

Source: Adapted by M. Borman from *Wound closure manual* (2007). (Ch. 3, Fig. 6, p. 46). Somerville, NJ: ETHICON, Inc.

The choice of needle eye is based on the location and type of tissue being sutured, the size of the suture being used, the availability of various needles, and considerations related to decreasing surgery time. The surgical FA must be familiar with the surgeon's needle eye preferences in all operative procedures where he or she assists.

Shaft   The shaft, or body, determines the needle's shape, size, and diameter. This area of the needle is grasped or held by the needleholder as the needle is passed through the tissue. The shaft may be straight (this may be a "Keith" needle, used for easily accessible tissue, such as in skin closure), curved, or partially curved. The various needle sizes are determined by measuring the chord length, needle length, and needle radius (Figure 6-6).

A needle may be oval, round, triangular, side-flattened, rectangular, or trapezoidal in design. Some needles are flat and ribbed in the area where they are grasped by the needleholder. This design reduces slippage of the needle in the needleholder during suturing.

Needle shape, size, and thickness must all be considered when selecting a needle (Figure 6-7). The choice of shape and size depend on the location and accessibility of the tissue being sutured, while thickness is determined by the type of tissue and size of suture being used. The needle should be as close to the size of the suture as possible.

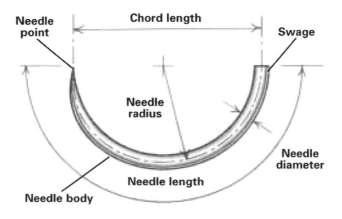

Figure 6-6

Anatomy of a suture needle.

Source: Wound Closure Manual (2007). (Ch. 3, Fig. 4, p. 44) by ETHICON, 2007, Somerville, NJ: Johnson and Johnson. Copyright 2007, ETHICON, Inc. Reprinted with permission.

SHAPE	APPLICATION
Straight 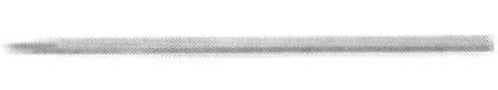	gastrointestinal tract, nasal cavity, nerve, oral cavity, pharynx, skin, tendon, vessels
Half-curved	skin (rarely used) laparoscopy
$1/4$ Circle 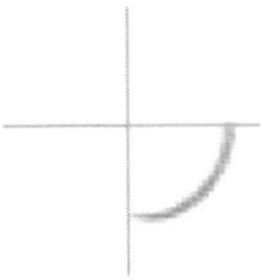	eye (primary application) microsurgery
$3/8$ Circle 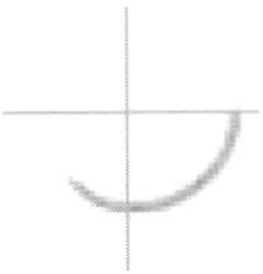	aponeurosis, biliary tract, cardiovascular system, dura, eye, gastrointestinal tract, muscle, myocardium, nerve, perichondrium, periosteum, pleura, skin, tendon, urogenital tract, vessels
$1/2$ Circle 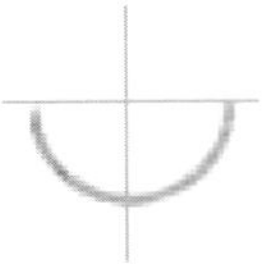	biliary tract, cardiovascular system, eye, fascia, gastrointestinal tract, muscle, nasal cavity, oral cavity, pelvis, peritoneum, pharynx, pleura, respiratory tract, skin, tendon, subcutaneous fat, urogenital tract
$5/8$ Circle 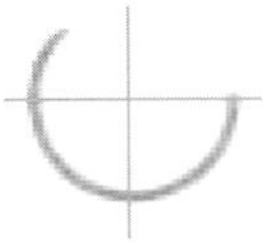	anal (hemorrhoidectomy), nasal cavity, pelvis, urogenital tract (primary application)
Compound Curved 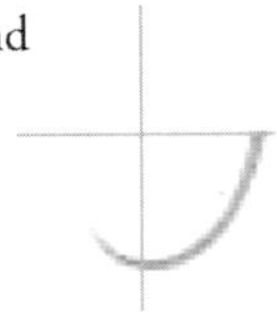	eye (anterior segment) laparoscopy

Figure 6-7

Needle shapes and uses.

Source: Wound Closure Manual (2007). (Ch. 3, Fig. 7, p. 47) by ETHICON, 2007, Somerville, NJ: Johnson and Johnson. Copyright 2007, ETHICON, Inc. Reprinted with permission.

Point The needle point is the end that first penetrates the tissue being sutured. The design of the point varies according to the type of tissue to be penetrated (**Figure 6-8**). The basic point designs are cutting, taper, and blunt.

Cutting needles are designed to penetrate tough tissue such as skin, tendons, fibrous or calcified tissue, and sternal bone. Variations in the cutting edges alter the direction of cutting and promote ease of tissue penetration.

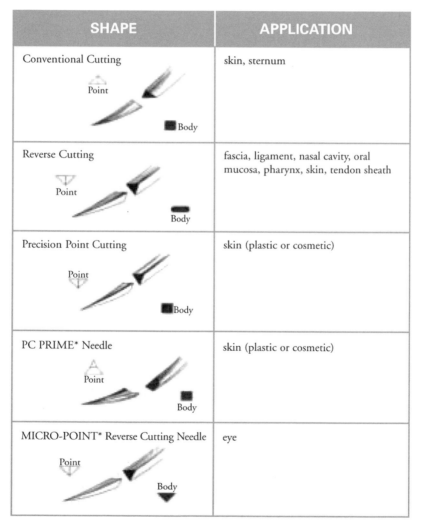

SHAPE	APPLICATION
Conventional Cutting	skin, sternum
Reverse Cutting	fascia, ligament, nasal cavity, oral mucosa, pharynx, skin, tendon sheath
Precision Point Cutting	skin (plastic or cosmetic)
PC PRIME* Needle	skin (plastic or cosmetic)
MICRO-POINT* Reverse Cutting Needle	eye

Figure 6-8

Needle points, shapes, and uses.

SHAPE	APPLICATION
Side-Cutting Spatula 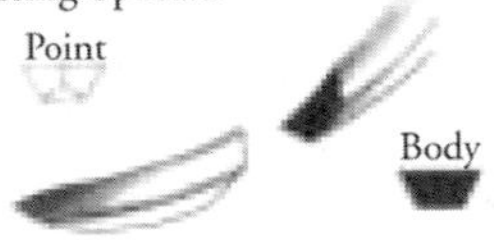 Point Body	eye (primary application), microsurgery, ophthalmic (reconstructive)
CS ULTIMA* Ophthalmic Needle 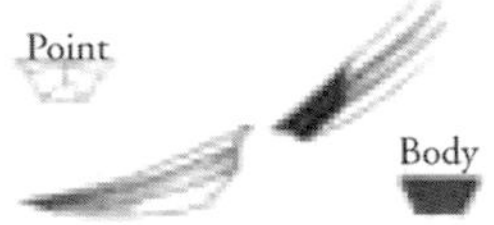 Point Body	eye (primary application)
Taper 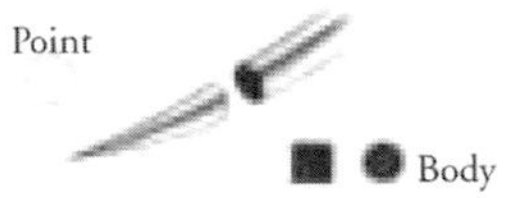 Point Body	aponeurosis, biliary tract, dura, fascia, gastrointestinal tract, laparoscopy, muscle, myocardium, nerve, peritoneum, pleura, subcutaneous fat, urogenital tract, vessels, valve
TAPERCUT* Surgical Needle 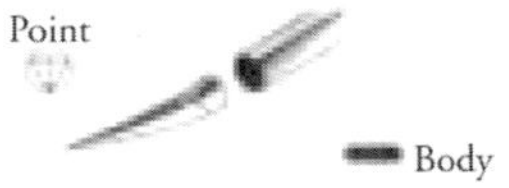 Point Body	bronchus, calcified tissue, fascia, laparoscopy, ligament, nasal cavity, oral cavity, ovary, perichondrium, periosteum, pharynx, sternum, tendon, trachea, uterus, valve, vessels (sclerotic)
Blunt 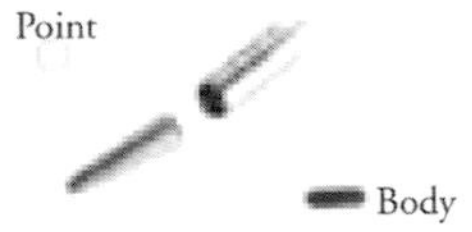 Point Body	blunt dissection (friable tissue), cervix (ligating incompetent cervix), fascia, intestine, kidney, liver, spleen

Figure 6-8 (*Continued*)

Source: Wound Closure Manual (2007). (Ch. 3, Fig. 8, p. 48) by ETHICON, 2007, Somerville, NJ: Johnson and Johnson. Copyright 2007, ETHICON, Inc. Reprinted with permission.

Taper needles, usually called "round" needles, cause minimal tissue trauma, but must be used on tissue that they can penetrate easily.

The *blunt needle* does not have a sharp point but basically dissects the tissue as it is pushed through, causing less trauma than the conventional sharp pointed needle. The risk of needlestick injury is also reduced. The Council on Surgical and Perioperative Safety (CSPS) has endorsed the use of blunt suture needles as a recommended safety measure (CSPS, 2007). Similarly, the National Institute for Occupational Safety and Health strongly encourages the use of blunt-tip suture needles to decrease percutaneous injuries to surgical personnel (NIOSH, 2008). Moreover, the American College of Surgeons (ACS) issued a statement on blunt suture needles in 2005, encouraging adoption of blunt suture needles as the first choice for fascial closure and recommending that surgery facilities stock blunt suture needles in various sizes for use in multiple surgical applications (ACS, 2005). The FA has an integral role to play in sharps safety in perioperative care.

If the FA punctures his or her glove with a surgical needle or another sharp object, the following steps (Maxwell, 2008) should be taken if the needle or sharp object is clean (i.e., not used on the patient):

- Remove the affected hand from the sterile field immediately so as not to contaminate any portion of the sterile field;
- Announce to the circulating nurse that you have contaminated your hand; note your glove size (double gloving is recommended) (AORN, 2009b; CSPS, 2007);
- Request assistance from the circulating nurse with removal of the contaminated glove(s); and
- Keep the exposed hand from moving over any portion of the sterile field, participate in assisted gloving with the scrub person.

If the FA experiences an injury from a needle that has been used on a patient, he or she should adhere to the institutional procedure for postexposure evaluation and follow-up, including postexposure prophylaxis.

SUTURING SKILLS

Assisting During Suturing

One of the first tasks for a proficient FA is to find out the surgeon's preferences for suturing materials and techniques before a surgical procedure. As wound closure approaches, the field should be cleared of sponges and extraneous instruments to prepare for counts. The wound should be inspected for bleeders. Any bleeders should then be controlled. Overhead lights may need to be adjusted and retractors repositioned for better visibility. The FA and the surgeon should have a plan for who will tie knots and who will cut sutures.

When tying a suture that is being used only once, the FA will take the needle and its suture, tie the first knot with the correct tension, then rapidly throw on the additional knots. Both ends of the suture are then presented for cutting. The needle and remaining suture are then returned to the scrub person. The FA prepares to tie the next suture as the surgeon places the next suture into the tissues.

When several stitches are to be made with the same suture, the assistant grasps enough of the short end to tie rapidly and accurately. As the knot is being tied, the surgeon repositions the needle on the needleholder for the next stitch. The suture is cut, the short end is discarded, and the long end is retained as the process continues. When the suture becomes too short for convenient tying, another is requested.

At times, the FA may be required to help grasp the needle as it exits the tissue. The FA may first use the tip of an unopened needleholder to provide a downward counterforce on the tissue (usually skin) where the needle exits. As the needle exits and the surgeon pauses to readjust the needleholder, the FA should grasp the needle with the needleholder behind the point of the needle, rotating the needle 90 degrees through a natural curve. These measures will bring most of the needle above the skin surface. Some portion of the needle should remain below the skin surface; this measure provides a position of stability for the surgeon to regrasp it. As the surgeon pulls the needle through, the FA reaches for the suture as it emerges behind the needle, and prepares to throw the first knot. This procedure is known as the *needle fixation and presentation* technique.

Suturing Instruments

Needleholders (also referred to as "needle drivers"), tissue forceps, and suture scissors are the basic instruments needed for suturing. Through experience, the FA becomes familiar with the various needleholders and tissue forceps, and their uses. Repeated use of these instruments requires mastery of new technical skills.

Needleholders   Needleholders are similar to hemostats. Most needleholders are designed with ring handles and ratchet locks. Some of the delicate needleholders are designed like tissue forceps and have spring locks (Figure 6-9). The tips of needleholders are usually short and blunt, but some are designed with very fine, pointed tips. Needleholders are available in various lengths and sizes (Figure 6-10).

Selection of a needleholder is based on the depth of the area where the sutures will be placed and the size of the suture needle. Using a light, fine needleholder on a heavy suture needle could damage the instrument by springing the jaws or damaging the jaw inserts. If the needleholder is too fine, the needle may slip and

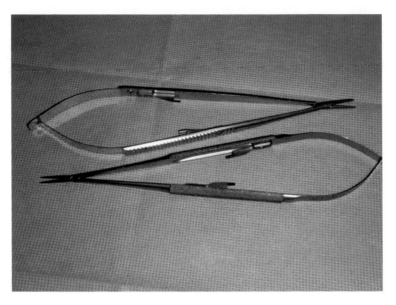

Figure 6-9

Castroviejo needleholder with spring lock.

Source: Photo courtesy of Winchester Hospital, Winchester, MA.

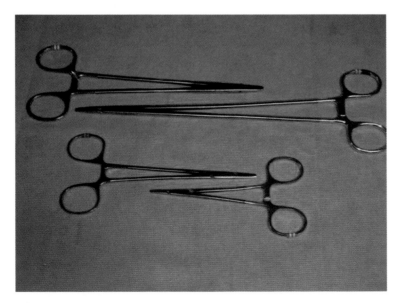

Figure 6-10

Examples of needleholders.

Source: Photo courtesy of Winchester Hospital, Winchester, MA.

cause tissue damage. Individual preference is another factor guiding selection, since there are numerous needleholders available. Needleholders are also available, usually by special order, for left-handed surgeons and FAs.

Needleholders must be inspected to insure that they function correctly. The jaws must hold the needle securely so that it will not slip as it is passed through the tissue. The jaw insert should be inspected for worn areas, and the security of the needle should be tested by gently attempting to move it with the fingers. The needleholder must open and close easily because too much resistance might result in inadvertent needle displacement in tissue.

Placement of the suture needle in the needleholder is important. The needle is grasped at a point approximately one-third to one-half the distance from the eye (or swaged) end (Figure 6-11). If the needle is grasped too close to the eye, it may bend as it is placed in the tissue. The needle may be placed at a right angle to the needleholder or at a slight angle (Figure 6-12). The needle is grasped at the tips of the needleholder jaws, and the needleholder is ratcheted one or two ratchets. If the needleholder tips are allowed to extend beyond the secured needle, they can interfere with suturing by pushing into the tissue. The needle can be damaged, notched, or bent if it is clamped too tightly in the jaws of the needleholder. If the needle is placed in the holder in the direction of use, it will not have to be repositioned.

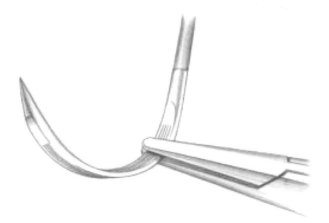

Figure 6-11

Needleholder with needle in correct position.

Source: Wound Closure Manual (2007). (Ch. 2, Fig. 9, p. 27) by ETHICON, 2007, Somerville, NJ: Johnson and Johnson. Copyright 2007, ETHICON, Inc. Reprinted with permission.

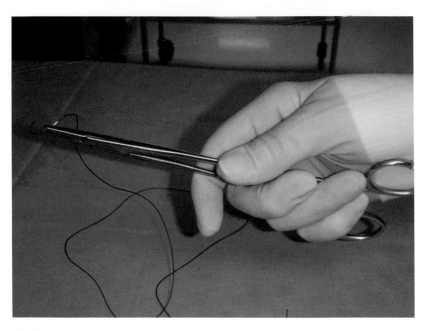

Figure 6-12

Needle slightly angled in needleholder.

Source: Photo courtesy of Winchester Hospital, Winchester, MA.

Needleholder Grips   The grip used on a needleholder depends on the amount of exertion required, the amount of control needed (i.e., delicate or firm), the location of the tissue being sutured, and the ease of suturing.

The *palmed grip* is used when suturing very dense tissue that is difficult to penetrate (e.g., the sternum). The needleholder is held in the palm of the hand and gripped on the shaft, close to the tip (Figure 6-13). This very secure grip is necessary when exerting a great deal of force on the needle. The direction of the needle is easily altered by rotating the needleholder in the hand. It is necessary to reposition the hand to release and reposition the needle.

The *thenar grip* is used for rapid, easy suturing. Precision is less exacting with this technique. The needleholder is grasped without inserting the thumb into the ring handle. The ball of the thumb (i.e., at its metacarpal joint) is pressed against the thumb ring of the needleholder for control. This position puts the needleholder in a direct line with the axis of the forearm and the motion of rotating the needleholder is simple and natural. It also provides the necessary leverage for opening and closing the needleholder (Figure 6-14). However, the sudden opening of the

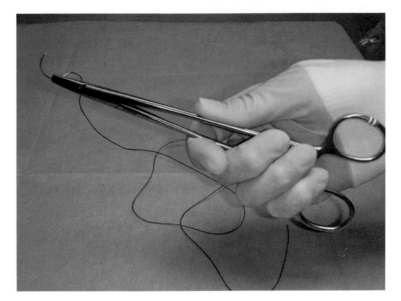

Figure 6-13

Palmed grip of needleholder.

Source: Photo courtesy of Winchester Hospital, Winchester, MA.

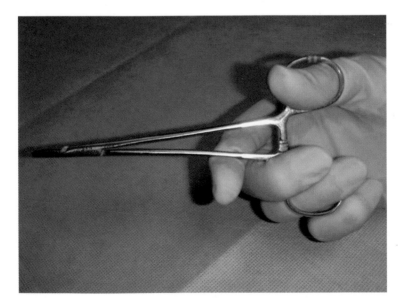

Figure 6-14

Thenar grip of needleholder.

Source: Photo courtesy of Winchester Hospital, Winchester, MA.

needleholder can cause movement of the suture needle, a potential problem that must be considered when using this technique.

The *thumb-ring finger grip* is the most traditional method of using a needleholder. This technique is more precise and affords easier control of the needle. Hand position does not have to be changed when opening and closing the needleholder (Figure 6-15).

The *pencil grip* is used for very fine, delicate needleholders that operate with a spring latch or are latchless. The spring latch can be closed and released with finger pressure. The needleholder is controlled by rotating it between the index finger and the thumb (Figure 6-16). However, rotation of the needleholder on its axis may require more complex movement of the hand, wrist and forearm.

Suture Scissors Suture scissors vary in length and size and may be straight or curved. Suture scissors must open and close smoothly. The blades must be sharp because dull or rough blades could snag the suture, causing it to be pulled loose, or possibly tear the tissue being sutured. The scissors are held in a position that

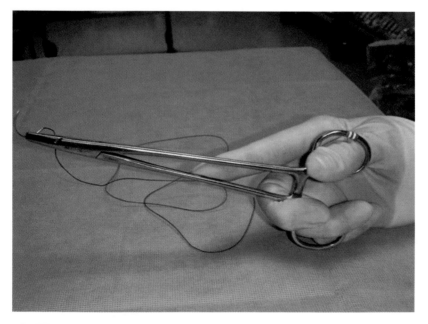

Figure 6-15

Thumb-ring finger grip of needleholder.

Source: Photo courtesy of Winchester Hospital, Winchester, MA.

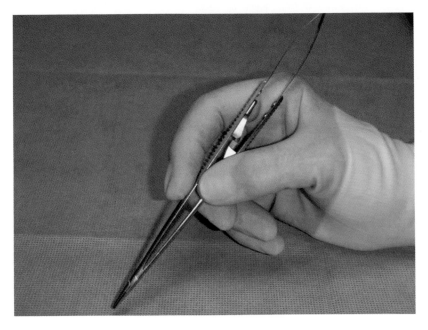

Figure 6-16

Pencil grip of needleholder.

Source: Photo courtesy of Winchester Hospital, Winchester, MA.

provides stability and control. The "tripod" position provides the best control. The thumb and ring finger are placed in the ring handles and the index finger is extended along the shaft of the scissor. The palm of the hand faces down. The position can be easily changed by rotating the wrist (Figure 6-17). When the FA must use the non-dominant hand for cutting sutures, a variation of the tripod position may be necessary (Box 6-1).

Good visualization is essential when cutting sutures. The suture knot must be in sight. The cutting distance can be estimated by looking through the opened scissor blades. Cutting with the tips of the scissors prevents inadvertent cutting of surrounding structures. Generally, the suture is cut as close to the knot as possible, but the length of the suture "tail" that is left is determined by the type of suture. Cutting the suture too short may decrease knot security. Additional support can be provided by resting the scissors hand against the other hand when cutting the suture. The suture is held taut as it is cut.

By anticipating the need to cut sutures, the FA can contribute to the efficiency of the operation. The FA should have the scissors ready when the suture is being tied. By observing and counting the number of throws the surgeon has placed, the astute FA will know when the suture is to be cut.

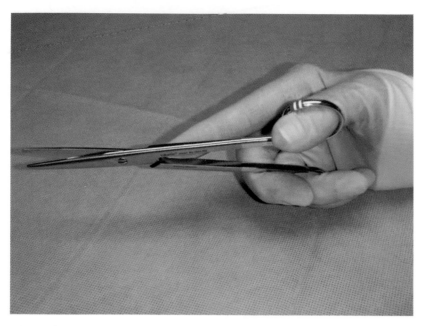

Figure 6-17

Position for using suture scissors.

Source: Photo courtesy of Winchester Hospital, Winchester, MA.

Box 6-1	Using Scissors in the Left Hand

There are occasions when a right-handed assistant will use the dominant hand to hold a retractor, making it necessary to use scissors to cut suture with the nondominant hand. Understanding the three interacting forces of cutting with scissors (closing, shearing and torque) helps the FA develop the right technique for use with a nondominant hand. Ordinarily, using the right hand (dominant hand), the assistant squeezes the rings of the scissors, transferring energy along the shanks of the scissors. This action ultimately results in the closing of the scissor blades. As the edge of one blade pushes flat against the other during closing, shearing occurs. During shearing, torque forces one blade edge against the other. These interacting forces act to cut either suture or tissue.

Allen recommends one of two techniques for using scissors in the left (nondominant) hand:

- Cut "flat": lay the scissors on the fingers and close the shanks without the fingers in the grips. Torque is created by the thumb pushing down on the grip; the fingers balance and stabilize the other blade.
- Pull with the thumb: use the scissors as one would in the dominant hand. With fingers in the grips, pull with the thumb as the shanks are squeezed together.

Source: Modified from Allen, G.J. (1999). The cutting edge: Using scissors in the left hand. *The Surgical Technologist*, January, 26–27.

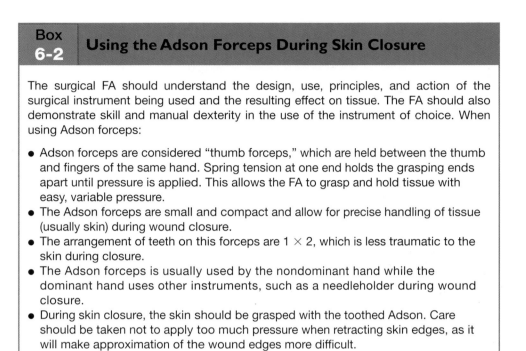

| Box 6-2 | Using the Adson Forceps During Skin Closure |

The surgical FA should understand the design, use, principles, and action of the surgical instrument being used and the resulting effect on tissue. The FA should also demonstrate skill and manual dexterity in the use of the instrument of choice. When using Adson forceps:

- Adson forceps are considered "thumb forceps," which are held between the thumb and fingers of the same hand. Spring tension at one end holds the grasping ends apart until pressure is applied. This allows the FA to grasp and hold tissue with easy, variable pressure.
- The Adson forceps are small and compact and allow for precise handling of tissue (usually skin) during wound closure.
- The arrangement of teeth on this forceps are 1 × 2, which is less traumatic to the skin during closure.
- The Adson forceps is usually used by the nondominant hand while the dominant hand uses other instruments, such as a needleholder during wound closure.
- During skin closure, the skin should be grasped with the toothed Adson. Care should be taken not to apply too much pressure when retracting skin edges, as it will make approximation of the wound edges more difficult.

Tissue Forceps   As with all surgical instruments, the FA must be familiar with the types of tissue forceps and their possible applications during the surgical procedure (Box 6-2). Tissue forceps are used in conjunction with the needleholder (for more information on forceps and their use, see Chapter 3, Tissue Handling and Chapter 4, Providing Exposure: Retractors and Retraction). Using the forceps in the opposite hand allows for tissue stabilization as well as providing exposure before the suture needle penetrates the tissue. The tissue must be handled gently to avoid unnecessary injury or trauma, which may interfere with healing. The forceps brace the tissue as the tip of the needle emerges on the exit side of the incision during closure. The teeth of the forceps should be set into the tissue only when necessary to avoid slippage. The tissue forceps can also be used to grasp and remove the suture needle after it has passed through the tissue. The forceps are then used to hold the needle while it is repositioned in the needleholder.

SUTURING TECHNIQUES

During suturing, cut tissues should be reapproximated to resume as near normal a position as possible. It is important to correctly identify the different tissue layers being sutured in order to reposition them properly. The width and depth of the stitch, choice of suture material, and needle type depend on the type of tissue

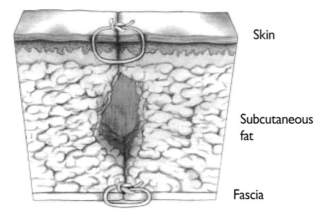

Skin

Subcutaneous fat

Fascia

Figure 6-18

Dead space in tissue.

Source: Modified from *Wound closure manual* (2007). (Ch. 1, Fig. 2, p. 5). Somerville, NJ: ETHICON, Inc. Reprinted with permission.

being sutured. Suturing provides support to tissues while they heal, so that gaps (or "dead space") will not delay healing (Figure 6-18). Dead space not only weakens the suture line, but it is also a potential site for collection of serum or blood, contributing to the risk of surgical site infection.

Whenever possible, the FA should sew toward himself or herself (Figure 6-19). This method is more comfortable and maximizes visibility. To begin suturing, the tissue is grasped with the forceps. With the hand in the prone position, the needle tip is inserted. The needle should enter a structure at a right angle to its surface. The hand is rotated at the wrist so that the needle is arced through the tissue. The tip of the needle should be readily accessible after it goes through the tissue. To withdraw the tip of a curved needle, the hand starts in a pronated position. The needle tip is withdrawn with the forceps or the needleholder and pulled through the tissue in a small arc that follows the needle's curve. During this maneuver, the hand turns 180 degrees to supination; this is a natural movement that involves only the forearm. Damage to the needle tip is avoided by grasping the needle on its body rather than on the tip itself. If the needle does not penetrate through the tissue, a larger needle is needed. The FA should not attempt to force the needle through because it may break. If the tissue layers are close together, both sides may be sutured with one placement of the needle. In many instances the suture needle is first passed through one side and then through the opposing side (Figure 6-20).

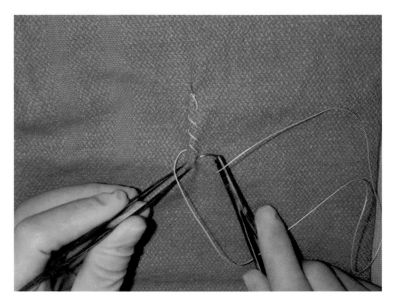

Figure 6-19

Suturing toward self.

Source: Photo courtesy of Winchester Hospital, Winchester, MA.

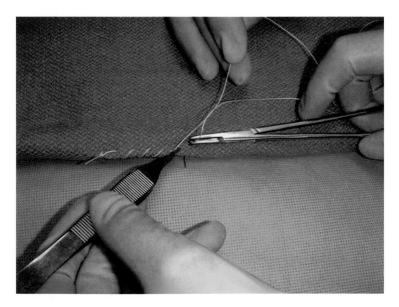

Figure 6-20

Placing suture in one side.

Source: Photo courtesy of Winchester Hospital, Winchester, MA.

Interrupted Sutures

Interrupted sutures are used when sutures will be under increased tension, such as for the bowel or for a fascial closure. Although this technique is somewhat slower than a continuous suture, it is safer if there is potential for the suture to break due to tension or tissue fragility. When the fascia is closed with interrupted sutures, late fascial dehiscence is usually less problematic than with a continuous suturing technique. Interrupted sutures also enable more precise approximation of tissues and thus are frequently used for plastic surgery, where minimal scarring is desired. When suturing with interrupted sutures, the FA must take care to avoid excessive tension on the tissue and must leave an adequate amount of suture on both sides for tying.

Continuous Sutures

In this faster suturing method, the FA pulls the suture through the tissue in one continuous motion after the needle passes through both sides of the wound. Care must be taken not to pull the suture too tight. If pulled too tight, the tissue can strangulate and possibly cause necrosis, or the suture may cut through the tissue. When a long, continuous suturing technique is used, the running suture may loosen, allowing the wound to gap in one area as the suture is being tightened at another. To prevent this problem, the suture should be followed by another assistant or oneself (**Figure 6-21**). To follow the suture oneself, the suture is grasped with the little finger in the hand holding the tissue forceps (**Figure 6-22**). This technique can be useful and easy to learn. (At times, a stapling device may be used instead of sutures. Key considerations in the safe use of stapling devices are presented in **Box 6-3**).

Following the suture for the surgeon using a continuous suture must be done carefully and correctly if it is to be effective. Direction and guidance from the surgeon during the operative procedure helps in learning this technique. The FA holds adequate tension on the suture to keep the tissue layers together without distorting or strangulating the tissues. Whenever possible, the suture is held from the exited side of the wound because there is less chance of tearing the tissue with the suture (see **Figure 6-21**). The suture should be held close enough to the wound to avoid shortening the suture length but not so close as to obstruct the placement of the needleholder and sutures. When releasing the suture, do not allow it to become entangled in drapes, instruments, or other sutures. Timing between the FA and the surgeon is important when releasing and grasping the suture. If tension is released prematurely, the suture line may loosen, resulting in poor approximation of the tissues, or the remaining suture may fall onto the suture site, obscuring the surgeon's view before he or she moves the needle to reload it.

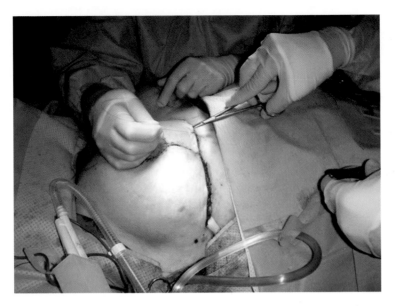

Figure 6-21

Technique for following surgeon's suture.

Source: Photo courtesy of Winchester Hospital, Winchester, MA.

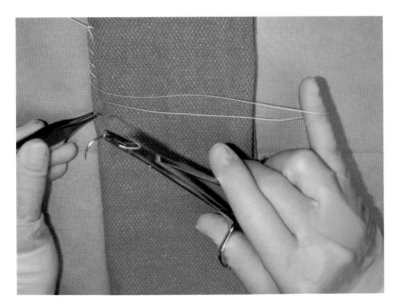

Figure 6-22

Following own suture.

Note: Suture is grasped by the little finger.

Source: Photo courtesy of Winchester Hospital, Winchester, MA.

Box 6-3	Stapler Safety and Helpful Hints for the FA

Often surgical staplers are used instead of or with conventional sutures during a surgical procedure. Staplers are designed and manufactured by several companies for use in laparoscopic and open procedures. Some staplers deliver staples and can also divide the tissues between the staple lines. These staplers are useful during procedures such as resection or anastomosis of bowel, stomach, lung, or blood vessels. It is imperative that surgical first assistants (FAs) be familiar with the products used in the facility where they practice to ensure safety during stapling.

- The FA should be knowledgeable about the choice of stapler and type of tissue that will be stapled or cut during each procedure.
- The FA should be familiar with open vs. laparoscopic staplers. Some staplers can be used in either open or laparoscopic procedures.
- The FA should inspect the integrity of the stapler.
- The FA should ensure there is a cartridge-reload in the device, as some staplers are not packaged with a staple load.
- The FA should be familiar with staple colors and their corresponding staple lengths. This knowledge is important because tissue has various thicknesses, and there are different reloads to accommodate the tissue appropriately. The FA should be familiar with how to load each stapler, how many reloads can be used before having to open a new device, and the steps for firing each stapler safely and effectively.
- The FA should be familiar with how to open and close each stapler on tissue.
- The FA should pass the stapler through the correct size trocar port and in a way that avoids firing the stapler unintentionally.
- The FA should be familiar with how to load buttressing tissue onto the device if necessary.
- The FA should visualize the stapling device ends before firing to minimize the chance of having to use another reload. At the same time, it is important not to overload the stapler.
- Before firing, the FA should ensure that only the tissue to be stapled and/or cut is in the jaws of the device. Ensure that the tissue is flat and not bunched, as this can result in a poor staple line and possible leakage at the staple line.
- Some devices are designed to compress tissue for better hemostasis. When using these devices, the tissue should usually be compressed and held for a period of time before firing.
- The FA should inspect the tissue's integrity and seal after the stapler has been fired and prior to closing.
- The FA should remove the used stapler cartridge and clean the jaws of the stapler by swishing the stapler jaws in sterile saline on the surgical field to clear the anvil of all staples after each use. Loose staples can become dislodged and have the potential to become tangled in future stapling, thus jeopardizing the seal of the staple line. They could also potentially catch on the knife blade as it is engaged, which could dull the cut through the tissue.

It may be necessary to grasp the suture with forceps rather than with fingers, for instance when the suture is too short to grasp with fingers or when the operative site is deep or restricted. When grasping the suture with forceps, the FA must not use a crushing type of forceps or grasp the suture too tightly. Damage to the suture could mean it will break immediately or weaken, causing it to break later.

Subcutaneous Sutures

Suturing subcutaneous tissue is often unnecessary. Unless there is a strong line of Scarpa's fascia running through the subcutaneous layer, this layer has little holding power. If the fascia and skin are closely approximated, the subcutaneous tissue is unlikely to have dead space. If it is necessary to close the subcutaneous layer, the suture used is usually absorbable. Sutures are placed vertically through the tissue from one side of the wound to the other. Horizontal sutures should not be used, as they can compromise the blood supply to the skin. Sutures must be placed close enough together to eliminate any gaps in the suture line. Tension on the sutures must be adequate to hold the tissue together, but must not be excessive, or the suture may pull through the tissue or strangulate the tissue itself.

Skin Sutures

The skin-suturing technique used in a procedure depends on the type of incision, its location, the patient's condition, the desired result, and the surgeon's or FAs preference. Suture materials used for the skin are nonabsorbable and must be removed postoperatively. Monofilament sutures are commonly used because they are less traumatic to the tissue. This type of suture is smooth and easier to remove. Braided materials may harbor infectious organisms and potentially cause superficial wound infection. More tissue reaction will occur with braided sutures. The suture selected should be as fine gauge as possible but still provide the necessary support to the skin edges as they are reapproximated.

Interrupted sutures provide a better cosmetic result as the wound heals. The simple interrupted suture technique is frequently used. Simple interrupted sutures are placed by entering the skin on one side of the wound edge and exiting on the other side. The entry and exit points are usually only a few millimeters from the incision site and should be approximately the same distance from the skin edges on each side to avoid distortion of the incision line. After the suture is tied, the knot is pulled to one side of the wound, close to the skin. This technique will adjust the tension and equalize the skin edges. Using simple interrupted suture results in a square-shaped suture that encloses an equal area of dermis on both sides and avoids inverting skin edges (**Figure 6-23**).

Mattress sutures may be needed when increased accuracy is necessary. Mattress sutures also provide more support to the suture line; such support may be needed in situations where there is increased strain on the suture line itself (see **Figure 6-23**). The horizontal mattress suture is more commonly used in fascia than on skin. The interrupted mattress suture is placed by entering and exiting the skin edges at a slightly greater distance than with the simple interrupted stitch. Once the first stitch is placed, the needle is passed back through the skin very close to the edges (approximately 2–5 millimeters) and then tied in place. Again, gentle loose tying to close the tissues allows for the slight edema that normally occurs during wound healing.

Continuous suture technique is frequently used on the skin because it can be done quickly, but the cosmetic result is not as good as with the interrupted techniques. To place the sutures, the FA begins on one side of the incision and exits on the other side at approximately the same distance from the skin edges on each side. The suture is tied, and the short end of the suture is cut. The suture is then used in a "running" fashion or in an "over and over" looping fashion until the wound is closed. A continuous mattress suturing technique can be used if needed (**Figure 6-24**).

Subcuticular suture technique provides an excellent cosmetic result, resulting in a very fine scar. Subcuticular sutures are most valuable for skin closure in parts of the body with a thick dermal layer or where skin is firmly attached to strong subdermal fascia. If the dermis is thin, subcuticular closure should be avoided. An absorbable suture is usually used; however, a nonabsorbable suture can be used and removed later. To remove the nonabsorbable suture, it is necessary to secure the ends of the suture at skin level, where they can be easily grasped for removal. Subcuticular stitches are placed in the lower part of the dermis. The first stitch is placed into the corner of the incision just below the dermal-epidermal junction. The stitches are placed in a horizontal fashion and alternated from one side to the other, with each stitch taking small epidermal bites. The stitches must be placed at the same depth on each side. If they are not, the wound will be uneven. When the suture line is completed, the suture is tightened by pulling the ends and an instrument tie completed on each end at skin level (**Figure 6-25**).

Skin staples are commonly used and are very versatile. The skin edges are everted and brought together with one or two tissue forceps (such as the Adson) as the

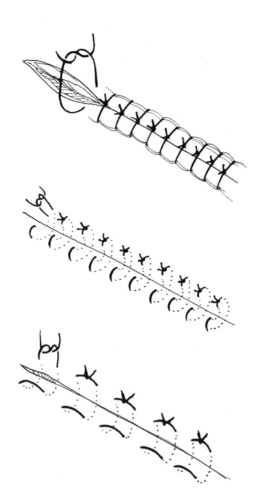

Figure 6-23

Interrupted skin suturing techniques. *Top to bottom:* Simple interrupted; Interrupted vertical mattress; and Interrupted horizontal mattress.

Source: Wound Closure Manual (2007). (Ch. 2, Fig. 3, p. 19) by ETHICON, 2007, Somerville, NJ: Johnson and Johnson. Copyright 2007, ETHICON, Inc. Reprinted with permission.

staple is applied. Staples cause minimal tissue trauma or compression and provide a superior cosmetic result when compared to continuous or interrupted skin sutures (Figure 6-26).

Skin adhesives can be used to glue the skin edges together when the wound edges can be closely approximated. They cannot be used if there is evidence of infection or if there is too much tension on the wound edges. This is a more rapid skin closure technique than suturing or stapling. If the patient is at high risk for poor healing (e.g., diabetic), a skin adhesive should not be used (Forsch, 2008).

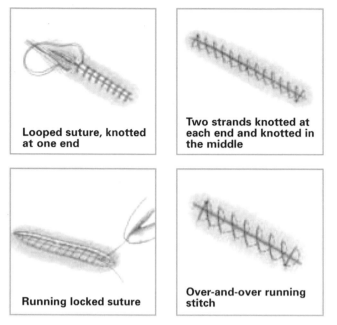

Looped suture, knotted at one end

Two strands knotted at each end and knotted in the middle

Running locked suture

Over-and-over running stitch

Figure 6-24

Continuous skin suturing techniques.

Source: Wound Closure Manual (2007). (Ch. 2, Fig. 2, p. 19) by ETHICON, 2007, Somerville, NJ: Johnson and Johnson. Copyright 2007, ETHICON, Inc. Reprinted with permission.

Figure 6-25

Subcutaneous suturing.

Source: Wound Closure Manual (2007). (Ch. 2, Fig. 6, p. 23) by ETHICON, 2007, Somerville, NJ: Johnson and Johnson. Copyright 2007, ETHICON, Inc. Reprinted with permission.

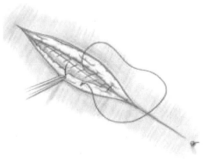

Adhesive tapes can be used for skin closure of the incision. They can be used to complement staples or suture closures but cannot be used in the presence of infection or where there is too much tension on the wound edges. When one is placing tapes, the wound edges should not be brought together by pulling on the tape. The

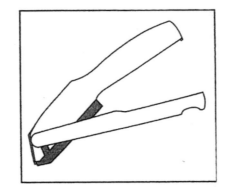

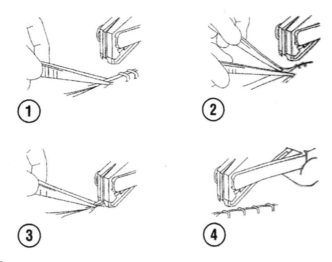

Figure 6-26

Procedure for applying skin staples using Proximate stapler.

Evert and approximate skin edges using either 1. one tissue forceps to pull skin edges together, or 2. two tissue forceps to pick up each wound edge individually and approximate the edges. 3. Align the arrow on the tip of the stapler with the incision. 4. Squeeze the trigger until the trigger motion stops. Release the trigger and remove the stapler from the fired staple.

wound edges should be placed side by side or in close proximity, using fingers or forceps.

Repairing Skin Lacerations The goals of this type of repair are to achieve hemostasis, avoid infection, restore function, and achieve optimal cosmetic effect. Wound assessment includes evaluating injury to muscle, tendons, nerves, bone, and blood vessels. Bleeding is controlled initially by direct pressure. The patient's history includes cause and time of injury and health information such as diabetes, HIV, allergies, and status of tetanus immunization. The wound is irrigated with saline or sterile water. Suturing is the preferred method to repair a skin laceration. The horizontal mattress technique is used for gaping or high-tension wounds or if the skin is fragile. The vertical mattress technique is used if the skin edges tend to invert. A continuous suturing technique can be used for long low-tension wounds. Tissue adhesives and adhesive strips may be used for selected low-tension wounds. Skin staples can be use for selected high-tension wounds or if the dermis is thick (e.g., the back or scalp) (Forsch, 2008).

Regardless of the type of skin-suturing technique used, some basic principles must be followed.

- Bleeding can distort the wound, disrupt the suture line, and create hematomas that may result in a potential for infection;
- Before the first bite of the needle is made, the wrist should be presupinated to cock the hand in a position that provides strength for driving the needle through the skin;
- Sutures are placed with as little trauma as possible;
- Tissue is handled carefully and gently, and crushing injury is avoided;
- Sutures are never pulled too tight because tissue can become strangulated and the blood supply compromised. Sutures should only be tight enough to hold opposing tissues together. Tissue edema in the postoperative period can increase the pressure of tissue against the sutures, resulting in hatch-mark scarring; this problem can be avoided by leaving sutures slightly loose when placed. To achieve this, the FA notes when the skin edges first make contact and the skin rises just slightly above the surrounding skin surface. This indication shows that there is the right amount of tension at the suture line and the knot can then be set;
- Skin edges are slightly everted as they are reapproximated; this results in better healing and a better-looking scar; and
- The skin edges are re-aligned as closely as possible to their original alignment.

Considerations During Laparoscopy

Laparoscopic surgical procedures raise additional considerations for the FA. Laparoscopic expertise in suturing and tying knots requires technical skills similar to, yet different from, open procedures. Both require competence and dexterity developed from repetitive practice over time. Fundamentals of Laparoscopic Surgery (FLS) programs are available to develop laparoscopic skills using box trainers (information on the FLS program may be found in Chapter 13, Resources). The FA should use these tools to hone laparoscopic suturing skills before assisting in laparoscopic surgical procedures. Box 6-4

Box 6-4	Key Points when Suturing or Tying Knots During Laparoscopic Procedures

There are numerous suture choices available for laparoscopic suturing as well as products which can be applied to the end of a suture to mimic a knot during a laparoscopic procedure. FAs should familiarize themselves with available products.

Assisting the Surgeon During Laparoscopic Suturing

- The FA can apply countertraction to the tissue being sutured using a laparoscopic grasper. This technique facilitates the ease of the suture passing through the tissue. Both hands of the surgeon are then free so he/she can grasp the needle using the laparoscopic instrument of choice.
- Holding the tissue or anatomical structure in close proximity to the area being sutured prevents too much tension on the anatomical structure when tying. This technique can also assist in preventing any slippage with the knot as it is being tied and secured.
- Endograspers may be utilized to hold running suture during closure (Figure 6-27).

Laparoscopic Suturing

- The FA should have clear visualization of all anatomical structures when suturing.
- The FA may sometimes need to pass the suture through one layer of tissue and then visualize the needle tip to ensure the needle has passed through the tissue layer safely. Then he or she can pass it through the other layer.
- Countertraction makes it easier to pass the needle through tissue.
- Grasping the middle of the needle prevents dulling of the needle tip.
- Passing the suture through the tissue should be accomplished with one fluid motion.

Assisting the Surgeon During Laparoscopic Tying

- The FA retracts surrounding structures to assist the surgeon and prevent entanglement of the suture material.
- The FA may need to hold the tissue which has been sutured to relieve tension during knot tying.
- When the suture is cut, the tips of the endoscopic scissors should be visible (Figure 6-28).

(continued)

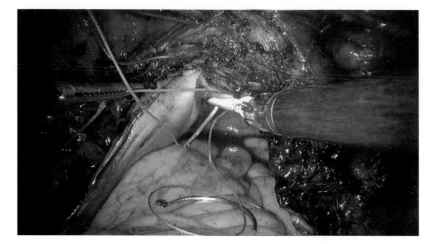

Figure 6-27

Holding running suture during laparoscopic surgery.

Note: Retracting suture during vaginal cuff repair: FA, noted using the endograsper to the left middle of photo, grasps and holds the running suture during an endoscopic robotic-assisted vaginal cuff closure. Note how the FA is using the endoscopic grasper effectively without interfering with the surgeon's visibility of the patient's anatomy. To prevent fraying, the FA grasps the suture using the end of the instrument tips.The FA places enough tension to retract tissue and the running suture without putting undo stress on the tissue or suture material. Endoscopic needle drivers could also be used.

Source: Photo courtesy of Winchester Hospital, Winchester, MA.

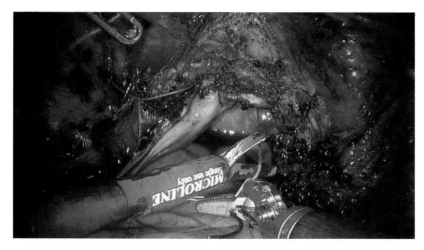

Figure 6-28

Cutting suture during laparoscopic surgery.

Note: When using the endoscopic scissors to cut suture intraoperatively, the FA should have both scissors tips visible and pointing upward. Clear visibility of all surrounding structures should be noted by the FA to ensure safety before cutting suture. The FA should confirm length of "tail" to be left with surgeon.

Source: Photo courtesy of Winchester Hospital, Winchester, MA.

Laparoscopic Knot Tying

- To secure the first throw, a surgeon's knot is used. A double wrap throw around the tip of the endoscopic needle driver is used to make the knot on the first throw. A Maryland laparoscopic grasper or another laparoscopic needle driver is recommended in the nondominant hand.
- It's easier to grasp and tie the knot if the "tail" of the other end of the suture is small in length; approximately 2 to 3 cm.
- Once the initial double throw is complete, the FA grasps the tail and pulls with even tension to secure the initial tie. It is easier to bring both needle drivers over to the "tail" end when grasping it to make another tie throw, as opposed to the tying procedure used during open surgery, in which the needle drivers would be pulled in opposite directions. This technique allows the FA to have better control over the suture material and decreases stress on the suture material.
- Once the first double throw is complete, several additional square knot throws are performed. The number of additional throws will depend on the suture material being used and the surgeon's preference.

outlines considerations for the FA to facilitate suturing and tying during laparoscopic surgery.

PREVENTING PERCUTANEOUS INJURY

Blood-borne diseases such as HIV, viral hepatitis B, viral hepatitis C, and bacterial infections can be transmitted to members of the surgical team through percutaneous injury. It has been estimated that over 384,000 percutaneous injuries occur annually among health care workers in the United States (Hotaling, 2009). In the perioperative setting, these injuries frequently occur to surgeons and first assistants, and suture needles are frequently cited as the common cause. Often, percutaneous injuries from suture needles are self-inflicted and can occur during the following events:

- loading or repositioning the needle on the needle holder;
- passing sutures between the scrub personnel and the surgeon or the FA;
- suturing, especially of muscle and fascia, or when the needle is being manipulated or guided with the fingers;
- retracting or stretching tissue with the hands;
- suturing when the surgeon sews toward his own hand or the assistant's hand; and
- tying the suture with the needle still attached.

Leaving a used suture needle unattended on the operative field or placing the needle in an overfilled sharps container heightens the risk of percutaneous injuries (AORN, 2009a; DHHS-NIOSH, 2008). The FA should avoid handling suture needles with the fingers and develop skills to manipulate the needle with a forceps and/or the needleholder.

Strategies for prevention of percutaneous injury include double gloving, blunt tip suture needles, hands-free technique, counting procedures, proper use of sharps containers, and effective teamwork.

Double gloving reduces the risk of exposure to the patient's blood due to glove tears or punctures, especially from suture needles. Both the American College of Surgeons (ACS) in its Statement on Sharps Safety (ACS, 2007) and the Association of periOperative Registered Nurses (AORN) in its Recommended Practice: Prevention of Transmissible Infections in the Perioperative Setting (AORN, 2009b) recommend the double-glove technique in order to reduce the risk of body fluid exposure. Although more overt tears and holes in gloves may be easier to detect, punctures from suture needles often go undetected. The use of puncture-proof or puncture-resistant gloves provides the same protection as double gloving. Wearing cloth outer gloves reduces punctures of the inner glove during orthopedic procedures (AORN, 2009b). Tactile sensation is reduced by double gloving or wearing heavier gloves, and it may be difficult to use these techniques in extremely delicate operative procedures. It is important to periodically check gloves for tears, holes and punctures before, during and after all procedures.

Blunt tip suture needles are available in a variety of suture materials and sizes that are used primarily for fascia and muscle suturing. The Department of Health and Human Services, NIOSH, Occupational Safety and Health Administration (OSHA), the ACS, and AORN all recommend the use of blunt tip suture needles on less-dense tissue such as fascia and muscle (DHHS/NIOSH, 2008; ACS, 2005; AORN, 2009a). The ACS Statement on Sharps Safety reports that the use of blunt tip suture needles reduces the number of sharps injuries from 38% to 6% or lower (ACS, 2007). As the technology for making blunt tip suture needles expands, the use of these needles on other tissues will become more common.

Hands-free technique (HFT) or use of a neutral zone can also reduce the risk of sharps injury during surgery. A specific area is designated as a neutral zone (e.g., a basin, a magnetic pad, etc.) where sharp items such as needles and scalpels are placed by the scrub person, surgeon and FA before and after use. Direct hand-to-hand passing of these items is avoided and the risk of injury is decreased. There should be verbal acknowledgement whenever sharps are being moved to and from the operative field. The HFT should be used, except in situations when the surgeon and/or FA must stay focused on the operative field for the safety of the operation. A partial HFT, in which the scrub person hands the sharp item directly to the surgeon and/or FAs hand and the sharp is returned to the scrub person by using the neutral zone, may be used in these situations (ACS, 2007; AORN, 2009c).

Counts of instruments, sponges, sharps, and other items that could be left behind in the patient are performed before starting the operation, before closing a cavity within a cavity, before wound closure, at the end of the operative procedure, and whenever there is permanent relief of either the scrub person or circulating nurse. AORN's Recommended Practice for Sponge, Sharp, and Instrument Counts (AORN, 2009c) provides detailed guidance on these procedures. Counting policies are established by the institution, and the FA must know and comply with these policies. All members of the surgical team have a collaborative duty to account for these items during the operative procedure.

Suture needles are frequently miscounted (Cima, 2008). There is disagreement regarding the need to count 17-mm and smaller needles because they cannot always be radiologically visualized (Giarrizzo-Wilson & Burlingame, 2008). AORN recommends that all needles should be counted in order to provide for safe patient care and a safe work environment (AORN, 2009c). Whenever the FA uses suturing materials, it is important to continually account for their location and to return used sutures and needles to the scrub person via the neutral zone. This continuous accounting for needles during the operative procedure is essential, and assures that all needles are retrieved.

Count discrepancies can occur. The accuracy of the counting process can be affected by the complexity of the surgery, whether the surgery is an emergent or urgent procedure, or the surgical team is fatigued or overworked (Egorova et al., 2008). Other factors to consider are unexpected changes in procedures as well as patient obesity. It is the responsibility of the surgical team to carry out all necessary steps to locate a missing item. Intraoperative x-ray may be indicated. Any and all count discrepancies must be documented (AORN, 2009c).

Sharps containers are mandatory for the proper disposal of needles and scalpel blades used during the operative procedure. Proper placement of these items in the container is essential. Many needlestick injuries occur when placing items in these containers due to inappropriate placement and design of the container and overfilling. A "letter-drop" style of container, as opposed to the "straight-drop," may help to decrease needlestick injuries (Hatcher, 2002).

Teamwork is an essential part of every operative procedure. John Monighan advocates that "operations should flow with a style and natural pace, rather like a well choreographed dance" (Oram, 2006, p. 61). All team members must be able to communicate and work together effectively. It is important to acknowledge and respect the contribution of all team members. The FA must recognize when it is necessary to clarify expectations. "Mind reading" is not a requirement of the FA position; the surgeon must communicate with the FA, and the FA must be willing to ask for direction. The FA must question or clarify the progress of the operative procedure with the appropriate team member/members. A successful outcome for the patient depends upon all team members working together. Improved teamwork and communication may have beneficial effects on both technical performance and patient outcomes (Catchpole, Mishra, Handa, & McCulloch, 2008).

Continual communication between all team members decreases the possibility of error or an untoward outcome for the patient. When the FA is relieved by another FA, the hand-off should include all pertinent information regarding the patient (i.e., condition, allergies, and medical history), the status of the procedure, all anticipated events, possible complications discussed during the preop briefing, and expectations regarding the operative procedure.

CONCLUSION

Regardless of the suturing material and method used, the FAs goal during any suturing activity is to achieve a wound that heals without complications. To achieve this goal, the FA makes educated choices about the type of suture material, suturing instruments, and suturing technique. Coupled with these cognitive abilities, the FA must be proficient in the manipulative skills of suturing. This combination of intellectual and manual dexterity results in effective and efficient patient care. Given that the FA is using sharp suture needles, the regular and thoughtful application of research findings in preventing percutaneous injury to self or other members of the surgical team is crucial.

REFERENCES

1. American College of Surgeons. (2005). [ST-52] Statement on blunt suture needles. Retrieved February 24, 2009 from www. facs.org/fellows_info/statements/st-52.html

2. American College of Surgeons. (2007). Statement on sharps safety. *Bulletin of the American College of Surgeons, 92*(10). Also available at www.facs.org/fellows_info/statements/st-58.html

3. Association of periOperative Registered Nurses (AORN). (2009a). AORN guidance statement: Sharps injury prevention in the perioperative setting. *2009 Perioperative standards and recommended practices* (pp. 275–280). Denver, CO: AORN.

4. Association of periOperative Registered Nurses (AORN). (2009b). Recommended practices for prevention of transmissible

infections in the perioperative setting. *2009 Perioperative standards and recommended practices* (pp. 475–485). Denver, CO: AORN.

5. Association of periOperative Registered Nurses (AORN). (2009c). Recommended practices for sponge, sharp, and instrument counts. *2009 Perioperative standards and recommended practices* (pp. 405–414). Denver, CO: AORN.

6. Catchpole, K., Mishra, A., Handa, A., & McCulloch, P. (2008). Teamwork and error in the operating room; analysis of skills and roles. *Annals of Surgery, 247*(4), 699–706.

7. Cima, R.R., Kollengode, A., Gartner, J., et al. (2008). Incidence and characteristics of potential and actual retained foreign object events in surgical patients. *Journal of the American College of Surgeons, 207*, 80–87.

8. Clinical Rounds. (2007). Keeping patients in stitches. *Nursing, 37*(5), 34.

9. Council on Surgical and Perioperative Safety (2007). The CSPS endorses that all measures to prevent sharps injuries will be used, inclusive of: Double-gloving, use of blunt suture needles, hands-free technique or neutral zone, and the universal adoption of all sharps safety measures in perioperative care is recommended. (Adopted 07.15.07) Retrieved February 5, 2009 from www.cspsteam.org/information/information1.html

10. Department of Health and Human Services (DHHS) and National Institute for Occupational Safety and Health (NIOSH) (2008). Use of blunt-tip suture needles to decrease percutaneous injuries to surgical personnel (DHHS/NIOSH Publication No.2008-132). Washington, DC: U.S. Government Printing Office.

11. Egorova, N., Moskowitz, A., Gelijns, A., Weinberg, A., Curty, J., Rabin-Fastman, B., et al. (2008). Managing the prevention of retained surgical instruments; what is the value of counting? *Annals of Surgery, 247*(1), 13–18.

12. Food and Drug Administration (FDA) (2003). Guidance for industry and FDA staff: Class II special controls guidance document: Surgical sutures; guidance for industry and FDA. Food and Drug Administration. Rockville, MD: FDA.

13. Forsch, R.T. (2008). Essentials of skin laceration repair. *American Family Physician. 78(8), 945–951.*

14. Giarrizzo-Wilson, S., & Burlingame, B. (2008). Counting small needles. *AORN Journal, 87*(6), 1231.

15. Hatcher, I. (2002). Reducing sharps injuries among health care workers: A sharps container quality improvement project. *The Joint Commission Journal,* July, 410–414.

16. Hotaling, M. (2009). A retractable winged steel (Butterfly) needle performance improvement project. *The Joint Commission Journal on Quality and Patient Safety, 35*(2), 100–105.

17. Maxwell, J.J. (2008). Tips for the student surgical technologist. *Association of Surgical Technologists Student Association News, 15*(4), page 3.

18. Martin, D., & Williams, S. (2003). Medical applications of poly-4-hydroxy-butyrate: A strong flexible absorbable biomaterial. *Biochemical Engineering Journal, 16,* 97–105.

19. NIOSH (2008). Use of blunt-tip suture needles to decrease percutaneous injuries to surgical personnel: Safety and health information bulletin: Publication No. 2008-101. Retrieved February 5, 2009 from www.cdc.gov/niosh/docs/2008-101/default.html

20. Nundy S., Mukherjee, A., Sexton, J.B, Pronovost, P.J., Knight, A., Rowen, L.C., et al. (2008). Impact of preoperative briefings on operating room delays. *Archives of Surgery 143*(11), 1068–1072.

21. Oram, D. (2006). Basic surgical skills. *Best Practice & Research Clinical Obstetrics and Gynaecology, 20*(1), 61–71.

22. *Quill SRS Techniques and Procedures: A Novel Approach to Soft Tissue approximation* (copyright *2008)*. Vancouver, BC: Angiotech Pharmaceuticals, Inc.

23. Rothrock, J.C. (2007). *Alexander's care of the patient in surgery* (13 ed.). St. Louis: Mosby Elsevier.

24. Texas Hospital Association (2008). Color-coded wristband standardization project. Retrieved January 5, 2009 from www.texashospitalsonline/org/Wristband/index.asp

25. Woo, E. (2008). Speak up about patient allergies. *Nursing, 38*(10), 13.

26. *Wound closure manual* (2007). Somerville, NJ. ETHICON, Inc, a Johnson and Johnson Company.

The Assessment and Diagnostic Process

Robert M. Blumm

There is an organized process by which the history and physical examination (H&P) and other assessment data contribute to the identification of a diagnosis. The word *process* also indicates a procedure that utilizes the points under discussion every time the clinician examines a patient (Figure 7-1). There is a beginning to this type of patient encounter, and there is a conclusion. A process implies that we will utilize the same steps, in the same sequence, regardless of the patient's demographic variables. The goal of using a process is to avert errors that can possibly harm the patient and to inform the other members of the surgical team about conditions that require special consideration in the perioperative period. Regardless of one's clinical title, this approach has been tested and will provide the first assistant (FA), surgeon, anesthesia provider, and nursing staff with essential personalized patient information.

PATIENT ADMISSION

The patient's admission to a health care facility begins with an assessment of the patient's status. The initial assessment may be brief (major problem, airway, hemodynamic status, level of consciousness). As more is learned about the patient, the new information is integrated into the patient's record and directs the clinician to more and more specific questions about the nature of the patient's problem. An admission note will include as much of the following information as available:

- Patient identification, date, and time
- Admission note (e.g., problem causing patient to seek care)
- Medical record/computer number
- Condition on admission

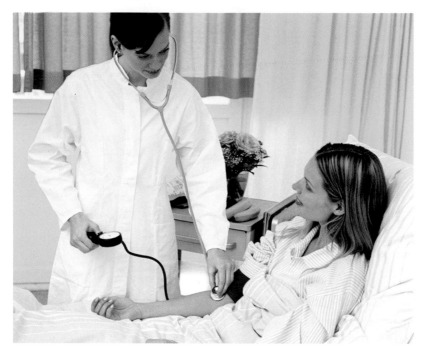

Figure 7-1

Taking the blood pressure.

Source: Courtesy of Phippen, M.L., Ulmer, B.C., & Wells, M.P. (2009). *Competency for safe patient care during operative and invasive procedures* (Chapter 18, p. 533). Denver: CCI.

- Preliminary diagnosis
- Vital signs (when taken?)
- Labs, special procedures indicated (e.g., x-ray films, ECG)
- Medications the patient is currently taking
- Diet (nothing by mouth [NPO]?)
- Oxygen requirement

In categorizing and organizing information, the clinician may use the *SOAP* format to document what is important to the patient's situation:

- S (subjective): How does the patient describe the condition in his/her own words?
- O (objective data): Refers to the physical examination, lab results, radiology, pathology, or results of other diagnostic studies.
- A (assessment): Includes a summary of the patient's condition, progress, or problems. If there are additional problems such as chronic obstructive

pulmonary disease (COPD), hypertension, or infection, each problem is separately numbered.

- P (plan): Based upon the findings and returned studies, what is the plan for this patient? Will medications be altered, changed, or eliminated? Will additional consultations be required? Should this patient remain on the present unit or be transferred? What about diet, intravenous lines, ambulation, sleep medications, and pain control?

Although only preliminary information will be available on admission, use of the SOAP format enables the clinician to organize data collection in a way that will result in a diagnosis and subsequent plan of care.

PATIENT HISTORY

The H&P can be thought of as a three-dimensional model. To define this approach, the FA can view one's responsibilities as a diagnostic workup, a preoperative evaluation, and a preoperative preparation (Way & Dougherty, 2006). It is essential that the clinician understand that the H&P is more than an obligatory document, but that it is a detailed and accurate communication between clinician and patient that involves the utilization of all five senses. The major focus is on the combined ability to listen and observe. We listen to acquire information that is translated by the patient's own words, and for this reason certain comments or responses should be placed in quotation marks. The process is akin to a medical autobiography, and the patient must be comfortable, approached in a warm and understanding manner, and given privacy (Sveitland & Cook, 2003). The appropriate approach is that of a detective who makes decisions or builds a case based upon a careful understanding of the comments of the person who is speaking. The medical professional speaks to the patient in a warm and friendly manner, demonstrating concern for the patient's history and chief complaint. The history should be conversational, and each question should be meaningful and directed toward obtaining specific information.

Whether as Physician Assistants (PA), Registered Nurse First Assistants (RNFA), Advanced Practice Registered Nurses (APRN), or another member of a professional group serving as an FA, we have acquired a medical vocabulary to communicate patient care concerns, but it is important to realize that the patient often is not aware of medical terminology and may be confused when clinicians use medical slang. The communication style should employ the language of the patient. If the patient cannot understand English, it becomes the reviewer's responsibility to use the proper system and have an interpreter present to assist us. Barbara Bates,

M.D., well known for her books on physical examination and history taking, was one of the first to suggest that the interviewer facilitate the patient's understanding with gestures or acknowledgements (Bates, Bickley, & Hoekelman, 1995; Bickley, 2008). One should maintain eye contact with the patient while writing scant notes that can be expanded after completion of the H&P. Other concepts include reflection, clarification if the response is confusing, empathetic responses, and asking patients how they feel about certain aspects of their history (Bickley, 2008).

Epstein and colleagues (2008) note that between 30% and 80% of patients' expectations are not met during routine primary care visits due to the physician's lack of awareness of the patient's worries, limited time for patients to express worries, limited involvement of patients in decision making, and rare expressions of empathy with the patient. As a result, patient compliance with recommended treatment may be poor. Epstein et al. (2008) stress that patient-centered communication succeeds when patients can discuss their true concerns and address their concerns in the order of priority—as identified by the patient. In other words, the first issue raised by a patient may not be the issue of greatest clinical importance. The authors' recommendations to allow patients to identify concerns, freely ask questions, seek clarification, and participate in decision making are pertinent to the FA engaging in preliminary and subsequent patient interactions.

The kind of interaction espoused by Epstein et al. (2008) may not suit all situations, such as those requiring emergency surgery. Surgery is defined commonly as *elective* or *emergent*, and this categorization affects the approach to the patient. Elective surgery is often patient-initiated or is a surgery of convenience. Elective surgery can be initiated by consulting physicians when they are either unsure of the diagnosis or when the procedure is not within their scope of practice. For example, a neurologist would not make a decision about a surgical procedure requiring the skills of a neurosurgeon but would refer to the appropriate surgeon. Some procedures are usually elective in nature (e.g., breast biopsy or inguinal hernia repair). Elective patients require certain examinations, laboratory tests, radiological and other diagnostic imaging studies, and confirmation of proper consent by the patient or guardian. This information contributes to the formulation of one or more diagnoses.

Emergency surgery may be associated with trauma or intestinal obstruction, subdural bleeding, or collapse of a lung; these conditions can be immediately life-threatening and require prompt treatment. The examination is therefore dictated by the condition of the patient and the patient's ability to understand and comply with the procedure. In an emergency, the history may be limited to one sentence, or there may be no history if the patient is unconscious and unaccompanied

(Dunphy, 2006). Elective patients are evaluated with a full history and physical examination, whereas emergent patients receive a focused examination. The initial assessment may be limited to the "ABCs": airway, breathing, and circulation.

Two common types of histories are those that are performed by nursing personnel (RNFA, APRN), and those performed by physicians and PAs. Often the history performed by an RNFA or APRN (e.g., nurse practitioner [NP]) incorporates an expanded assessment that includes psychosocial information that is helpful to other clinicians involved in the patient's care. The medical model physical exam is somewhat focused on systems that are important. However, it may lack a psychological or mental health assessment in addition to general observations related to diet, lifestyle, activity level, and other factors that are helpful to nursing staff as well as providers from other departments (e.g., physical therapy, occupational therapy, rehabilitation, radiology, chaplaincy services, social work, and discharge planners).

The history performed in the medical model used by a PA (Labus, 1998; Labus, 2004; Seidel et al., 2006) includes the following components:

- Patient identification
- Chief complaint (CC): the reason for medical attention in the patient's own words
- Present problem
- Past medical history: immunizations, serious injuries, medications, allergies, past surgery, anesthesia or transfusion reactions, prior hospitalization
- Past family history
- Personal and social history
- Review of systems (ROS)

The approach often used in the Nursing Model (Allen et al., 2007; Cundy, 2004; Goldman, 2008; Weber, 2007) includes:

- Identification and biographical data (patient name, identification number, date of visit, date of birth, age, sex, race, language, religion, occupation, and marital status)
- Allergies
- Chief complaint
- Symptoms: severity, duration, location, aggravating factors, relieving factors
- Current medications (prescription, over-the-counter, herbal)
- Medical history (including responses to previous treatments)

- History of present illness
- Childhood illnesses
- Previous hospitalizations
- Health problems
- Emergency contact list
- Obstetrical (OB) history
- Psychosocial history
- Feelings of safety
- Religious and cultural observances
- Activities of daily living
- Health maintenance history
- Family medical history
- Review of systems

There are a number of textbooks that help one to formulate a systematic approach to the patient for the H&P. Utilizing a consistent and systematic approach to the patient H&P will increase competency. Clinicians who are overworked, overburdened, distracted, understaffed, or attempting to perform too many tasks may increase the risk of error. Studies by the Institute of Medicine (Kohn, Corrigan, & Donaldson, 2000) revealed that over 100,000 patients may die annually in hospitals throughout the United States and over four million patients may suffer an adverse situation because of iatrogenic causes. Clinicians can help to reduce these statistics by using a systematic approach that evaluates both expected and unexpected findings and communicates them clearly and concisely to patient care colleagues (Seidel et al., 2006). For example, it is important to note the patient's use of a hearing aid and document the person's hearing impairment. If a person cannot hear properly, directions may not be followed properly. Similarly if a patient wears strong prescription glasses, it is important to note visual deficits in the record so that current and subsequent caregivers can plan for additional resources to enhance vision.

Additionally, the clinician should be aware of age-specific differences. Patients of different ages will have special needs related to growth and development, motor/sensory function, psychodynamic needs, cognitive development, education, pain, and physiologic changes (D'Alfonso, 2006).

OBTAINING THE HISTORY

Obtaining the history is a complex process. Spoken and unspoken cues include body language and interpretation along with communication skills that work interdependently to produce the desired information. The history does not start off with the patient but with the clinician's own personal hygiene, fresh attire, clean equipment (e.g., sanitized stethoscope), and a positive mental attitude. Because much of the physical exam requires being close to and physically touching the patient, personal cleanliness is important. Hair and nails should be impeccably clean with the nails cut properly to assist in palpation and auscultation.

Before greeting the elective patient, the FA should review the available medical records and become familiar with the patient: age, presenting complaint, recorded history, and any other essential information that may have been documented by the primary care provider. Reviewing the nursing notes is valuable for noting certain essentials (such as sensory impairments) that will help the FA to communicate or to establish two-way dialogue.

Other essential information includes laboratory tests and imaging studies (Dorsey, 2009). Appendix I and Appendix II outline common tests that may be ordered before surgery. The FA should review the test results and integrate them into the examination. Additional tests may be recommended after the patient's examination, based on the findings of the H&P.

Another source of essential information is the patient's medication history. The Joint Commission (TJC, 2006, 2009) requires that a list of medications taken by the patient at home, including complementary and alternative drugs (Barclay & Murata, 2008), be available. Although at this time TJC (2009) is reviewing and refining the medication reconciliation standard, medication reconciliation remains an important patient safety consideration. Table 7-1 provides information useful to the medication reconciliation process. Figure 7-2 shows a Medication Reconciliation form used in the author's facility.

Additional medication-related safety risks include the use of abbreviations that may be misread or misunderstood, and the misnaming of medications that have names that sound like other drugs. Table 7-2 lists Do-Not-Use Abbreviations from The Joint Commission (2009); avoiding these abbreviations can reduce prescribing and administration errors. Table 7-3 lists some examples of "look-alike sound-alike" drugs.

After reviewing the patient's record and test results (and before entering the patient's room or preoperative area), the FA should sanitize the hands to minimize the transfer of bacteria. The FA should enter the patient's room or preoperative area with a pleasant expression and should first identify the patient using two identifiers (TJC, 2008). Identifiers may include asking the patient to state his or her name, and checking the patient's identification band for the name, date of birth, and medical record number. The clinician may say "Good Morning, I am Mary Smith and I am the surgeon's assistant. I am here as part of Dr. Jones' team to perform your history

Table 7-1   Medication Reconciliation Considerations

Medication reconciliation is the process of comparing a patient's medication orders to all of the medications that the patient has been taking. Reconciliation is done to avoid medication errors such as omissions, duplications, dosing errors, or drug interactions. It should be done at every transition of care in which new medications are ordered or existing orders are rewritten.

- Collect current list of medications taken at home or in current health care setting, including the following information:
  - Dose
  - Frequency
  - Allergies
  - Drug intolerance
  - Immunization history
- Validate list with patient; if the patient is unable to verify, a surrogate may be required.
- Ensure medication list available to surgeon(s) when writing orders.
- Develop a list of medications to be prescribed.
- Compare medications on the two lists.
- Make clinical decisions based on the comparison.
- During patient care transitions, communicate the new list to the patient and to the appropriate caregiver; transitions include changes in setting, service, practitioner, or level of care.

On discharge from the facility (ambulatory, inpatient), in addition to communicating an updated list to the next provider of care, provide the patient with the complete list of medications to be taken after discharge from the facility. Be sure to include instructions about how to continue taking any newly prescribed medications, and how long to take them. Encourage the patient to carry the list with him or her and to share the list with any providers of care, including primary care and specialist physicians, nurses, pharmacists, and other caregivers.

Source: Adapted from The Joint Commission. (2006, Feb.9). *Sentinel Event Alert #35, using medication reconciliation to prevent errors.* Retrieved January 1, 2009 from http://www. jointcommission.org/ sentinelevents/sentineleventalert/sea_35.htm

and physical examination. Would you please tell me your name? May I look at your identification band and check your medical record number?"

After confirming the patient's identity, the FA can take the opportunity to explain his or her role (depending on whether one is an RNFA, NP, or PA) and briefly educate the patient about his or her profession and skills. This brief discussion helps patients to feel more comfortable in their surroundings. FAs and their colleagues play an important role in strengthening the patient's sense of security and trust.

Standard Register ®

NEW ISLAND HOSPITAL

Medication Reconciliation List

PHYSICIAN'S ORDERS

Please complete at Triage or on Hospital admission
Information Obtained by:

Date: Time:

DRUG SENSITIVITIES:

Source: ☐ Patient   ☐ Family   ☐ Provider List
☐ Other

Ht: Wt:

Medications are to be reconciled by the LIP on admission

DATE ORDERED	TIME	MEDICATION	DIRECTIONS (Dose, Route, Frequency)	LAST DOSE Date & Time	CONTINUE MEDICATIONS On Admission		See Other Physician's Order Sheet
					Yes	No	√
		Example: Aspirin	81 mg. orally 1 x /day	Yesterday			
		1					
		2					
		3					
		4					
		5					
		6					
		7					
		8					
		9					
		10					
		11					
		12					
		13					
		14					

If above not completed, RN to contact LIP and review <u>each</u> item listed for a telephone order.

Telephone order: _____ / _____ RN ☐ VBRB

Date: _____ Time: _____

Physician/LP Signature: _____

Print name & ID# _____ Date: _____ Time: _____

New 6/06   NIH 237

Figure 7-2   Sample medication reconciliation form.

Likewise, telling the patient that you have sanitized your hands also fosters trust because patients increasingly are aware of hospital-acquired infections as well as errors publicized in the press. This period of interaction is a pivotal moment because the FAs approach will dictate just how receptive the patient will be to the treatment plan developed by the FA and the other staff who are members of the surgical team.

Table 7-2   "Do-Not-Use" Abbreviations

According to The Joint Commission, the current list of abbreviations, acronyms, symbols, and dose designations to be avoided (and preferred use) include the following.

AVOID	USE INSTEAD
U, u	(write *unit*)
μg	(write *microgram*)
IU	(write *International Unit*)
Q.D., QD, q.d., qd	(write *daily*)
Q.O.D., QOD, q.o.d, qod	(write *every other day*)
Trailing zero (e.g., X.0 mg)	(write *X mg*)
Lack of leading zero (e.g., .X mg)	(write *0.X mg*)
MS	(write *morphine sulfate*)
MSO_4	(write *morphine sulfate*)
$MgSO_4$	(write *magnesium sulfate*)
The symbol "@"	(write *at*)
the symbols ">" and "<"	(write *greater than* or *lesser than*)

Note: A trailing zero may be used only when required to demonstrate the level of precision of the value being reported, such as for laboratory results, imaging studies that report the size of lesions, or catheter/tube sizes. It may not be used in medication orders or other medication-related documentation. All abbreviations for drug names should be discontinued.

The facility's implementation of the "do not use" list of abbreviations, acronyms, symbols, and dose designations applies to all orders and all medication-related documentation that is handwritten or entered as free text into a computer.

Note: For a complete list, go to: The Joint Commission. (2009, March 3). *The official "Do Not Use" list.* Retrieved April 7, 2009 from http://www.jointcommission.org/NR/rdonlyres/2329F8F5-6EC5-4E21-B932-54B2B7D53F00/0/dnu_list.pdf

Source: Adapted from The Joint Commission (2008). Retrieved January 1, 2009 from http://www. jointcommission.org/NR/rdonlyres/4BAD7889-79DE-493F-A6FD-CEB9F003434D/0/CAH_NPSG. pdf and http://www.jointcommission.org/NR/rdonlyres/433B9886-F95E-40B8-B25A-FE521D34E936/0/ PhysiciansandTheJointCommission.pdf

The beginning of the history starts with data collection (Seidel et al., 2006):

- *Date of history*
- *Identifying data:* Name, medical record number, age, sex, race, preferred language, place of birth, marital status, occupation, dominant hand, religion and any impediments related to hearing or vision.
- *Source of referral:* Primary care physician (PCP), specialist, surgeon, NP or PA, none

Table 7-3   "Look-alike/Sound-alike" (LASA) Medications

The Joint Commission (TJC) has identified *look-alike/sound-alike* (LASA) medications that pose a risk for inaccurate prescribing and delivery. According to TJC, health care facilities must choose 10 pairs of look-alike/sound-alike medications from this list that are currently in use and take action to prevent errors. Comprehensive lists of LASA drugs are available on the web sites of the Institute for Safe Medication Practices (http://www.ismp.org/) and the U.S. Pharmacopoeia (http://www.usp.org/). Clinicians should use special precautions to ensure that the correct medication is prescribed and delivered when prescribing or administering the following drugs:

- Concentrated liquid morphine products versus conventional liquid morphine concentrations
- Ephedrine and epinephrine
- Hydromorphone injection and morphine injection
- Hydroxyzine and hydralazine
- Insulin products
  - Humalog and Humulin
  - Novolog and Novolin
  - Humulin and Novolin
  - Humalog and Novolog
  - Novolin 70/30 and Novolog Mix 70/30
- Lipid-based daunorubicin and doxorubicin products versus conventional forms of daunorubicin and doxorubicin
- Lipid-based amphotericin products versus conventional forms of amphotericin
- Metformin and metronidazole
- OxyContin and oxycodone
- Vinblastine and vincristine

Note: For a complete list, go to The Joint Commission. Retrieved April 7, 2009 from http://www. jointcommission.org/AccreditationPrograms/HomeCare/Standards/09_FAQs/NPSG/Medication_safety/ NPSG.03.03.01/look_alike_sound_alike_drugs.htm

Source: Adapted from The Joint Commission. (2008). Retrieved January 1, 2009 from http://www. jointcommission.org/NR/rdonlyres/4BAD7889-79DE-493F-A6FD-CEB9F003434D/0/CAH_NPSG.pdf and http://www.jointcommission.org/NR/rdonlyres/C92AAB3F-A9BD-431C-8628-11DD2D1D53CC/0/ LASA.pdf

- *Source of the history:* Self, parent, spouse, adult child, relative, other.
- *Reliability of the history:* Is the patient lucid, alert to the surroundings, aware of the procedure, and able to give detailed information?
- *Chief complaint(s)(CC):* This represents the problem, the symptoms or the reason for the procedure.

- *History of present illness (HPI):* Here is your opportunity to be a medical detective. This *aspect is of high importance* as you are speaking to a patient prior to a procedure and have the opportunity to elicit much information under reduced stress.

Components of the history are outlined in Appendix 7-1.

A clear and chronological narrative or sequence of events includes the onset of the problem, the first symptoms, the approximate time and date, determination of whether the problem is intermittent or continuous (you may have to interpret words such as *intermittent* for the patient's understanding), what makes the pain better, what makes the symptoms worse, and how this affects lifestyle or ability to function. The principal symptoms should be described in terms of Bates' "seven basic attributes" (Bates, Bickley, & Hoekelman, 1995):

1. Location
2. Quality
3. Quantity
4. Timing (onset, duration, frequency)
5. Setting
6. Factors that aggravate or relieve
7. Associated manifestations

A visual pain scale (**Figure 7-3**) is a useful tool for eliciting the patient's perception of the level of pain.

THE REVIEW OF SYSTEMS

After completion of the history, the clinician performs a Review of Systems (ROS). The ROS can be separate from the actual physical examination or can be accomplished in tandem. As input is received from the patient, it becomes significantly easier to examine that body part; thus, performing the two together provides a logical continuation of questions and the hands-on aspect of a physical assessment. With experience and practice, the FA will combine the ROS and the physical examination; however, for the purposes of this chapter, the ROS and the physical examination will be discussed separately. In general, the ROS is performed moving from head to toe. Depending on the patient's identified problems, the reviewer will focus more on specific parts, but an entire review is performed. For example, an individual complaining of acute abdominal pain may have a focused review of the gastrointestinal system. However, the clinician would not omit a review of the cardiovascular system because some vascular lesions (e.g., abdominal aortic

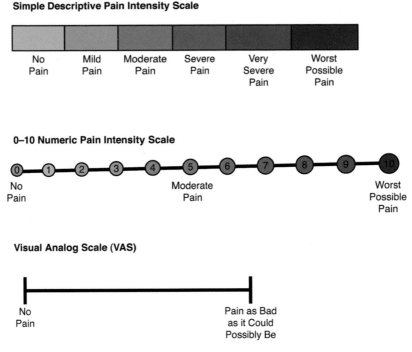

Figure 7-3

Pain intensity scale.

Source: Courtesy of Phippen, M.L., Ulmer, B.C., & Wells, M.P. (2009). *Competency for safe patient care during operative and invasive procedures* (Fig. 18-2, Pain Scale, p. 560). Denver: CCI.

aneurysm) may produce symptoms of abdominal pain. Appendix 7-2 reflects the common components of the ROS.

THE PHYSICAL EXAMINATION

The subjective information obtained from the history and the ROS is balanced by the objective information acquired from the physical examination (PE). A PE requires utilization of all the senses as well as a developed sense of intuition based on extensive experience. Performing a PE is a skill that requires practice; FAs should be life-long learners to keep up with new knowledge and techniques as they become available.

It is important to note that to inspect or visualize a patient, the FA should use a setting that has appropriate lighting and a comfortable room temperature; the patient should be disrobed but wearing a gown so that only the area to be visualized and examined is exposed. From time to time, a determination needs to be made as to whether an assistant or chaperone is required. Cultural or religious beliefs of the patient may guide the clinician. These judgment decisions are made in tandem with adherence to facility regulations. Each facility has its own established policies and procedures which outline the guidelines for clinicians. It is the FAs responsibility to know the guidelines and to adhere to them. This adherence to policies enhances patient safety and reduces legal challenges that can damage the FAs—or the institution's—reputation. FAs must also be mindful of regulatory guidelines that prescribe (and limit) their individual scope of practice. Readers should be aware of their own state's rules and regulations that affect their practice role, whether as PA, RN, or other professional.

Skills required for the examination include four modalities: *inspection, auscultation, percussion,* and *palpation.*

Inspection   This involves using our sense of sight. In addition to seeing, there is the aspect of critical observation. Some observers may not see the larger picture because they focus on details, thereby missing important cues that enable one to distinguish normal from abnormal. For example, this author stresses to his students that they should examine hundreds of breasts, or prostate glands, to differentiate between a normal variant and that which is abnormal. This holds true also for all other organs. The person inspecting should ask, "What am I looking at? How does it differ from others I have seen? Is this a normal variant?" Asking these questions invariably leads to additional questions.

Of particular importance during inspection is looking for *asymmetry.* Asymmetry must have a cause, and this is where the other aspects of the exam enter.

Auscultation   A stethoscope is required to properly auscultate a patient. If you are going to auscultate on a frequent basis, it is imperative that you purchase the best stethoscope you can afford. Although some may be lighter or more colorful than the standard black model with a diaphragm and a bell, they may not function as well and may provide inaccurate information. Daily use of the stethoscope mandates that the earpieces be comfortable and fit properly. Select a soft earpiece that fits the ears, diminishes the sounds of the outside world, and enhances the sounds of the diaphragm and the bell. Whether listening for breath sounds, cardiac rhythms, or bowel sounds, it is important that the FA hear the quality, the rate, and the soft and harsh sounds. The purpose of this chapter is not to achieve expert use of the stethoscope; this can be accomplished only with frequent practice and study.

Percussion   Percussion is a technique used to gather tactile information. Percussion allows the examiner to use his fingers as a sonar device through tissues, and to distinguish between the hollow sounds of a viscous area and the thud or deep sound of a solid organ. It is in this manner that one can map out the size of a liver or a spleen,

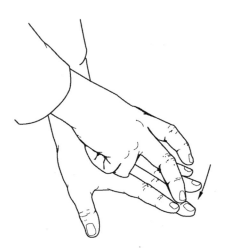

Figure 7-4

Technique of percussion.

Source: Adapted from Rothrock, J.C. (Ed.). (1999). *The RN First Assistant: An expanded perioperative nursing role* (3rd ed., Fig. 9-4, p. 206). Philadelphia: Lippincott.

as well as gather information about thoracic and abdominal organs (Figure 7-4). Many basic textbooks elaborate on this art, and one should become familiar with the didactic and technical aspects and practice as often as possible to become proficient and expert (Bates, Bickley, & Hoeklman, 1995; Bickley, 2008; Seidel et al., 2006).

Palpation   To palpate is to use one's fingers and hands to feel both superficially and deeply. One should not first palpate in the area of pain because this will cause involuntary guarding by the patient, which will alter the findings. In palpation, clinicians use their fingers, and in particular, the finger pads, to feel the area for masses, accumulation of fluids, foreign bodies, fluid waves, tumors and masses, and to distinguish that which is freely mobile from that which is firm and fixed. The hands of an examiner should be warm (first, rub them together briskly), and the nails should be well groomed or manicured. There is no place for sharp fingernails in the examination of a patient.

Before beginning the PE, it is important to assemble the required equipment, supplies, and instrumentation to perform an excellent examination and evaluation of the patient (Seidel et al., 2006). The examiner's "Toolbox" can include:

- Stethoscope
- Sphygmomanometer: hand inflatable rather than digital
- Ophthalmoscope/otoscope
- Penlight
- Cardiac caliper
- Paperclips
- Cotton balls
- Tuning forks for Weber-Rinne (hearing) tests (Seidel et al., 2006)
- Snellen (visual acuity) chart

- Metric ruler (clear)
- Gloves
- Lubricant
- Nasal and vaginal speculums
- Hemoccult card and solution
- Tape measure
- Tongue blades
- Thermometer

The physical examination builds on the history and the ROS, and employs the modalities of inspection, auscultation, percussion, and palpation. Appendix 7-3 outlines the areas to be examined.

DIAGNOSTIC EXAMINATIONS

After completing the physical examination, additional diagnostic tests may be indicated. Depending on the initial, admitting diagnosis, certain diagnostic examinations may define further the nature and extent of the lesion (see Appendix II). Patients with vascular pathology may require specific vascular imaging studies (e.g., sonography, computed tomography [CT], angiography); patients with auditory complaints may require audiometry or other related tests. Patients complaining of abdominal pain may undergo radiographic tests (with or without contrast material), CT, and/or ultrasound. Table 7-4 shows an example of a history and PE of a female complaining of abdominal pain. Note that the clinician has identified a number of possible diagnoses (*differential diagnosis*); selection of the most likely diagnosis requires additional testing to *rule out* (i.e., eliminate or exclude) the unlikely diagnoses. Clinicians should become familiar with the tests commonly performed on their patients: why the tests are ordered, what they show (and do not show), how they are interpreted, and their limitations.

The physician (or licensed independent practitioner such as PA or advanced practice nurse) will apply the information from the assessment to write a preoperative order. The order includes the following:

- Patient name
- Date and time
- NPO (nothing by mouth)
- Laboratory tests ordered
- Diagnostic studies ordered
- Consents for surgery (Figure 7-5)
- Medical Clearance/H&P

Table 7-4   Sample Format for Surgical History and Physical Examination (H&P) for a Female with Abdominal Pain

Patient Information:

- Name
- Address
- Date
- Time
- Age: *70 years*
- Sex: *female*

Chief Complaint (CC): *acute onset of abdominal pain and nausea 10 hours ago.*

History of Present Illness (HPI): *sudden onset right upper quadrant pain about 1 hour after lunch of fried food; constant severe pain, exacerbated by movement.*

Past Medical History (PMHx): *appendectomy 10 years ago; hysterectomy at age 45 years; no tuberculosis, diabetes, rheumatic fever, asthma, epilepsy, myocardial infarction, or hypertension*

Family History (FHx): *Father died from myocardial infarction age 75 years; Mother died from "old age" at 85 years; no family history of cancer or other illnesses.*

Medications: *ibuprofen 400 mg, twice a day for hip pain.*

Allergies: *no known drug allergies.*

Review of Systems (ROS):

- Cardiovascular system (CVS): *no chest pain, palpitations, orthopnea.*
- Respiratory System (RS): *slight shortness of breath on exertion, no cough.*
- Gastrointestinal System (GI): *(see HPI).*
- Genitourinary System (GU): *no dysuria, hematuria; menopause at age 50 years.*
- Central Nervous System (CNS): *no transient ischemic attacks (TIA), headaches, fainting, or paresthesia.*
- Musculoskeletal System (MS): *arthritis affecting hips and lower back.*
- Abdominal System (AS): *appendectomy, hysterectomy, indigestion after fatty food intake.*
- Social History (SHx): *lives with husband in first floor apartment; nonsmoker, occasional glass of wine.*

Physical Examination (PE):

- General: *moderate distress secondary to abdominal pain; lying still; Temperature 37.5°C, Blood Pressure 110/80 mmHg, Heart Rate 110, Respiratory Rate 22 (shallow).*
- CVS: *pulse 110 beats per minute, regular rate and rhythm, normal S1, S2, no murmurs or extra sounds.*

(continued)

Table 7-4   (Continued)

- RS: *20 breaths per minute, shallow; trachea midline; chest expansion Right = Left; air entry: Right = Left; breath sounds vesicular with scattered rhonchi.*

- AS: *abdomen is flat, nondistended, hysterectomy and appendectomy scars; diffuse tenderness and involuntary guarding in the upper abdomen, no organomegaly, decreased bowel sounds, digital rectal exam within normal limits, guaiac negative.*

- CNS: *alert and oriented; cranial nerves intact; reflexes: Right = Left; tone/power/sensation: Right = Left, normal.*

Impression: *70-year-old Caucasian woman with sudden onset of severe epigastric pain, nausea and vomiting after ingestion of fatty food. History of indigestion and fatty food intolerance; no history of pancreatitis or ulcer disease.*

Differential Diagnosis	*Acute cholecystitis*
	Pancreatitis
	Perforated peptic ulcer
	Myocardial Infarction
Studies	*Ultrasound of gallbladder*
	Electrocardiogram to rule out acute myocardial infarction
	Upright chest radiograph to rule out perforation
	Complete blood count and metabolic panel, lipase, amylase
Plan	*Manage pain with intravenous analgesia*
	NPO (nothing by mouth)
	Intravenous fluids
	Further management depending on study results

Source: Adapted from Adamas-Rappaport, W., & Brannan, S. (2005). *Surgery.* St Louis: Elsevier Mosby.

INFORMED CONSENT

Informed consent refers to a patient's agreeing (consenting) to allow the surgeon to perform surgery based on information provided to the patient. It is a physician's legal requirement to disclose the risks and benefits of the proposed procedure to the patient. Consideration must be given to the patient's age, education, and ability to understand the information (mental competence). The consent form (Figure 7-5)

NEW ISLAND HOSPITAL

CONSENT FOR SURGERY

1. I authorize and request the performance upon Patient's Name: _____
    under the direction of Doctor: _____ and/or other physicians associated
    with them in the practice of the following operation (state nature and extent of
    operation):_____

    and also the performance of additional or different operations and procedures including those
    which may affect my reproductive capacity which the above named doctor or his associates
    or assistants may consider necessary or advisable in the course of the operation because of
    known or unknown or additional conditions which may be revealed during the operation or
    treatment.

2. The nature and purpose of the proposed surgery, the possibility of blood transfusion, other
    possible methods of treatment, the risks, benefits and alternatives involved, and the
    possibility of complications have been explained to me to my satisfaction. No guarantee or
    assurance has been given by anyone as to the results that may be obtained.

3. The hospital authorities may dispose of any tissues or parts removed.

4. I am over eighteen years of age.

I HAVE READ THE ABOVE CONSENTS AND UNDERSTAND THEM

Patient's Signature: _____ Witness Signature: _____

Date: _____ Time: _____ A.M./P.M.   Relationship to Patient: _____

**To be signed by patient if over 18 years of age or if patient is married. Otherwise, a parent
of the patient should sign.**

*   The patient is unable to consent because: _____
    _____

    I, therefore, consent for the patient: Print Name: _____ Signature: _____

    Relationship to Patient: _____ Date: _____ Time: _____ A.M./P.M.

*   Attestation if not documented elsewhere in the Medical Record.

    I have explained the above information to the patient or the patient's representative.

    Signature of
    Practitioner: _____   Date: _____ Time: _____ A.M./P.M.

Reviewed 5/02   Consent for Surgery   NIH 102

Figure 7-5

Consent for surgery.

provides evidence of this agreement (Rothrock, 1999). The following are essential elements of the informed consent (ECRI Institute, 2008):

- Diagnosis
- Nature of the proposed treatment
- Likelihood of success of the proposed treatment (including risks and benefits)
- Available alternatives (including risks and benefits)
- Possible consequences of not receiving treatment

If the FA (or other team member) believes that consent was not obtained or information provided to the patient was inadequate, it is the legal and ethical duty of the clinician to ensure that both the consent and the supporting information are obtained by the physician. The informed consent process protects a patient's right to self-determination. Moreover, the process requires that the patient understands the advantages and disadvantages of consenting, is not coerced, and is capable of giving consent (Rothrock, 1999).

THE AMERICAN SOCIETY OF ANESTHESIOLOGISTS SCALE (ASA, 2008)

The results of the FAs assessment, history, and physical examination provide a basis for calculating the risk to patients undergoing anesthesia and surgery. The American Society of Anesthesiologists Physical Status Classification System (ASA, 2008; Andrews & Cascarini, 2008) was devised to alert the anesthesia provider that various comorbidities may increase risk to the patient. Thus, the patient's ASA Class creates awareness for the surgeon, the assistant, the anesthesia caregiver, and other team members regarding the potential problems that may arise during the procedure. (See Chapter 10 for more information on anesthesia care.) Information about the ASA Class also enables the members of the operating room (OR) team to prepare for potential emergencies or sudden changes to the patient's status during the operative procedure. For example, if members of the OR team know in advance that a patient has a family history of malignant hyperthermia (MH), then the circulator can collaborate with the anesthesia personnel to have the MH crash cart in the room. The circulating nurse can be mentally and physically prepared to meet a possible MH emergency.

The American Society of Anesthesiologists Physical Status Classification System (2008), also known as the ASA scale, is a measure of physiologic well-being. Mortality risk increases as the ASA scale number increases. Surgical team members should be aware of the patient's ASA classification.

- ASA 1: a healthy patient without comorbidities that could affect the patient during surgery
- ASA 2: one systemic disease, well controlled; does not affect daily activity (predicts minimal mortality)
- ASA 3: multisystem disease, well controlled but limits activity
- ASA 4: severe incapacitating disease, with poor control, constant threat to life (greatly increased mortality predicted)
- ASA 5: moribund patient not expected to survive 24 hours with or without surgery
- ASA 6: brain dead, organ donor
- Subclass E: indicates emergent procedure; emergent surgeries can have double the mortality of elective procedures

CONCLUSION

This chapter has discussed assessment techniques of history taking, the review of systems, and the physical examination. Laboratory and imaging studies (Appendix I and Appendix II) provide information that, in conjunction with the FAs assessment, will suggest a diagnosis. The results of the history and PE also assist anesthesia providers to classify potential patient risk.

Based on the assessment information and data, the identification of a specific diagnosis is confirmed with the surgeon, who will develop a plan of care consistent with the FAs findings. Paige et al., (2008) suggest that a preoperative briefing protocol be established to improve accuracy and enhance teamwork among members of the surgical team. Communication among team members is also stressed by the Agency for Healthcare Research and Quality (AHRQ, 2007). Through clinical skill, communication, and collaboration, the FA plays a critical role in optimizing the patient's surgical experience.

GLOSSARY

Cremasteric reflex: superficial neural response caused by stroking skin of upper, inner aspect of the thigh in a male; normally results in brisk retraction of testis on the stroked side.

Differential diagnosis: determination of which one of two or more diseases with similar symptoms is the one from which a patient is suffering based on an analysis of the clinical data.

Diplopia: double vision.

GERD: gastroesophageal reflux disease; backflow of stomach contents into the esophagus.

Hyperhidrosis: excessive perspiration.

Hyperresonance: increased resonating sound of air when an area is percussed.

Impaction: generally refers to tightly wedged material such as ear wax or feces in the colon.

Intertrigo: superficial dermatitis in the folds of the skin.

Lagophthalmos: incomplete closure of the eyelids.

Mastopexy: surgical correction of a pendulous breast.

Mediterranean anemia: see *Thalassemia*.

Murmur: sound resulting from blood moving through the heart or blood vessels.

Normocephalic: having normal head size and shape.

Patella–femoral tracking: method of imaging the patella to test weight bearing and knee flexion in relation to the femoral bone; used to test for "runner's knee."

Pathognomonic: referring to a sign or symptom that is specific to a disease.

Pleurisy: inflammation of the lungs.

Prostate-specific antigen (PSA) test: blood test to detect prostate cancer.

Ptosis: drooping of one or both eyelids.

Red light reflex: observing symmetrical and equal intensity reflexes from the retinae; a test for retinoblastoma.

Rheumatoid disease: referring to inflammatory condition of the joints, ligaments, or muscles.

Rule in (R/I): commonly used medical term, meaning to confirm a diagnosis.

Rule out (R/O): commonly used medical term, meaning to eliminate or exclude a diagnosis from consideration (e.g., the albumin cobalt binding [ACB] test helps rule out a heart attack in the differential diagnosis).

Scaphoid abdomen: having a sunken anterior wall.

Sickle-cell anemia: a condition in which abnormal hemoglobin distorts erythrocytes.

Striae: streaks or linear scars often seen on postpartum abdomens.

Tactile fremitus: palpable vibration of the chest wall.

Thalassemia: inherited disorder of hemoglobin synthesis, causing a form of anemia; also known as *Mediterranean anemia*.

Tinnitus: tinkling or ringing in the ear(s).

Varicose veins: tortuous, dilated vein with incompetent valves.

Viscous area: sticky, gummy.

Viscus: refers to an internal organ enclosed within a cavity (e.g., thorax, abdomen).

Weber–Rinne test(s): test(s) used to measure hearing with a tuning fork.

REFERENCES

1. Adamas-Rappaport, W., & Brannan, S. (2005). *Surgery.* St Louis: Elsevier Mosby.
2. Allen, K.D., Broome, B.S., Franges, E.Z., Lester, V.D., Riegle, E.A., Womsley, M., et al. (2007). *Health assessment made incredibly visual* (chap. 1, pp. 1–90). Ambler, PA: Lippincott Williams & Wilkins.
3. American Society of Anesthesiologists. *ASA Physical status classification system.* Retrieved December 27, 2008 from http://www.asahq.org/clinical/physicalstatus.htm
4. Andrews, S., & Cascarini, L. (2008). *Principles of surgery: Everything you need to know but were frightened to ask!* Shrewsbury, UK: tfm Publishing Limited.
5. Agency for Healthcare Research and Quality (AHRQ). (2008). *TeamSTEPPS.* Retrieved December 28, 2008 from http://teamstepps.ahrq.gov/
6. Barclay, L., & Murata, P. (2008). AAP addresses use of complementary and alternative medicine. *Medscape Medical News.* Retrieved December 17, 2008 from http:///www.medscape.com/viewarticle/584824
7. Bates, B., Bickley, L., & Hoekelman, R.A. (1995). *A pocket guide to physical examination and history taking* (2nd ed.). Philadelphia: Lippincott.
8. Bickley, L.S. (2008). The Health History. In *Bates' pocket guide to physical examination and history taking* (pp. 3–10). Philadelphia: Lippincott.
9. Cundy, J.A.B. (2004). Assessment techniques: Nursing assessment skills.
   In S.L. Allen (Ed.), *RNFA study guide & practice resources.* Denver: Competency & Credentialing Institute.
10. D'Alfonso, J. (2006). *Age specific care.* Denver: Competency & Credentialing Institute.
11. D'Alfonso, J., & Sapinoso, E. (2005). *Delivering culturally competent care.* Denver: Competency & Credentialing Institute.
12. Doherty, G.M. (2006). *Current surgical diagnosis and treatment* (12th ed., chap. 1). New York: Lange Medical Books/McGraw-Hill.
13. Dorsey, C. (2009). Preparation of the patient for the procedure: Physical, psychological and emotional considerations. In M.L. Phippen, B.C. Ulmer, & M.P. Wells, (Eds.), *Competency for safe patient care during operative and other invasive procedures* (pp. 85–129). Denver: Competency & Credentialing Institute.
14. Dunphy, J.E. (2006). Approach to the surgical patient. In G.M. Doherty, & L.W. Way, (Eds.), *Current surgical diagnosis & treatment* (12th ed., pp. 1–5). New York: Lange Medical Books.
15. ECRI Institute. (2008). Informed Consent. *Healthcare risk control: Executive summary, laws, regulations, and standards 4, 2.* (Vol. 2). Retrieved April 6, 2009 from https://www.ecri.org/Documents/Sample_HRC_Informed_Consent_Report.pdf
16. Epstein, R.M., Mauksch, L., Carroll, J., & Jaén, C.R. (2008). Have you really addressed your patient's concerns? *Family Practice Management, 15,* 35–40.

17. Goldman, M.A. (2008). *Pocket guide to the operating room* (3rd ed.). Philadelphia: F.A. Davis Company.

18. The Joint Commission. (2009). *Do-Not-Use abbreviations ("The official Do-Not-Use list")*. Retrieved April 7, 2009 from http://www.jointcommission.org/patientsafety/donotuselist/

19. The Joint Commission. (2008). *Look-alike/sound-alike drugs*. Retrieved April 7, 2009 from http://www.jointcommission.org/AccreditationPrograms/HomeCare/Standards/09_FAQs/NPSG/Medication_safety/NPSG.03.03.01/look_alike_sound_alike_drugs.htm

20. The Joint Commission. (2006). Medication reconciliation. *Sentinel Alert* (Issue 35). Retrieved January 4, 2009 from http://www.jointcommission.org/sentinelevents/sentineleventalert/sea_35.htm

21. The Joint Commission. (2009). *Medication reconciliation to be reviewed, refined* (February 5, 2009). Retrieved February 7, 2009 from http://www.jointcommission.org/sentinelevents/sentineleventalert/sea_35.htm

22. The Joint Commission. (2008). *Universal protocol for preventing wrong site, wrong procedure, wrong person surgery*. Retrieved December 28, 2008 from http://www.jointcommission.org/PatientSafety/UniversalProtocol/

23. Kohn, L.T., Corrigan, J.M., & Donaldson, M.S. (Eds.). (2000). *To err is human: Building a safer health system*. Washington, DC: National Academy Press.

24. Labus, J.B. (2004). *The physician assistant medical handbook*. Philadelphia: W.B. Saunders.

25. Labus, J.B. (1998). *The physician assistant surgical handbook* (pp. 1–18). Philadelphia: W.B. Saunders.

26. Mann, B.D. (2009). *Surgery: A competency-based companion*. Philadelphia: Elsevier Saunders.

27. Pagana, K.D.S., & Pagana, T.J. (2009). *Mosby's diagnostic and laboratory test reference* (9th ed.). St Louis: Mosby.

28. Paige, J.T., Aaron, D.L., Yang, T., Howell, D.S., Hilton, C.W., Cohn, I., et al. (2008). Implementation of a preoperative briefing protocol improves accuracy of teamwork assessment in the operating room. *The American Surgeon, 74*, 817–823.

29. Phippen, M.L., Ulmer, B.C., & Wells, M.P. (2009). *Competency for safe patient care during operative and other invasive procedures*. Denver: Competency & Credentialing Institute.

30. Rothrock, J.C. (1999). The diagnostic process. In J.C. Rothrock (Ed.), *The RN First Assistant: An expanded perioperative nursing role* (3rd ed.). Philadelphia: Lippincott.

31. Seidel, H.M., Ball, J.W., Dains, J.E., & Benedict, G.W. (2006). *Mosby's physical examination handbook* (6th ed., pp. 1–18). St Louis: Mosby.

32. Sveitland. H., & Cook, J. (2003). Clerking a surgical patient. In *Crash course: Surgery* (pp. 87–93). New York: Mosby.

33. Way, L.W., & Doherty, G.M. (2006). *Current surgical diagnosis and treatment* (12th ed., pp. 1–5). New York: Lange Medical Books/McGraw-Hill.

34. Weber, J., & Kelley, J. (2007). *Health assessment in Nursing* (3rd ed.). Ambler, PA: Lippincott Williams & Wilkins.

Additional Resources

The Joint Commission. Updates. Retrieved April 7, 2009, from http://www.jointcommission.org/Library/WhatsNew/med_rec.htm

APPENDIX 7-1   COMPONENTS OF THE HISTORY

- *Past medical history (PMH):* in patient's own words because this technique can elicit a patient's concern, apathy, or hopelessness.
- *General state of health:* indicates exposure to caustic environments, gases, radiation, or surgeries.
- *Adult illnesses:* can include all diseases that are in a Review of Systems (ROS). Many diabetic patients may fail to mention their diabetes or conditions that are affected by cardiac disease. When a patient has had a medical illness for an extended period of time, the illness may be perceived to be part of one's normal routine; therefore, it may be omitted. This is an area to which the FA may have to return, usually after reviewing the patient's current medications. For example, the FA may ask, "Oh, you take metformin (glucophage)? What are you taking metformin for? Oh, I see, you have a history of diabetes."
- *Psychiatric/social:* includes depression, mood swings, forgetfulness, feelings of incompetence, inability to socialize because of a physical problem, such as hearing loss.
- *Accidents and injuries:* demonstrates frequency of accidents and may correlate with attention span; indicates areas that have been traumatized; may indicate previous procedures that have been performed such as splenectomy, tracheostomy, chest tube insertion, or other past interventions.
- *Operations:* include all procedures both major and minor, complications, infections, problems relating to anesthesia, and problems relating to bowel motility. What was the diagnosis? Were there any pulmonary problems that increased your hospital stay?
- *Hospitalizations:* Why were you admitted to the hospital? What was the diagnosis? Who were your physicians? Did you have any problems? What was your length of stay?
- *Current health status:* How do you feel? Do you have limitations? What is your quality of life?
- *Vaccinations:* includes influenza or pneumonia for adults as well as standard pediatric immunizations (Weber, 2007).
- *Allergies:* To what medication? Describe the allergic reaction. Do you recall the treatment?
- *Medications:* past medications, current medications and dosage and strength, home remedies, vitamins and minerals, herbal medications, and borrowed medications. Have you stopped these medications? When? Why? Is your surgeon aware? Are you taking aspirin or vitamin E? Do you have medication problems? Drug allergies?

- *Transfusion reactions:* including date, type of reaction, number of units.
- *Alcohol:* How many drinks do you consume per week or per day? What type of alcohol do you consume?
- *Smoking:* What type of tobacco do you smoke? How much per day? If cigarettes, filter or nonfilter? How many years have you been smoking? How many years since you stopped smoking?
- *Diet:* such as low fat, low carbohydrate, high protein, and rationale for this diet.
- *Preventative medicine maintenance:* breast exam (mammography, computed tomography [CT] scan of breasts), prostate exam (prostate-specific antigen [PSA]), colonoscopy, immunizations for influenza or pneumonia, stools for occult blood, yearly blood work, 24-hour urine.
- *Personal habits:*
    - Sleep profile: Do you require sleeping pills, or are you using a sleep apnea device?
    - Exercise profile.
    - Exposure to environmental toxins in the workplace.
- *Family history:* including status of family members: Are they living or deceased? If deceased, at what age and from what disease? Have any family members had a crisis during or immediately after anesthesia? Age of living parents and siblings. Can you recall any diseases that your family members may have had such as cardiac disease, cancer (e.g., breast, colon), lung disease or asthma, psychiatric disease, gastrointestinal disease, renal disease, arthritis or anemia?
- *Psychosocial:* Have you or are you now suffering from depression or anxiety? Have you experienced this in the past and did you receive medication for treatment? Are you still taking this medication on a daily basis? What is your current outlook on life in general and on your medical problem specifically? Do you have a spouse or a friend that you can share your problems with? Do you suffer from fears and anxiety about life in general or your medical condition specifically? Do you have a religious affiliation and is this a positive factor in your dealing with life problems?
- *Cultural:* How is wellness/illness/death/pain perceived? What family relationships and support are important during illness? Are there specific taboos related to touch, interaction (e.g., between members of different sex)? What are important spiritual beliefs and customs? How is communication affected by language, literacy level, spokesperson (patient, family representative, other)? Are there special cultural dietary needs? (D'Alfonso & Sapinoso, 2005).

APPENDIX 7-2   THE REVIEW OF SYSTEMS (ROS)

- *General characteristics:* Is the patient suffering from fever, chills, night sweats, weakness, fatigue, loss of balance, loss of strength in hands, inability to grasp objects that were easily grasped before, sleeplessness, anxiety, or fear? Has the patient sustained any gait disturbance, loss of memory, or difficulty in thinking or speaking?
- *Diet:* Are there any specific dietary needs? Are these for nutrition or for religious reasons? Can the patient describe a usual daily diet? Does the patient use salt? How much? Sugar? How often? Sweeteners as a sugar substitute? How many glasses of water are consumed daily? Alcohol? Sodas? Juices? Dairy products?
- *Hair, skin and nails:* Is the hair thick and coarse (possible hypothyroidism) or thin and fine (possible hyperthyroidism); is the patient bald? Does the patient use hair coloring or have scaling or itching and excoriations which may be a result of using hair products? Have there been recent changes in the skin such as rashes, dryness, or excessive sweating? Are there any new lumps, changes in color, or new moles or lesions? Has the patient seen any changes in the nails such as thickness or brittleness?
- *Head:* Has the patient had any recent headaches? Ask for a description, frequency, and location. Has the patient recently or in the past experienced any head trauma necessitating hospitalization, CT scans, or observation? Is there a history of a concussion?
- *Eyes:* What is the patient's vision? Does the patient use contact lenses, and if so, what type? Does the patient wear glasses or require reading glasses? Has the patient had a recent eye examination, and is this an annual exam? Have there been changes in vision such as diplopia, floaters, eye pain, pressure, dryness, excessive tearing, flashing lights, or redness? Does the patient have a history of glaucoma, cataracts, or ocular surgery?
- *Ears:* Are there any hearing deficits that make the patient feel uncomfortable? Has the patient experienced constant or intermittent ringing in the ears (tinnitus)? Had recent earaches? Used Q-tips in cleansing the ears (possible impaction)? Has there been any discharge from the ears, or have they been infected recently?
- *Nose:* Does the patient have a history of nasal bleeding, stuffiness, obstruction, surgery, allergy, itching, or sinus problems? Has the patient taken over-the-counter (OTC) or prescription medicines to alleviate this problem? Are these medications being taken now, and if so, what medicine?

- *Mouth and throat:* Has the patient had recent sores in the mouth, or does the patient have a history of mouth sores when having manipulations such as oral surgery or dental work in general? Does the patient complain of bleeding gums or loose teeth? Is there a partial bridge or removable teeth? (This is important information for the anesthesia provider to know, especially if the patient suffers a respiratory event and obstruction.) Does the patient suffer from frequent sore throats, sore tongue, or hoarseness? Does the patient have gastroesophageal reflex disease (GERD) or experience excessive vomiting?
- *Neck:* Has the patient noticed any changes in the neck such as stiffness or inability to turn to the right or left? Have there been any lumps, goiters, thyroid problems, swallowing problems, or pain?
- *Breasts:* Have there been any changes of the breasts such as color, texture, lumps, asymmetry, inversion of the nipple, pain, swelling, or discharge (what color)? Has a breast exam been performed recently and by whom? Has the patient had mammography or CT scans of the breast, or previous breast surgery such as biopsy or mastectomy, augmentation or reduction, or mastopexy? Does the patient perform self-breast exam and how often?
- *Respiratory:* Has the patient experienced frequent coughing? Is the cough productive? What color is the expectorant? Does the patient currently suffer from or have past experiences with shortness of breath, wheezing, coughing up blood, or chest pain? Has there been a diagnosis of bronchitis, pneumonia, asthma, emphysema, tuberculosis, or pleurisy? Have chest x-rays or pulmonary function tests been performed?
- *Cardiac:* Does the patient see a cardiologist? What is the name of the cardiologist? Has the patient ever had cardiac testing such as yearly electrocardiograms (ECG), echocardiogram, stress tests, angiography, or any invasive cardiac testing? Is the patient aware of cardiac diseases such as past heart attack, tachycardia, bradycardia, palpitations, changes in rhythm such as atrial fibrillation, murmurs, orthopnea, shortness of breath (SOB), rheumatic fever, valvular problems, previous heart surgery, or chest pain (variants of angina)? Does the patient take heart medicine or medication for his blood pressure?
- *Gastrointestinal:* Have there been changes in appetite? Does the patient suffer from heartburn, swallowing disorders, vomiting, or nausea? How often does the patient have bowel movements, and are they normal or loose? Have the patient describe the color and size or shape of stools. Does the patient have dark tarry stools or suffer from constipation or diarrhea? Is there any rectal bleeding and if so, is this noticed as blood in the toilet bowl

or blood on toilet tissue? Is the blood dark or bright red? Does the patient have frequent abdominal discomfort, excessive belching, or flatulence? Has the patient ever had problems relating to the liver, gallbladder, or common duct? Has the patient ever had jaundice or a history of hepatitis? If positive for hepatitis, what type? Does the patient see a gastrointestinal specialist? Had a colonoscopy?

- *Urinary:* How many times during the day does the patient urinate? What color is the urine? Has the patient noticed foamy or bubbling urine? Seen blood in the urine? Has a male patient noticed a weakness in the urinary stream or involuntary stopping of flow and then restarting? Does the patient awaken several times during the night to urinate? Has a male patient ever had a digital rectal exam in which the prostate was examined? Is the exam done yearly? Is a prostate-specific antigen (PSA) specimen drawn prior to the examination? Is there a history of urinary tract infections and has the patient been medicated for this? Has the patient had a cystoscopy? Ever had a catheter in the bladder? Is there a history of "kidney stones"? Has there ever been a loss of bladder control (incontinence)?

- *Male genital:* Is the patient sexually active? Does the patient have one partner or multiple partners? Does the patient have sex with females and/or males? Does the patient use a condom? Has he ever had a sexually transmitted disease (STD)? Has he been diagnosed with human immunodeficiency virus (HIV) or acquired immunodeficiency syndrome (AIDS)? Does he have any sores on the penis? Is there any penile discharge and if so, describe the color and consistency? Is he suffering from weak erections or erectile dysfunction?

- *Female genital:* When did the menses begin? Are the periods considered regular or irregular? What is the duration of the normal period and does she suffer from unusually painful periods? When was the last menstrual period; has she reached menopause? Is there a history of breakthrough bleeding? Is the patient sexually active and does she have one or multiple partners? Does she use barrier methods, condoms, contraceptive devices, or spermicides? Has she ever been diagnosed with an STD or with HIV/AIDS? Does she have any vaginal discharge, itching, lumps or sores, ulcers or rashes? Has the patient ever been pregnant? How many times? Has she had any spontaneous abortions or lost a baby during pregnancy? How many live births has she had? Did she deliver vaginally or by C-section? Has she ever had an abortion, dilatation and curettage (D&C), or any gynecologic (GYN) surgery? What is the frequency of GYN exams and pap tests?

- *Vascular:* Has the patient been diagnosed with peripheral arterial disease (PAD)? Are there varicose veins? Does the patient suffer from leg cramps, pain, or pain after exercising or walking? Has there been vascular surgery such as a vein stripping?
- *Musculoskeletal:* Does the patient suffer from muscle or joint pain, arthritis, rheumatoid disease, backache, neck pain, stiffness in fingers, or carpal tunnel syndrome? Can the patient describe pain, limitations, and symptoms? Has the patient ever had a fracture? Where? Was it corrected with a cast or splint or with surgery? Are prostheses used? Are any medications taken for discomfort and if so, which medications and how frequently?
- *Hematologic:* Has the patient ever been diagnosed with a blood disease? Does the patient take iron supplements? Is there a familial history of Mediterranean anemia or sickle-cell anemia? Has the patient ever had a blood transfusion? Suffer from any transfusion reactions? If yes, what was the reaction? Does the patient bleed or bruise easily and frequently?
- *Neurological:* Is there a history of fainting, seizures, blackouts, dizziness, tingling of fingers or toes, weaknesses that are of new onset, headaches, migraines, or any history of neurosurgery? Does the patient have tremors, areas of numbness, or balance problems?
- *Endocrine:* Does the patient suffer from excessive hunger, thirst, or urination? Has there ever been a diagnosis of diabetes and if so, how long ago was the diagnosis and what type of treatment is the patient currently taking ? Is there heat or cold intolerance? Has there ever been a diagnosis of thyroid problems? What was the diagnosis and what medications are being taken? Is there a history of thyroid or parathyroid surgery?
- *Psychiatric:* Does the patient suffer from anxiety, depression, mood disorders, despondency, or feelings of hopelessness? Has the patient ever had suicidal thoughts or ever attempted suicide? How many times? Does the patient see a medical professional and what medications, if any, are being taken for this problem?

APPENDIX 7-3   PHYSICAL EXAMINATION

General Survey: name, date of birth (DOB), sex, height, weight, vital signs (temperature, blood pressure, pulse, respirations, and the 5th vital sign—pain scale), chief complaint, allergies, attending physician, admitting diagnosis, date, and time of admission.

Mental status: mini-mental exam, alertness, level of consciousness, cognitive ability, posture, dress, mood.

Skin: color, moisture, lesions, temperature, scars, rashes, mobility, turgor.

Nail: color, shape, lesions, evidence of cyanosis, characteristics, brittleness, or infections.

Hair: distribution, color, quantity.

Head: inspect and palpate (normocephalic, irregular, depressions or deformities), facial symmetry, brow position, evidence of neurologic disease, lesions, or scars.

Eyes: color, vision, lesions, inflammation, conjunctiva and sclera; evidence of ptosis or lagopthalmos; full fundoscopic examination. Are pupils equal, and responsive to light and accommodation? Six cardinal positions of vision (testing specific ocular muscles and cranial nerves); convergence, red light reflex.

Nose: characteristics, previous surgery, septal position, symmetry of nares, turbinates boggy or pale, inflamed or hypertrophic? Is there evidence of septal perforation?

Ears: size, position; hearing deficits noted by presence of "lip reading" (watching speaker's mouth for formation of words) or lack of response to interviewer whispering, or rubbing fingers together. Weber-Rinne exam, tympanic membrane and mobility, evidence of infection, perforation, mass, light reflex, cerumen, pain on manipulation, impaction, sinus pain.

Mouth and pharynx: lips and symmetry, oral mucosa, teeth, gums, hard and soft palate, floor of mouth for lesions, tongue for lesions and fasciculations, tonsils, inflammation.

Neck: Inspect the neck, ability to rotate, flex and hyperextend. Trachea position, ability to swallow, palpation of thyroid for masses, goiter, nodes; examination and palpation of lymph nodes.

Chest: Inspect for symmetry, excursion on inspiration, anterior-posterior (A/P) diameter, retractions, rate, rhythm, depth, and effort of breathing as well as accessory muscle use. Ascultate and listen for wheezing or stridor with and without stethoscope. Palpate for masses, edema, tactile fremitus, areas of pain, thoracic expansion. Percuss for fluid levels, areas of dullness or tympani, resonance or hyperresonance. All areas of chest both anterior and posterior must be examined bilaterally. Listen for bronchial breath sounds through transmitted sounds that you ask your patient to repeat.

Breast and axilla: This is an area of great importance and should not be deferred due to the embarrassment of the clinician or the patient. FAs should not omit breast, vaginal, male genitalia, rectal, or prostate exams on their patients because clinicians cannot achieve competency unless they have repeated these exams multiple times and have achieved a thorough understanding of normal and abnormal findings. Inspection: look at the patient's (male or female) breast while the hands are at the side. Observe symmetry, retractions, irregular contours, lumps, skin color, inflammation, and texture. Then have the patient raise the hands and repeat the visual exam. Repeat this sequence one more time while the patient has the hands on the hips. At this time, inform the patient what is being observed and provide education about breast self-examination; in women, the exam should be performed one week after the menses. The date can be marked on the female patient's calendar for this ritual. The self-examination may identify lesions which can be treated early and gives patient a feeling of control over her body.

For breast palpation, start at the nipple/areola junction and observe the size, shape, retraction, inversion, discharge (color), ulcerations and the direction in which the nipple is pointed. Express the nipple for any discharge, making note of the color or presence of blood or excessive pain. Feel for excessive thickening of the nipple. Gently move your fingers in a circular motion around the nipple, then the areola, and then in ever widening circles. Do this to the entire breast up to the axilla. Feel the axilla for any enlarged lymph glands or masses, lumps, inflammation, or the presence of hyperhidrosis. As you palpate, examine for consistency, lumps, depressions, tenderness, and nodes. If there are nodes or lumps, they are palpated and their location, size, consistency, and tenderness are noted. Then mark the area with a marking pen so that these findings may be reviewed with the attending physician. Perform the same examination on males, who can also develop breast cancer.

Cardiovascular system: The examination of the heart and greater vessels should be accomplished while the patient is sitting and again while supine. The examination starts with palpation of all pulses, establishing the rate and the amplitude. Figure 7-6 illustrates peripheral pulse sites. A Doppler stethoscope (Figure 7-7) may be required to locate peripheral pulses.

The blood pressure (see Figure 7-1) should be taken while the patient is sitting and again while supine. While the patient is sitting, look for any areas of palpitation and observe the carotid artery; palpate the artery for thrills and ascultate for murmurs and obstructive signs. Then have the patient assume a supine position and use tangential lighting so that first you may inspect the chest for the apical point (in a thin person, look for a small area of rhythm). Palpate the pericardium.

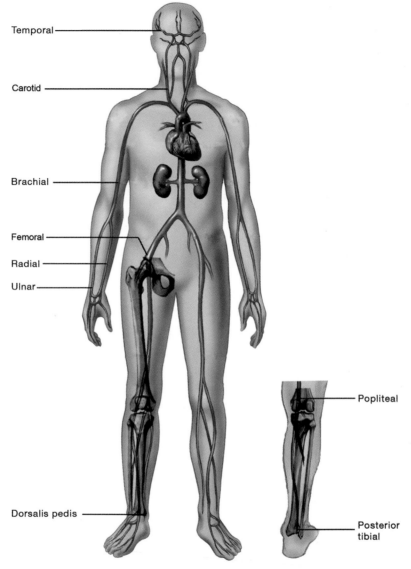

Temporal

Carotid

Brachial

Femoral

Radial

Ulnar

Popliteal

Dorsalis pedis

Posterior tibial

Figure 7-6

Peripheral pulse sites.

Source: Courtesy of Phippen, M.L., Ulmer, B.C., & Wells, M.P. (2009). *Competency for safe patient care during operative and invasive procedures* (Fig. 5-2, p. 102). Denver: CCI.

Gently feel for the apical pulse, which should be at the fifth intercostal space in the midclavicular line. Are there any scars on the chest that provide evidence of cardiac or thoracic surgery?

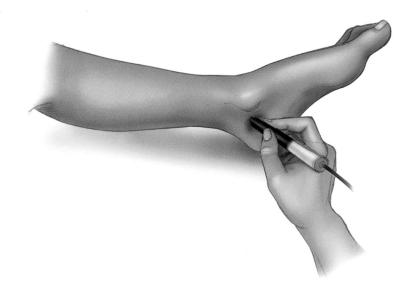

Figure 7-7

Doppler stethoscope to measure Dorsalis pedis pulse.

Source: Courtesy of Phippen, M.L., Ulmer, B.C., & Wells, M.P. (2009). *Competency for safe patient care during operative and invasive procedures* (Fig. 11-3, p. 303). Denver: CCI

Cardiovascular auscultation is performed by the clinician by auscultating the four cardiac areas and noting the findings. Listen in the areas of the second right interspace known as the aortic area, the second left interspace known as the pulmonic area, the lower left sternal border known as the tricuspid space, and the fifth interspace known as the apex of the heart or the mitral area. Listen first with the diaphragm of the stethoscope and then with the bell. Listen for S-1 and S-2; the presence of S-3 or S-4 are pathognomonic for cardiac conditions. The exam is repeated in the sitting position and may require the patient to sit forward in order to hear murmurs.

Measure the jugular venous pressure. This exam is not complete until one has assessed the patient's extremities to look for varicosities, ulcers, pigmentation, loss of hair on the dorsum of the feet, and coldness and other signs of peripheral vascular disease.

Abdominal exam: The abdominal exam starts with inspection: are there any abdominal scars that would indicate previous surgery or trauma? What is the body type? The abdomen can be scaphoid, flat, normal, obese, or morbidly obese. Look at the skin to determine presence of striae, inflammation, rash, intertrigo, or superficial veins. Is there bulging that is normally associated with hernia, tumor, or lipoma? Is the umbilicus protruding or is it depressed? Are areas of fluid or peristalsis visible? Do any of the organs look enlarged? Are there pulsations of the large vessels?

Percussion of the abdominal organs is performed to elicit evidence of fluid or rebound hollowness, and the size of the liver and spleen. Using one's hand, determine if the patient has a fluid wave indicating ascites. Is the abdomen generally tympanic or solid? After percussing the areas, examine the same areas by palpation. Map the abdomen into four quadrants and visualize the organs lying directly below the area being palpated or percussed.

If the patient is being examined preoperatively for an emergency surgery, the FA may need to perform special procedures and tests that are specific to diseases such as diverticulitis, appendicitis, ruptured ovarian cyst, bladder tumor, and bowel obstruction. Always palpate the area of tenderness last. For example, in a patient with suspected acute appendicitis, palpate the lower right quadrant last.

Rectal: The rectal exam can be done in the left lateral decubitus position unless it is being done simultaneously with a pelvic exam in females. The examiner observes the condition of the skin, looking for indications of ulceration, rash, skin tags, external hemorrhoids, bulging from a tumor or cancer, inflammation, drainage, pilonidal cysts, excoriations, fistulas, or fissures. Be aware also of bleeding from the anus or evidence of STDs such as warts or vesicles, which may not have been mentioned during the history. Look for evidence of pressure injuries, particularly in patients coming to surgery from long-term care facilities.

With a gloved and well-lubricated finger, feel for internal hemorrhoids, obstruction, bulging or loss of integrity of the colon, impaction, sphincter strength; note pain or tenderness. In the male, palpate the prostate, a walnut-sized organ that will be anterior to the rectum on the exam. Feel for size, consistency, lumps or masses, symmetry and pain.

Male genitalia: The examination of the male will include the penis and the scrotum and its contents. Is the penis circumcised or uncircumcised? Are there any lesions, warts, pustules vesicles, or sores to indicate a possible sexually transmitted disease? Is there any discharge from the penis after milking? If so, what is the color, and is blood evident? Is the scrotum normal-looking with symmetric testes, or is one lower than the other? Is the testicle firm and placed anterior or posterior with an intact nonpainful epididymis? Is there evidence of an inguinal hernia? Is it reducible? Is this a direct or indirect hernia? Is there a femoral hernia? Elicit the cremasteric reflex bilaterally by stroking the skin of the male's upper, inner thigh.

Female genitalia, vaginal exam: Inspect the hair distribution. Is there evidence of external lesions such as chancres, warts, or vesicles? Is the anatomy such as the clitoris, the labia majora, and minora normal on observation? Is the hymen intact? Is there any evidence of bleeding or discharge, and if so, note whether it has an odor. What kind and what color is the discharge? Palpate the Bartholin gland as well as the Skenes glands. Inspect for bulging and urinary incontinence. Inspect the perineum for scars from vaginal delivery or episiotomy. Palpate the cervix and press firmly on the lower abdomen to palpate the ovaries. Please allow the female the opportunity to urinate before this exam because there will be pressure over her bladder. Utilizing a warmed speculum, gloves and a well-lubricated finger, examine the introitus and the texture of the vaginal walls by having the patient bear down to rule out (R/O) a rectocele or cystocele. Insert the speculum and visualize the cervix for color, position, size, shape, discharge, and size and shape of the cervical os. A pap smear may be required during this exam; the necessary equipment should be available.

Neurologic exam: The neurologic examination is not meant to be complete but requires, at the minimum, an evaluation of the cranial nerves 1 through 12 and an assessment of the patient's balance, gait, motor function, vibratory sense, deep tendon reflexes (DTR), muscle tone and strength in comparison to the contralateral side. A mini-mental status may be required.

Musculoskeletal exam: Observe stature and symmetry by comparing the contralateral side, contour, and alignment. Table 7-5 identifies considerations for assessing the patient's posture, gait, and mobility. Note the gait as the patient walks or enters the room. Be aware of the ease of motion or any difficulty in rising, sitting, bending, or twisting. Palpate the neck for masses or tenderness. Have the patient flex, hyperextend, perform lateral bending, and rotation. Be aware of any limitations of movement. The patient will be required to elevate the arms and press against the examiner to test for strength bilaterally. Have the patient adduct and abduct the arms. Test the flexion of the elbows and the ability to rotate. Palpate for nodes on the elbows or tenderness at the epicondyles. Assess the wrists and flex, hyperextend, and rotate each wrist. Check bilaterally for strength. Palpate the fingers for pain or nodes to R/O arthritis. Check for the ability to bring the thumb and fifth finger together, as well as spreading of fingers against resistance and closing the fist while the examiner attempts to open it. Check the hip for range of motion and ability to abduct and adduct. Perform a knee exam with emphasis on patella-femoral tracking, extension and flexion, joint stability, presence of fluid on knee and special exams depending on the diagnosis and reasons for surgery. Assess the feet and ankles, looking for strength in greater toes, bottoms of feet for

Table 7-5   **Assessing Posture, Gait, and Mobility**

Posture	• Evaluate the patient's body build and alignment when standing and walking. • Look for curvature of the spine: lordosis, scoliosis, or kyphosis. • Inspect the extremities for length, shape, and symmetry.
Gait	• Evaluate the patient's balance and steadiness. • Determine the patient's ease and length of stride. • Look for limp or other asymmetrical leg movements or deformities. • Determine the patient's need for ambulatory assistive devices.
Mobility	• Assess the patient's ability to perform activities of daily living. • Determine the extent of range of motion by having the patient demonstrate active movement of major joints.

Source: Adapted from Ignatavicius, D., & Workman, M.L. (2006). *Medical-surgical nursing: Critical thinking for collaborative care.* 5th ed. St. Louis, Elsevier Saunders. Reprinted with permission from Phippen, M.L., Ulmer, B.C., & Wells, M.P. (2009). *Competency for safe patient care during operative and invasive procedures* (Table 5-13, p. 111). Denver: CCI.

rash, excoriations, dry skin, evidence of athletes' foot, and ability to flex, extend, and rotate. Perform a Thompson's test on both Achilles tendons to R/O rupture. Note any lesions, nail deformities, or evidence of fungal infection of the toenails. Use the opportunity to educate the patient about the proper technique of nail cutting and the prevention of an ingrown toenail.

8

Planning and Providing Care

Patricia C. Seifert
Julie Mower

In Chapter 7, the patient interview, history, review of systems, and physical examination were discussed as sources of subjective and objective information. Additional data provided by laboratory tests and imaging studies (see Appendices I and II) provide a foundation for the diagnosis and subsequent plan of treatment to achieve the therapeutic goal (Rothrock, 1999a).

The plan of care includes:

- Priorities
- Establishment of goals
- Identification of desired outcomes
- Specific actions and interventions

Planning saves time and resources and enhances multidisciplinary collaboration. A plan of care should be communicated to other members of the surgical team.

PRIORITIES

Setting priorities enables the first assistant (FA) to identify life-threatening or potentially harmful events. For example, managing the patient's airway has a higher priority than inserting an intravenous (IV) line during an emergency situation, although both airway and IV procedures may be conducted simultaneously with sufficient personnel. Setting priorities requires an understanding of the "normal" chronological progression of a procedure (e.g., the actions and instrumentation needed for each step of a given procedure) as well as knowledge and experience in dealing with unexpected events (e.g., sudden hemorrhage).

ESTABLISHMENT OF GOALS

Goals may be subjective (patient's goals) or objective (surgical goals), and the patient and the surgeon may share the same goal(s). Goals may be related to improved psychosocial status (e.g., cosmetic surgery), improved ability to engage in activities of daily living (e.g., coronary artery bypass graft [CABG]), or improved functional status (e.g., hip replacement). It is important that the FA discuss goals and identify those goals desired by the patient (Epstein et al., 2008).

IDENTIFICATION OF DESIRED OUTCOMES

Goals and outcomes may be similar, particularly from the patient's perspective. However, in addition to patient-specific desired results, outcomes also refer to specific and general results. For example, specific results for a particular patient may include improved functional status, removal of a life-threatening lesion, or cessation of chronic pain. General outcomes may relate not only to a "success-ful" surgical result (e.g., heart valve replacement) but also to achieving national benchmarks and performance standards such as infection rates, ventilator-assisted pneumonia, stroke, and other morbidity/mortality statistics. Outcomes may also include cost considerations (cost per case), regulatory compliance, and quality improvement initiatives. FAs can play a leading role in achieving desired outcomes, given their familiarity with the patient, staff, environment, and procedures. Facilitating a collaborative environment promotes positive outcomes and increases staff satisfaction.

SPECIFIC ACTIONS

The manner in which goals and outcomes are achieved for each patient depends on the needs of that patient (biopsychosocial), the skill of the team, the knowledge and experience necessary to accomplish the selected procedure, and the resources available. The FA should understand the reasons for each action, its intended effect, and potential hazards. Keeping the procedure as simple as possible by minimizing unnecessary and wasteful actions should be the goal of each member of the surgical team (Oram, 2006).

FORMING A PLAN

Novice FAs typically develop the patient plan according to a structured methodology: by body system (neurologic, cardiac), surgery type (craniotomy), or underlying disease/pathology (tumor). The plan is not static, but a dynamic process

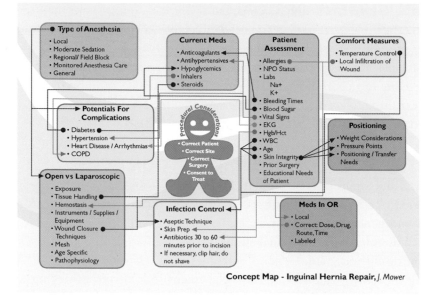

Concept Map - Inguinal Hernia Repair, J. Mower

Figure 8-1

Concept map.

Source: Designed by Julie Mower.

that is best achieved by frequent and careful analysis of the multiple systems affected simultaneously by a single event. A concept map (Figure 8-1) developed for the patient undergoing inguinal hernia repair illustrates the interrelationships of patient assessment, anesthesia type, potential for complications, procedural considerations, and other factors to be considered. The headings within the concept map apply to most surgical procedures, although specific factors within the headings would differ for individual patients. The map reflects not only a variety of factors but also the importance of relationships among members of the surgical team.

Expert FAs should not simply react to an event, but should be able to anticipate potential adverse outcomes and take measures to prevent such events from occurring. Before a definitive diagnosis and plan are established, a number of potential patient problems must be assessed. For example, an elevated liver enzyme on a lab report may put the patient at risk for increased bleeding and alterations in drug metabolism; it may also be a side effect of a drug taken by the patient. Alternatively, it may be a symptom of alcohol or drug abuse, or an underlying hepatic inflammatory disease process. It is important that the FA not rely solely on information "in the chart," but to interpret the results and determine the influence these additional factors may have on the surgical experience. For the patient with abnormal liver enzymes, the FA may anticipate the need for additional hemostatic agents or devices, platelets, or possibly instrumentation for a liver biopsy. Liver enzyme derangements may necessitate a longer time for both anesthetic induction and emergence. The patient also may be at increased risk for infection, diminished effectiveness of pain medication, and increased risk for postoperative bleeding. Some of the critical strategies that FAs can implement to improve recovery include strict aseptic technique, gentle handling of tissue, and effective use of OR time to limit exposure to anesthetic agents.

Another example involves a 52-year-old male patient in the Emergency Department (ED) with a history of squeezing chest pain relieved by nitroglycerin. Examination and further studies reveal hypertension, inverted T waves on electrocardiogram, cardiomegaly on chest x-ray, and elevated cardiac enzymes. According to the family history, the patient's father died of a myocardial infarction (MI) at the age of 52 years. The clinician synthesizes this information and generates a problem list that includes the following admitting diagnoses:

1. Coronary artery disease (CAD)
2. Subendocardial MI
3. Hypertension

If the patient also complains of back pain, gastroesophageal reflux, or other problem, this is added to the problem list.

Admitting orders are written to direct care and elicit additional information. They should be concise and be written in a logical sequence. One mnemonic for writing orders is shown in Table 8-1. This format can be adapted for postoperative care.

The initial plan for treating the patient's CAD may include medications, telemetry monitoring, cardiac stress test, and cardiac catheterization. If cardiac catheterization demonstrates coronary artery obstructive atherosclerotic lesions of 70% or greater in three main coronary arteries, the patient may be referred to a cardiac surgeon for CABG. The progression from the initial patient complaint of "squeezing chest pain" for 8 hours before admission to planning for CABG surgery is based on the subjective and objective data and "cues" that direct the clinician to diagnostic studies, which support the treatment plan indicated for a specific patient.

Table 8-1 A.D.C.A.VAN DISML: Mnemonic for Writing Orders

Letter	Word	Examples
A	Admit	Admitting team, attending physician, person legally responsible for patient, room number
D	Diagnosis	Admitting diagnosis or procedure (post-op orders)
C	Condition	Stable, critical
A	Allergies	Sensitivity or reaction to food, drugs, environmental allergens (e.g., latex, adhesive tape)
V	Vital signs (VS)	Temperature, pulse, respirations, blood pressure, weight, central venous pressure, etc.; determine frequency of VS
A	Activity	Bed rest, ambulate 4 times per day, etc.
N	Nursing procedures	Bed position: elevate head of bed 30°
		Preps: pre-op shower, scrub
		Respiratory care: incentive spirometry
		Wound care: dressing changes twice a day
		Notify House officer if temperature above _____
D	Diet	Nothing by mouth (NPO); clear liquid, low salt, diabetic
I	Intravenous infusions, Ins & Outs	Amount of all 'tube' drainage, daily intake and output, intravenous fluids: type and rate
S	Specific orders	Oxygen, glucose checks, fall precautions
M	Medications	Pain, sleep, laxative, or other medications as needed or indicated (antibiotic, diuretic, cardiac)
L	Labs	Blood, urine; imaging studies; times to be drawn

Sources: Adapted from Gomella, L.G., & Haist, S.A. (2007). *Clinician's pocket reference* (11th ed.). New York: McGraw-Hill. Retrieved May 7, 2009 from http://books.google.com/books?id=7NNhk3hgddQC&pg=PA25&lpg=PA25&dq=A.A.D.C.+VAAN+DISSL:++++Mnemonic+for+Writing+Orders&source=bl&ots=Kup6v6IKty&sig=gYMajlPafQmLAmMQuG6o_VOc-Lw&hl=en&ei=SvACSuLhBqmDl AewjZ3uBA&sa=X&oi=book_result&ct=result&resnum=1#PPA28,M1; Tulane School of Medicine. *Writing orders*. Retrieved May 7, 2009 from http://www.mcl.tulane.edu/courses/clinicaldx/Writing%20Orders.htm

Decision Processes

FAs and their medical colleagues employ a variety of processes to arrive at the patient's diagnosis and plan. "Cues" refers to things that are said or done that elicit a particular thought or action. Cues may include sex, skin color, age, history of chest pain (and its relief), family history, and other factors that suggest a diagnosis.

In the case of the patient presenting to the ED, cues suggest a cardiac-related condition.

Woolever (2008) states that there may be a number of paths that lead to the same decision and that physicians should use the thought processes that work best for them. One of the author's first recommendations is to use the clinical experience and knowledge of colleagues who treat the same population. Pattern recognition is also important. In the example described above, a diagnosis of coronary artery disease is consistent with the pattern of the patient's signs and symptoms; but if a 30-year-old woman with a new baby complained of chest pain, her symptoms might be attributed to maternal anxiety before a myocardial infarction was considered. However, whether a physician is determining a medical diagnosis or a nurse practitioner is identifying a clinical problem, caution must be used in assuming that a young female patient would not be experiencing a heart attack and that an older man without specific cardiac-related signs and symptoms (S&S) would not be suffering an anxiety attack.

Woolever (2008) also recommends using the scientific method (problem, hypothesis, collection and analysis of data, confirmation or rejection of hypothesis). Symptoms of a fever and productive cough may suggest pneumonia. Although the temperature is elevated and rhonchi are auscultated, the additional information supplied by a chest x-ray is needed to confirm (i.e., "rule in") the initial hypothesis. The diagnosis of pneumonia indicates that the patient's problem is not influenza or a lingering cold. Subsequently, these problems may be "ruled out" (excluded).

Considering probabilities helps to narrow the spectrum of options and rule out unlikely problems. When multiple diagnostic laboratory tests are ordered that do not focus on a particular problem, too much competing information may delay identification of a problem. For example, in a patient with cardiac symptoms, it is probable that the person has a cardiovascular-related problem, and testing would focus on the status of the cardiovascular system. Tests of renal, neurologic, or musculoskeletal problems would not be done initially. If the results of the cardiovascular system tests are equivocal, additional testing would be performed to narrow the underlying causes of the presenting symptoms. Additionally, invasive tests—such as a biopsy—would not typically be performed until less invasive tests have indicated a need for the biopsy.

The cues, patterns, and probabilities seen in the patient initially admitted to the ED with chest pain, and subsequently confirmed by diagnostic testing, suggest planning for CABG surgery. Components, considerations, and outcomes for CABG surgery are shown in Table 8-2. It should be stressed that any plan may be modified depending on the particular patient's needs.

Table 8-2 Planning for Coronary Artery Bypass Grafting: Components, Considerations, Outcomes

Components	Considerations	Outcomes
Coronary artery disease (CAD) lesions	One, two, three vessel CAD Left main CAD Left ventricular function	Complete revascularization; absence of coronary ischemia
Anesthesia	Induction risks (e.g., loose teeth; left main/severe CAD) Medications (cardioactive)	Absence of anesthetic complications
Antibiotics	Appropriate antibiotic infused within one hour of incision Maintenance dose	Infused/maintained per standard; absence of infection
Intraoperative monitoring	Peripheral arterial blood pressure (B/P) line, femoral arterial B/P line, pulmonary artery catheter; electrocardiogram; transesophageal echocardiography (TEE) Tissue oxygenation Cerebral monitoring Glucose, electrolyte levels Urine output (U/A)	Hemodynamic stability maintained; absence of lethal dysrhythmias Capnography; pulse oximetry within normal limits Adequate sedation/anesthesia maintained Glucose/electrolyte levels maintained within desired range; U/A greater than 30 cc per hour, adequate renal function
Position	Supine Lateral (minimally invasive approach?) Padding Positioning equipment	No positioning injuries; adequate exposure provided
Incision	Sternotomy (redo) Thoracic minimally invasive surgery (MIS)	Hemostasis achieved Adequate access to mediastinal structures
Grafts/conduits	Internal mammary artery (IMA; right, left, bilateral); Diabetes— generally a contraindication for bilateral internal mammary artery bypass graft Greater saphenous vein (varicosities, previous venectomy) Radial artery (arterial grafts for young pt with severe disease);	Appropriate grafts harvested; graft integrity maintained; hemostatic anastomotic graft and harvest sites

	adequate perfusion of ulnar artery (confirmed by Allen's test or Doppler ultrasonography)	
	Other conduits	
Cardiopulmonary bypass (CPB)	On pump	Adequate cardiac output, B/P maintained
	Off pump	Heart weaned from CPB
	Plan for converting to CPB (if needed)	
	Myocardial protection	
Temperature	Active warming (e.g., forced warm air device) to maintain pre-, postbypass normothermia	Normothermia pre- and postbypass
Anastomoses	IMA	Anastomoses completed, hemostasis of graft sites
	Vein	
	Other	
Hemostasis	Repeat sternotomy (increased bleeding)	Bleeding repaired; coagulation studies within normal limits
	Anastomotic leaks	Conduits hemostatic
	Bleeding from conduit arterial branches and venous tributaries	
Chest drainage	One, two, three chest tubes	Chest/pleural drainage tubes patent
	Pericardial, pleural drainage	Drainage within normal limits
Pacing	Atrial (A)	Pacing provides adequate cardiac output; dysrhythmias controlled
	Ventricular (V)	
	Atrioventricular (AV) pacing	
	Generator function	
Dressings	Dressings for lines, incision, chest tube, and pacing wire insertion sites	Dressings intact and secure to all sites
Closure	Sternal closure	Stable closure, hemostatic
	Need for sternal reinforcement in frail chest	
Transfer/handoff	Report to receiving unit complete	Continuity of care maintained; missing information identified and provided; process improvement needs identified and rectified
	Debrief session with surgical team	
	FA accompanies patient to unit	
	Normothermia maintained during transfer	Normothermia on transfer to receiving unit
	Ensure all connections secure (lines, catheters, drains)	Connections secure and intact

PROVIDING CARE

After forming a plan, the FA considers factors important to the initiation of surgical treatment and facilitation of successful outcomes. Among these factors are infection prevention and safety considerations related to patient care, communication, and the technical aspects of surgery.

Infection Prevention

Health care-associated infections (HAIs) are the most common complication of hospital care. According to the Agency for Healthcare Research & Quality (AHRQ) and the Centers for Disease Control and Prevention (CDC), nearly 1.7 million HAIs occur yearly in the U.S., leading to approximately 99,000 deaths annually (AHRQ, 2009). Although infections have historically been perceived by clinicians as an inevitable hazard of hospitalization, recent efforts have demonstrated that relatively simple measures can prevent the majority of common HAIs. Consequently, hospitals and other health care providers are under intense pressure by consumers, regulators, and others to reduce the burden of these infections.

Four specific infections together account for more than 80% of all HAIs (AHRQ, 2009):

- Surgical site infections (SSI)
- Catheter-associated urinary tract infections (CAUTI)
- Central venous catheter–related bloodstream infections (CRBSI)
- Ventilator-associated pneumonia (VAP)

Although all surgical patients may have one (or more) of these infections, SSIs are discussed in this section.

Surgical Site Infection (SSI)   SSIs can be categorized as superficial, deep, or organ/space, and occur within 30 days after surgery. A superficial SSI affects the skin or subcutaneous tissue; a deep SSI involves the fascia and muscle; and an organ/space SSI involves any portion of the anatomy below the incision (in organs such as the liver or pancreas, or spaces such as the peritoneum or thoracic cavity).

Haridas and Malangoni (2008) studied SSIs in a series of more than 10,000 vascular and general surgery procedures. They found the great majority of infected patients demonstrated superficial infections (83.6%); deep infections were found in 7.3% and organ/space infections appeared in 9%. The authors found the following factors associated with SSI development:

- History of previous surgery (i.e., poorly vascularized scar tissue)
- Prolonged surgery time (i.e., more time/opportunity for pathogens to infect tissue)

- Hypoalbuminemia (i.e., poor cellular repair due to protein deficiency)
- History of chronic obstructive pulmonary disease (COPD) (i.e., impaired gas exchange produces fatigue and dyspnea, which retards healing)

Hypoalbuminemia and a history of previous surgery, in particular, were associated with increased risk for organ/space SSI (Haridas & Malangoni, 2008).

Kaye et al. (2009) performed a retrospective study of 561 older (≥ 65 years old) patients who had acquired SSIs. The authors noted additional risk factors associated with SSI:

- Wound class category (i.e., a "dirty" wound is more likely to become infected) (Table 8-3)
- American Society of Anesthesiologists (ASA, 2003) score (i.e., patients with lower physiologic reserve may have fewer defense mechanisms against pathogens) (see Table 10-3 in Chapter 10)
- National Nosocomial Infections Surveillance System (NNIS) risk index score (e.g., patients at greater risk are more likely to become infected) (Culver et al., 1991; Mews, 2009)
- Type of surgical procedure (e.g., bowel surgery may increase risk of infection)

Kaye and colleagues' (2009) findings are important because the growing aging population may possess intrinsic risk factors for SSI, such as comorbidities, poor diet, and pulmonary disease.

Table 8-3   Classification of Surgical Wounds

Classification	Description
Clean	Nontraumatic No inflammation No break in aseptic technique Respiratory, gastrointestinal (GI), genitourinary (GU) tracts not entered Primary closure Drainage by closed system
Clean-contaminated	Respiratory, GI, GU tracts entered under control (no spillage)
Contaminated	Fresh, traumatic wound Gross spillage
Dirty/infected	Acute inflammation Traumatic wound with retained, devitalized tissue Perforated viscera

Source: From Rothrock, J.C. (1999). Wound healing. In J. Rothrock (Ed.), *The RN First Assistant: An expanded perioperative nursing role* (3rd ed., pp. 259–286). Philadelphia: Lippincott.

The four categories of surgical wound classification are based on the risk of infection for each wound type (see Table 8-3). This assessment is completed at the time of the surgical procedure. *Clean wounds* comprise approximately three-quarters of all surgical wounds. They are made under sterile conditions without any break in aseptic technique. In addition, they are made without entering epithelial lined structures (e.g., respiratory, alimentary, or genitourinary tracts). *Clean-contaminated wounds* contain the usual and normal flora from incisions on epithelial-lined structures. Any controlled entry into a viscus is also considered a clean-contaminated wound. *Contaminated wounds* have sufficient microorganism contamination to cause infection after a period of incubation (i.e., within about six hours). They include fresh traumatic wounds, wounds with acute inflammation, wounds with gross spillage of gastrointestinal contents, wounds exposed to infected bile or urine, and wounds involving procedures with a major break in aseptic technique. *Dirty wounds* are severely contaminated or infected wounds prior to operative intervention. Old traumatic wounds with devitalized tissue, abscess wounds, and wounds exposed to contents from a perforated viscus fall into this category (Phippen et al., 2009).

Common Organisms The most common organisms isolated from clean, clean-contaminated, and contaminated surgical sites are *Staphylococcus aureus, S. epidermidis, Pseudomonas,* coagulase-negative staphylococci, and enterococci. The likelihood of infection is strongly influenced by the type and virulence of the contaminating organism. Table 8-4 lists these and other organisms.

Table 8-4   Organisms Associated with Surgical Site Infections

Organism	Considerations
Staphylococci	Gram-positive, non-spore-forming microbes
	S. aureus is the most common pathogen in SSIs
	S. aureus is most common in the anterior nares, but other sites, such as the hands, axilla, perineum, oropharynx, and nasopharynx, may be involved
	S. epidermidis, once considered nonthreatening, is increasingly methicillin-resistant
	S. epidermidis has become more common as the causative agent in clean wound infections, especially during implant surgery (e.g., prosthetic joints, valves, and other implanted medical devices)
	Infected and colonized patients are the most important sources

Transmission primarily via the hands of health care workers, which can become contaminated through contact with infected or colonized body sites

Toxin-producing strains of *Staphylococcus* can cause toxic shock syndrome under certain conditions (e.g., nasal and vaginal packing)

Staphylococcal organisms are resistant to destruction by heat and chemical disinfectants

Streptococci

Gram-positive cocci, non-spore-forming and pyogenic

Common Group B streptococci sites are the vaginal mucosa, the male urethral meatus, the throat, and the rectum

Streptococci spread by hand-to-hand contact, aerosolized droplets, or as dust-borne bacteria

They infect a wound in association with other organisms

Usually implicated in SSIs following cesarean birth or gynecologic procedures, or in systemic infection in immunocompromised patients

Commonly present in lower gastrointestinal surgery, in diffuse cellulitis, and in vascular stasis ulcers and gangrene in diabetic patients

Group A streptococci may cause cutaneous infections, while Group B streptococci can cause significant infections in neonates

Streptococcus pneumonia a common pathogen in hospitalized adults with community-acquired pneumonia

Enteric bacilli; enterococci

Gram-negative, non-spore-forming, aerobic organisms endogenous to the gastrointestinal tract

Types include *Escherichia coli, Proteus mirabilis, Klebsiella,* and *Enterobacter*

Enteric bacilli in SSIs are often result of autoinfection by endogenous flora

Wound usually necrotic and purulent

Infections frequently seen following bowel surgery without a prep, with ruptured appendix, and with diverticulitis presenting as a diffuse peritonitis

Can also cause infection following instrumentation of the gastrointestinal tract, and septicemia in the necrotic tissue of burn patients

Can be destroyed by heat and chemical methods of sterilization but have developed resistance to vancomycin

(continued)

Table 8-4   (*Continued*)

Organism	Considerations
Pseudomonas	Gram-negative and non-spore-forming
	Found in water, soil, and decomposing organic matter
	Often a secondary organism in SSI
	Has characteristic bluish-green discharge with an acrid, musty odor
	Susceptible to routine sterilization techniques but may emerge in SSIs during prolonged use of broad-spectrum antibiotics
Clostridia	Anaerobic, gram-positive, spore-forming organisms
	Species include *C. difficile, C. tetani, C. welchii, and C. sordelli*
	Common in the soil and the intestinal tract
	Causative agent in tetanus and gas gangrene
	Due to spore formation, are resistant to routine disinfectants and some sterilization methods
Mycobacterium tuberculosis	Non-spore-forming, aerobic bacillus
	Transmitted directly by discharge from respiratory tract, and indirectly via contaminated articles
	Bacilli can remain dormant for many years
Multidrug-resistant organisms (MDRO)	Predominantly bacteria that are resistant to antimicrobial agents
	MRSA—methicillin-resistant *S. aureus*
	VRSA—vancomycin-resistant *S. aureus*
	VRE—vancomycin-resistant enterococci

Sources: Adapted from King, C. (1999). Infection control. In J. Rothrock (Ed.), *The RN First Assistant: An expanded perioperative nursing role* (3rd ed.). Philadelphia: Lippincott; Mundy, L.M., Doherty, G.M., & Cobb, J.P. (2006). Inflammation, infection, & antimicrobial therapy. In Doherty, G., & Way, L. (Eds.), *Current surgical diagnosis & treatment* (12th ed., pp. 97–126). New York: Lange Medical Books/McGraw-Hill; Dorsey, C. (2009). Handle specimens and cultures. In Phippen, M., Ulmer, B., & Wells, M. (Eds.), *Competency for safe patient care during operative and invasive procedures* (pp. 447–464). Denver: Competency & Credentialing Institute.

Prevention Strategies   Recommendations for reducing SSIs include strategies that address risk factors associated with the environment, health care personnel, and the patient. Environmental considerations include appropriate attire, traffic control, and sterilization of instruments and supplies used for surgery. Personnel factors include good personal hygiene, using personal protective equipment (PPE): e.g., hats, masks, eye wear, gloves, gowns when contacting infected patients, and employing standard precautions for all patients regardless of infection status. Hand washing continues to be a critical strategy and should be performed often. Whether using

Table 8-5 "Standard Precautions"

Standard Precautions incorporate universal blood and body fluid precautions and body substance isolation measures. Apply to all patients regardless of diagnosis.

To be used for:

- **Blood**
- **All body fluids,** secretions, and excretions, regardless of whether visible blood is present
- **Nonintact skin**
- **Mucous membranes**

1. **Wash hands** before and after contact with potentially infectious material (blood, body fluids, secretions, excretions, and contaminated items) even if you are wearing gloves.
2. **Wear gloves** any time exposure to potentially infectious materials is likely.
3. **Use personal protective equipment.** Wear fluid-repellent gowns, protective eyewear, and masks when splashes or sprays of potentially infectious material are likely.
4. **Avoid recapping needles.** Use a neutral zone for placing sharps. No two people should touch the same sharp at the same time.
5. **Clean blood spills.** Use gloves and personal protective equipment. Confine spill and clean with a hospital-grade disinfectant.
6. **Patient placement.** Place patients who may contaminate the environment in private/isolation rooms.
7. **Handle used, contaminated patient care equipment/articles carefully.** Limit traffic in the OR to essential personnel.

Source: From King, C. (1999). Infection control. In J. Rothrock (Ed.), *The RN First Assistant: An expanded perioperative nursing role* (3rd ed., p. 97). Philadelphia: Lippincott.

soap and water or alcohol-based cleansers, FAs should be vigilant about washing their hands and encourage other caregivers to clean their hands often (Table 8-5).

Patient factors such as preexisting disease, intestinal surgery, or immunosuppression may be significant risk factors for SSI's (Mews, 2009). Technical/clinical strategies critical in minimizing the risk of infection. Ranji et al. (2007) identify three main interventions:

1. Perioperative antibiotics
   a. Use appropriate antibiotic medication
   b. Administer within one hour before skin incision
   c. Discontinue within 24 hours (48 hours for cardiac surgery patients)
2. Avoidance of operative site shaving
   a. Leave hair intact if possible
   b. Use clippers or other method of hair removal

3. Control of perioperative glucose levels
   a. Maintain blood glucose at recommended levels (< 180 mg/dL)
   b. Strict control of blood glucose levels (81–108 mg/dL) has demonstrated increased mortality among adults in the intensive care unit

Aseptic Technique   The use of aseptic practice is among the best infection prevention techniques. Asepsis—the absence of germs, infection, and septic matter—is an underlying principle of infection prevention. Once skin integrity is violated, the patient is exposed to potentially infectious agents from endogenous and exogenous sources. To achieve an infection-free outcome, the FAs actions focus on aseptic technique and methods known to reduce the risk of contamination during the operation. Components of surgical asepsis include rigorous environmental control, maintaining the sterility of the field and associated supplies and equipment, and continuous monitoring of both the patient and the surgical environment (King, 1999; Mews, 2009).

Surgical Care Improvement Project (SCIP)   One of the best-known initiatives developed to address SSIs and other surgical complications is the Surgical Care Improvement Project (SCIP), which is a multiyear national campaign to reduce surgical complications through collaborative efforts by organizational stakeholders. The goal is to reduce the incidence of surgical complications by 25% nationally by the year 2010. SCIP was initiated in 2003 by the Centers for Medicare and Medicaid Services (CMS, 2009) and the CDC. The SCIP partnership is coordinated through a steering committee of 10 national organizations including the American College of Surgeons (ACS), the Association of periOperative Registered Nurses (AORN), and the American Society of Anesthesiologists (ASA). More than 20 organizations provide expertise to the steering committee through a technical expert panel. FAs can work with surgeons, anesthesia providers, surgical technologists, perioperative nurses, pharmacists, infection control professionals, and hospital executives to make surgical care improvement a priority (Hall, 2007; The Joint Commission, 2008a; MedQIC, 2009).

The SCIP Process and Outcome Measures related to infection include (MedQIC, 2009):

- SCIP infection 1: prophylactic antibiotic received within one hour prior to surgical incision.
- SCIP infection 2: prophylactic antibiotic selection for surgical patients.
- SCIP infection 3: prophylactic antibiotics discontinued within 24 hours after surgery ends (48 hours for cardiac surgery patients).

- SCIP infection 4: cardiac surgery patients with controlled 6 a.m. postoperative blood glucose.
- SCIP infection 6: surgery patients with appropriate hair removal.
- SCIP infection 7: colorectal surgery patients with immediate postoperative normothermia.
- SCIP cardiac 2: surgery patients with immediate postoperative normothermia.

Never Events   In addition to the SCIP measures, other initiatives have focused on reducing costs associated with complications occurring in high-risk, high-volume, and high-cost procedures. The Centers for Medicare and Medicaid Services (CMS, 2009) have identified a number of hospital-acquired conditions (HACs) that can be sharply reduced by implementing evidence-based guidelines. Hospitals and other health care providers will no longer receive additional Medicare reimbursement from CMS for selected HACs, commonly known as "Never Events" (CMS, 2009; Catalano, 2008) (Table 8-6).

Table 8-6   "Never Events": Hospital-Acquired Conditions No Longer Receiving Additional CMS Reimbursement

- Blood incompatibility
- Foreign objects inadvertently retained in surgery
- Deep vein thrombosis or pulmonary embolus
- Air embolus
- Pressure ulcers
- Surgical site infections
  - Coronary artery bypass grafting
  - Bariatric surgery
  - Spinal fusion
  - Shoulder and elbow surgery
- Falls and trauma injuries
  - Burns
  - Fractures
  - Dislocations
  - Intracranial and crushing injuries
  - Other injuries due to external causes
- Signs of poor glycemic control
- Vascular catheter-associated bloodstream infection
- Catheter-associated urinary tract infection

Source: Centers for Medicare and Medicaid Services (CMS). (2009). *Hospital acquired conditions.* Retrieved April 26, 2009 from http://www.cms.hhs.gov/HospitalAcqCond

SAFETY CONSIDERATIONS

The Joint Commission's Universal Protocol™

Infection prevention is one element of patient safety. Surgical safety also focuses on preventing complications related to performing the wrong procedure or performing surgery on the wrong site or wrong patient. The Joint Commission's (2008b) "Universal Protocol"™ was instituted to reduce error during surgery and other invasive procedures. Components of the protocol include preoperative verification of the patient, the planned surgical site and procedure, required documentation, and availability of imaging studies, laboratory results, and necessary supplies or implants. Required documentation should be in the patient's record: history and physical examination (H&P), nursing assessment, preanesthesia assessment, and all necessary procedural consent forms (Table 8-7). Although the Joint Commission (TJC) and other organizations that promote quality care may annually revise standards, guidelines and other requirements, the following considerations remain important safety measures for patient care.

Table 8-7   Implementation Expectations for the Universal Protocol for Preventing Wrong Site, Wrong Procedure, and Wrong Person Surgery™

Preoperative Verification Process

Verification of the correct person, procedure, and site should occur (as applicable):
    At the time surgery/procedure is scheduled.
    At the time of admission or entry into the facility.
    Any time the responsibility for care of the patient is transferred to another caregiver.
    With the patient involved, awake, and aware, if possible.
    Before the patient leaves the preoperative area or enters the procedure/surgical room.

A preoperative verification checklist may be helpful to ensure availability and review of the following, prior to the start of the procedure:
    Relevant documentation (e.g., H&P, invasive procedure consent, general consent, blood product consent, laboratory values, and anesthesia consent).
    Relevant images properly labeled and displayed.
    Any required implants and special equipment.

Marking the Operative Site

Marking the operative site can take place in the preoperative holding area or the admission area.

Make the mark at or near the incision site. Do NOT mark any non-operative site(s) unless necessary for some other aspect of care.

The mark should be unambiguous (e.g., use initials or "YES" or a line representing the proposed incision; consider that "X" may be ambiguous).

The mark should be positioned to be visible after the patient is prepped and draped.

The mark should be made using a marker that is sufficiently permanent to remain visible after completion of the skin prep. Adhesive site markers should not be used as the sole means of marking the site.

The method of marking and type of mark should be consistent throughout the organization.

At a minimum, mark all cases involving laterality, multiple structures (fingers, toes, lesions), or multiple levels (spine). Note: In addition to preoperative skin marking of the general spinal region, special intraoperative radiographic techniques are used for marking the exact vertebral level.

The person performing the procedure should do the site marking.

Marking should take place with the patient involved, awake, and aware, if possible.

Final verification of the site mark should take place during the "time out."

A defined procedure should be in place for patients who refuse site marking.

Exemptions

Single organ cases (e.g., Cesarean section, cardiac surgery).

Interventional cases for which the catheter/instrument insertion site is not predetermined (e.g., cardiac catheterization).

Teeth—BUT indicate operative tooth name(s) on documentation OR mark the operative tooth (teeth) on the dental radiographs or dental diagram.

Premature infants, for whom the mark may cause a permanent tattoo.

Time Out Before Starting the Procedure

Conduct "time out" just before starting the procedure. It should involve the entire operative team (including the surgeon, anesthesia provider, circulator, and scrub person) using active communication, and should be briefly documented, such as in a checklist and/or visible item, such as a board. Organization should determine the type and amount of documentation, which should include:

Correct patient identity.

Correct side and site.

Agreement on the procedure to be done.

Correct patient position.

Availability of correct implants and any special equipment or special requirements.

Allergies.

Medications on sterile field and prophylactic antibiotics.

The organization should have processes and systems in place for reconciling differences in staff responses during the time out.

(continued)

Table 8-7   *(Continued)*

Procedures for non-OR Settings (Including Bedside Procedures)

Site marking should be done for any procedure that involves laterality, multiple structures or levels (even if the procedure takes place outside of an OR).

Verification, site marking, and time out procedures should be as consistent as possible throughout the organization, including the OR and other locations where invasive procedures are done.

The site marking requirement may be exempted in cases in which the individual doing the procedure is in continuous attendance with the patient—from the time of decision to do the procedure and patient consent to the time of procedure. The requirement for a time out final verification still applies.

Source: Adapted from The Joint Commission. (2008). *Implementation expectations for the universal protocol for preventing wrong site, wrong procedure, and wrong person surgery.* Retrieved April 11, 2008 from http://www.jointcommission.org/NR/rdonlyres/DEC4A816-ED52-4C04-AF8C-FEBA74A732EA/0/up_guidelines.pdf

Just before the start of the procedure, a "time out" is implemented to confirm that the requirements for the Universal Protocol™ have been met. Although it is every team member's responsibility to conform to the Universal Protocol™, the FA plays a significant role in ensuring patient safety by bringing in-depth knowledge and experience to the time out process.

Patient Identification   The FA has often had the opportunity to interact with the patient and thus plays an important role in confirming the patient's identity. Previous communication with the patient also alerts the FA to special patient needs and desires. At least two identifiers (e.g., medical record number, patient wrist band) should be used to confirm the patient's identity; the patient's room number should never be used as an identifier. The required identification process should be completed before every invasive procedure, even if the FA has been in frequent contact with the patient.

Patients themselves play a vital role in assuring correct site/procedure/patient surgery. FAs and other team members interacting with patients should encourage patients (capable of communicating) to ask questions and discuss concerns with the team member. When patients are unable to communicate, a patient surrogate or family member should be asked about patient (or family) concerns or questions.

Correct Site/Side   As the surgeon's assistant, the FA is aware of the specific site to be operated upon. In cases where laterality is an issue (e.g., carotid endarterectomy, kidney surgery, thoracotomy), the FAs knowledge of the patient is crucial to avoiding wrong-side surgery. Knowledge of imaging studies further strengthens the FAs role in avoiding error, given the FAs ability to read images accurately and confirm that the images and other diagnostic studies match the proposed surgical site and side.

Correct Procedure   The FA's communication with the surgeon about the proposed operative procedure helps ensure that the correct procedure is performed, and also enables the FA to coach the surgical team in planning for specific aspects of the procedure. The FA's knowledge and experience also allows the FA to discuss with team members potential alternate operative techniques if anatomic anomalies are found during surgery or the extent of the underlying lesion mandates an alternative operative plan.

Correct Position   The FA can guide the surgical team in correctly positioning the patient by instituting surgeon preferences for exposure. For example, some vascular surgeons have special requirements for positioning the head during carotid surgery (e.g., a donut under the head). Thoracic surgeons may request special positioning accessories during chest surgery (e.g., "bean bag," over-arm apparatus). Orthopedic surgeons may prefer a particular fracture bed position. The FA's special insights into surgeon preferences and the surgery type are important.

Necessary Implants, Devices, and Supplies   The FA can help staff make available the specific implants and other supplies required for the particular type of surgery, special patient requirements, and surgeon preferences. The FA's knowledge of the patient can be used to alert staff about potential cultural or religious objections to certain prostheses. For example, Muslim patients may wish to avoid a porcine heart valve; Hindu patients may not wish to have bovine heterografts used for vascular surgery. Patients may not object to the use of such implants, but the FA's knowledge of the patient enables the potential concern to be addressed and clarified.

Allergies   The FA may have knowledge of a potential allergy not obvious to staff. For example, suture allergies (see Chapter 6) may preclude use of certain suture materials. Potential allergens should be investigated and ruled out.

Latex sensitivity and allergy has become an increasing problem for patients and clinicians alike. Reactions to latex may range from mild irritation to anaphylactic response. Therefore, patients should be questioned about their sensitivity to latex, and if a latex sensitivity is confirmed (or highly suspected), the individual should avoid contact with latex products. A number of institutions have removed latex-containing items from their inventory, but where this has not been done, the FA should collaborate with the surgical staff to create a latex-safe environment (Reines & Seifert, 2005) by avoiding latex-containing gloves and other supplies. It is important for all team members to be aware of the possible presence of latex in items such as urinary drainage catheters, endotracheal tubes, blood pressure cuffs, and electrode pads.

Antibiotic Prophylaxis   The FA can confirm with anesthesia providers (and other colleagues) that the appropriate and necessary antibiotics have been infused within the recommended time frame.

Medications   During surgery FAs serve as another level of error prevention in the use of medications and irrigating solutions. For example, topical antibiotics should not be suctioned into an autotransfusion device because salvaged blood can mix with medications not intended for intravenous infusion. The FA plays an important role in preventing medication errors and using equipment appropriately.

Diagnostic Images and Laboratory Tests   Many FAs have expertise in "reading" imaging studies such as x-ray films, computed axial tomography (CAT) scans, and echocardiographic images. Having the appropriate image(s) is critical to verify the lesion, the proposed surgery, and the correct patient. The FA (and all team members handling images) should confirm that the name on the images is the same as the name of the patient. Reviewing the images provides an excellent opportunity to educate other team members about the purpose of the diagnostic study and the information that it provides.

The implications of laboratory testing results are critical to patients. Tests that indicate a possible need for platelet replacement (i.e., a preexisting abnormal platelet count) should be discussed among the team members (including the circulating registered nurse) in anticipation of possible platelet replacement. Additional required blood products (e.g., packed red blood cells) should be made available promptly.

Fire Precautions   Fire safety has become an important component of surgical safety. All team members should know the evacuation route in case of fire, the location and proper use of fire extinguishers, and the appropriate response to a fire. A common acronym for responding to a fire is *RACE: R*, rescue; *A*, announce the fire and pull the fire alarm; *C*, close doors to contain the fire and smoke; and *E*, extinguish the fire (if it can be done safely).

Additional fire concerns relate to electrical safety and potential patient burns during surgery. All team members should follow safe practices during the use of electrosurgical energy. The ESU pencil or active electrode should always be placed in a holder when not in use. Unattended laser probes and endoscopic light cords are other potential causes of fire or burns. FAs should follow the institution's policies for fire safety related to instruments and equipment that carry the potential for heat injuries.

The World Health Organization Surgical Safety Checklist

In addition to the efforts of the Joint Commission, the World Health Organization (WHO) introduced the Surgical Safety Checklist as part of its global "Safe Surgery Saves Lives" program to reduce surgical complications (Haynes et al., 2009; WHO, 2008).

The checklist specifies actions during the three phases of surgery: before anesthesia induction (Sign In), before the skin incision (Time Out), and before the patient leaves the OR (Sign Out). In a prospective study performed between October 2007 and September 2008 in eight countries, researchers found that using the WHO checklist reduced both deaths (from 1.5% to 0.8%) and surgical complications (from 11% to 7%) (Haynes et al., 2009).

The WHO Sign In period is similar to the Joint Commission's preoperative requirements for confirmation of the patient's identity and procedure. In addition, the WHO checklist emphasizes preparation and planning for a difficult airway or significant blood loss (WHO, 2008).

During the Time Out period, surgical team members discuss patient-specific concerns and possible critical or unexpected events, and confirm the availability and sterility of surgical instruments and supplies. The value of a comparable preoperative briefing protocol to review the major steps of a procedure was described by Paige et al. (2008), whose findings suggested that the briefing protocol improved an individual surgical member's behavioral skills related to team function. Moreover, the briefing protocol also increased the accuracy of an individual's self-assessment of skills (Paige et al., 2008). A team member's candid self-assessment is an important component of a culture of safety in which individuals can focus on patient needs rather than personal ego needs. Mentoring, coaching, and teaching are more likely to thrive in such an environment.

In the Sign Out period, team members review key concerns about the recovery and management of the patient. This component of the WHO (2008) checklist promotes continuity and is especially helpful to the FA who may be involved with the postoperative care of the patient. Participation in the procedure itself, the postprocedure briefing, and the transfer of the patient to the receiving unit strengthen the FAs overall ability to understand and guide the patient's progress.

Additional Safety Considerations

Checklists have enhanced patient safety, but additional safety considerations are also important to the FA. Among these are medication safety, correct counts, and prevention of venous thromboembolisms, inadvertent hypothermia, and pressure injuries. These are briefly described.

Medication Safety Medication safety is frequently listed as one of the Joint Commission's National Patient Safety Goals (TJC, 2008c). Strategies for improving medication safety include managing "look alike - sound alike" medications properly, avoiding abbreviations that increase the risk of error, and reconciling a patient's medications. More information on these strategies is available in Chapter 7.

Reducing patient harm from anticoagulation therapy has received increased scrutiny, and TJC specifies that a written plan be available for individualizing anticoagulation therapy for each patient. The plan should include patient involvement, the use of standardized practices, and should be specifically designed to reduce the risk of adverse drug events associated with the use of heparin (unfractionated), low-molecular-weight heparin (LMWH), warfarin, and other anticoagulants (TJC, 2008d). FAs play an important role in this process due to their knowledge of the patient, institutional pharmacy practices, equipment available to deliver anticoagulants (e.g., standard IV systems, "smart pumps"), and other environmental factors affecting the delivery of care.

Retained Foreign Objects and Correct Counts Generally considered the joint responsibility of the circulating nurse and the scrub person (surgical technologist or registered nurse) only, ensuring that the "counts" are correct is a shared duty because the FA has immediate knowledge and awareness of the location of "countable" items within the surgical field. This applies not only to sponges but also to items such as vessel loops, bulldogs, aneurysm clips, and a myriad of other small items that have the potential to become retained foreign bodies. This is not to suggest that the FA needs to perform the counts but that the FAs awareness of the placement and subsequent removal of an item (e.g., a bulldog) plays an important role in ensuring patient safety. The FA also relies on available evidence, such as the 2003 classic study by Gawande et al., concerning risk factors for the retention of foreign objects: emergency operations, unplanned procedure changes, and higher body mass index. Awareness of these risk factors helps the FA to anticipate an increased potential for error and employ preventive strategies.

Venous Thromboembolism Venous thromboembolism (VTE) includes deep vein thrombosis (DVT) and pulmonary embolus (PE). More than 100,000 Americans die from VTE each year (Rathbun, 2009). DVT is a condition in which blood clots form in the deep veins (commonly in one leg), break off, and embolize to the heart and lungs (causing PE). Patients undergoing surgery are at risk for VTE, and it is important for both patients and clinicians to recognize the signs and symptoms of VTE (Rathbun, 2009).

The SCIP campaign, the Joint Commission, and other organizations have addressed VTE and recommended prevention strategies. The SCIP campaign has added two measures related to VTE prevention (MedQIC, 2009; The Joint Commission, 2008a):

- SCIP VTE 1: Surgery patients with recommended VTE prophylaxis ordered.
- SCIP VTE 2: Surgery patients who received appropriate VTE prophylaxis from 24 hours prior to surgery to 24 hours after surgery.

Prophylaxis includes anticoagulation (see medication safety above) and mechanical methods of thromboprophylaxis such as intermittent pneumatic compression devices and graduated compression stockings (Geerts et al., 2008; Rathbun, 2009). FAs should be familiar with acquired risk factors (e.g., obesity, cancer, smoking, exposure to hormone therapy), and look for signs and symptoms of DVT (e.g., recent swelling, pain, or tenderness of one leg) and PE (e.g., sudden shortness of breath, sharp chest pain, coughing blood, sudden collapse). The FA works with the physician to initiate a treatment plan. FAs should encourage patients to stay active and remain well hydrated (Rathbun, 2009).

Inadvertent Hypothermia Between 60% and 90% of perioperative patients become inadvertently hypothermic (Hegarty et al., 2009; Kiekkas et al., 2005). An important study by Kurz et al. in 1996 highlighted the importance of maintaining normothermia in patients undergoing colorectal surgery. Their study compared normothermic and hypothermic patient groups; patients in the hypothermic group experienced increased SSI and prolonged hospital stays. The authors theorized that mild perioperative hypothermia, which can occur during surgery that lacks active warming interventions, may promote surgical wound infection by triggering vasoconstriction, which decreases subcutaneous oxygen tension. Reduced levels of oxygen in tissue impairs neutrophil function and decreases the strength of the healing wound by reducing collagen deposition (Kurz et al., 1996). More recently, Hegarty et al. (2009) reviewed the hypothermia literature and identified additional adverse consequences of inadvertent perioperative hypothermia. Among these were postoperative shivering, impaired medication metabolism, DVT, and increased blood loss.

Current interventions to avoid inadvertent hypothermia (as opposed to induced hypothermia for patients undergoing cardiac and other surgeries) include active devices such as forced warm air blankets, increased ambient temperature, covering exposed skin, and warmed intravenous solutions when large volumes of fluid are being transfused. FAs can help maintain normothermia of tissue within the surgical site or operative field by placing sterile towels over the exposed skin that is no longer part of the field (e.g., exposed leg after saphenous vein removal for CABG surgery), irrigating with warm fluids, and monitoring the patient and OR temperature.

Pressure Injury   During an extended surgical procedure, a pressure ulcer can develop secondary to reduced blood flow to the skin and the underlying tissue. Unrelieved pressure and a cumulative lack of oxygen and nutrients to the area can lead to tissue breakdown if blood flow is not restored. Injury to the skin and subcutaneous tissue can produce a pressure ulcer, one of the "never events" (see Table 8-6). Parts of the body at increased risk include areas with bony protrusions, such as the heels, hips, coccyx, and sacrum, especially in patients who are malnourished, paralyzed, or physically deformed. Risk factors in surgical patients also include older age, prolonged operative time, impaired oxygen supply (e.g., patients with coronary artery disease), use of vasoactive drugs, reduced hemoglobin and hematocrit, hypotension, low albumin levels, and corticosteroid use (Feuchtinger et al., 2005).

Pressure injury can also occur at points where devices (e.g., electrocardiographic pads) are attached to the skin for extended periods. Skin that is moist is also more susceptible to breakdown. Because fluid on skin for a prolonged period can increase the risk of a pressure injury, surgical team members should be especially cautious to ensure that prepping agents and other fluids do not accumulate under dependent areas of the body during surgery.

A severe pressure injury may not be evident immediately after an operative procedure; however, significantly reduced blood flow to dependent areas may produce a pressure ulcer postoperatively. One literature review highlighted a study that revealed a 45% pressure ulcer rate in patients undergoing surgical procedures that lasted more than ten hours (Sewchuk et al., 2006). Recommended actions that perioperative staff can implement to prevent pressure ulcers in high-risk patients include (Feuchtinger et al., 2005; Sewchuk et al., 2006):

- Inspection and documentation of the skin condition
- Use of moisture barriers
- Avoidance of skin injury from friction or shear forces through the use of appropriate positioning, transferring, and turning techniques
- Use of positioning devices and pressure-reducing mattresses to reduce skin injury caused by immobility, friction, or shear force
- Staff educational programs on assessment, prevention, and treatment protocols

- Communication of relevant information to the postoperative receiving unit about the patient's risk for development of a pressure ulcer and status of any existing pressure ulcers

Operative Considerations

Previous chapters provide in-depth discussions of surgical skills employed by FAs:

- Positioning (Chapter 1)
- Skin preparation and draping (Chapter 2)
- Tissue handling (Chapter 3)
- Exposure (Chapter 4)
- Hemostasis (Chapter 5)
- Suture (Chapter 6)

Readers should refer to individual chapters for in-depth discussions on the topic of interest.

This section discusses the management of a surgical procedure based on a teamwork system called TeamSTEPPS™ (AHRQ, 2006; Clancy, 2007). The system was developed by the Agency for Research and Quality in collaboration with the Department of Defense to improve patient outcomes by enhancing knowledge, performance, and attitudes. Four trainable skills comprise the system and are designed to improve communication and teamwork among health care professionals:

1. Leadership
2. Communication
3. Situation monitoring
4. Mutual support

A basic competency (knowledge) in situation monitoring and communication enables clinicians to develop a shared vision more effectively. Improved patient outcomes encourage greater proficiency (improved performance and teamwork skills) and foster a desire to be a part of the team (attitudes). The reciprocal relationships among knowledge, skills, and outcomes are strengthened to the benefit of both patients and clinicians.

Leadership The FA plays an important leadership role within the surgical team. The FA's preoperative patient interaction often provides information and knowledge that can facilitate an effective and efficient surgical plan. This knowledge should be shared with the surgical staff to assist them in preparing for the patient.

The FA's relationship with the surgeon is another important factor because the surgeon's operative plan may not always be communicated fully to staff; the FA is an important liaison between surgeon and staff (who may have questions about set-up, special instrumentation, or changes to the original operative plan). Developing team knowledge and skills is a leadership responsibility (Clancy, 2007), and the FA is a pivotal player in directing and coordinating the activities of the team.

An FA's planning and organizing skills are especially valuable when a new procedure is planned or when an emergency occurs. These situations require innovation, reliance on comparable past experiences, and knowledge of general principles. For example, an FA should always use caution around nerves and blood vessels. Applying this principle in an endoscopic surgical site—versus an "open" site—tests the FA's ability to combine known principles and apply new (endoscopic) skills. In this situation, the FA not only brings new knowledge but also improves performance and facilitates positive attitudes.

Communication   Optimal communication and teamwork skills between FAs and team members reduce error and optimize patient outcomes. A preoperative briefing by the FA can provide an opportunity to impart information and also answer the questions of both novice and experienced team members. This is especially critical during the Time Out period when all staff members' concerns should be respected and promptly investigated. The FA plays a key leadership role in patient safety by actively and proactively participating in the surgical pause to confirm that surgery is being performed on the right patient, with the right procedure, and on the right side/site. The FA also can—and should—ask these questions:

- Is the appropriate instrumentation available? If not, is there an acceptable alternative?
- Are necessary accessory items available? If not, does the surgery need to be cancelled or does another option exist?
- What supplies and equipment are needed that are not on the surgeon's preference/procedure card? Are any items listed on a preference card outdated or incorrect?
- Are special implants and/or devices required? Are there special supplies required for implantation?

If required items are unavailable (or the wrong item has been selected), the FA can correct the omission or request the appropriate item by communicating what is needed and why it is needed. These are "teachable" moments that promote team excellence through the FA's sharing of expert knowledge, skill, and experience.

Both novice and experienced FAs can also learn from staff who have expertise in working with a particular surgeon or specialty area. Information should be freely shared among team members.

Situation Monitoring Situation monitoring relates to supervising performance, developing common understanding among team members, and using effective strategies to anticipate and avoid potential errors and complications. Monitoring the sterile field is important to prevent intraoperative and postoperative complications. Complications recognized during surgery include unanticipated organ injuries (e.g., liver laceration), acute medical problems (e.g., sudden hemodynamic collapse), and technical problems that alter the operative outcome (e.g., converting a minimally invasive technique to an open procedure). Knowledge of the anatomy of the surgical site and the surrounding area is crucial to safeguarding the patient.

Each specialty has its unique "danger" zones, and the FA must be alert to the potential for injury. For example, the FA is not only concerned about the aorta during repair of an abdominal aortic aneurysm, but is also aware of potential injury to the inferior vena cava, the renal arteries and veins, the bowel, and other anatomic sites near the aorta. During inguinal hernia repair, the surgeon and the FA are cautious to avoid injury to the spermatic cord. Every procedure carries its own attendant risks, and the FA will need a thorough knowledge of the involved anatomy. This is also critical in situations where previous surgery has left scar tissue that obscures the "normal" landmarks.

Ensuring correct identification and labeling of the obtained specimens is another important safety consideration (Dorsey, 2009). This is especially critical when there are multiple specimens. The FA can assist the circulating nurse by clarifying the identity and source of the specimen, as well as specific positional considerations (e.g., left or right margin), and tests necessary for pathology review (e.g., culture and sensitivity, frozen biopsy).

Other situations to anticipate are those that have the potential for conversion from a minimally invasive procedure to a traditional open procedure. Laparoscopic conversions to open procedures may be due to extensive adhesions, anatomic anomalies, failure to maintain a pneumoperitoneum, or hemorrhage requiring exploration to achieve hemostasis (Antonacci et al., 2008). Contingency planning in these situations may avert complications. For example, preoperative diagnostic imaging may indicate the extent of adhesions or anatomic abnormalities. Important preventive measures include confirming equipment function (e.g., insufflator that creates the pneumoperitoneum), ensuring that endoscopes are displaying clear images, and checking instruments to ensure integrity and function. In the event that a conversion to an open procedure is indicated, the instruments and supplies needed for the open procedure should be made available promptly. Preparation for a conversion is best accomplished before the need arises.

When a complication occurs, the FA's contingency plan is likely to be based on personal knowledge of the patient and the staff, the involved anatomy, similar surgical procedures, and the surgeon's likely response to the situation. For example, when sudden bleeding occurs (e.g., laceration of a large vein), the surgeon may want immediate suction, packing, a finger placed over the source of the bleeding, or none of these actions. The FA needs to be an independent thinker ("What are my options?") and still be able to take direction from the surgeon ("Suction!"). These situations exemplify the interdependence between the FA and the surgeon, and among all team members. Complications cannot always be avoided through anticipation, but the seriousness of the complication and any lasting effects can be ameliorated through a prompt, effective response that limits injury. Thus, sudden bleeding that can be controlled quickly is less likely to cause long-term injury than copious bleeding that persists because suction was inadequate or a suture ligature was not promptly inserted.

Mutual Support   Back-up behaviors make up the fourth element of TeamSTEPPS™: the ability to anticipate others' needs and to achieve a workload balance (Clancy, 2007). Mutual support fosters teamwork, which in turn positively affects patient safety and improves clinical outcomes. An important way to demonstrate mutual support is to create an environment where individuals can learn from their mistakes rather than be punished for them.

Errors and other adverse events are rarely due to a single cause. Different types of errors can occur: errors in judgment, technique or diagnosis; systems errors; and misjudgment about the nature of the underlying disease. Underreporting of errors, near-misses, surgical complications or other adverse events may be due to fear of punishment, time constraints, concerns about lawsuits, or embarrassment (Bilimoria et al., 2009). In a culture in which underreporting occurs, identifying possible causes of the error and strategies for improvement is more difficult than in a supportive culture that identifies opportunities for improvement rather than excuses for punishment.

Patient Report, Hand-Off, and Debriefing   In addition to the positive effects of the TeamSTEPPS™ program on collaboration and effective teamwork, there are other activities that benefit both patients and staff. Among these are the postoperative report, the transfer ("hand-off"), and the postprocedure briefing.

The postoperative report to the receiving unit is generally performed by the circulating nurse. The information transferred includes the patient's personal information (name, age, sex), the surgical procedure, tubes and drains, monitoring lines, intravenous lines, medications, hemodynamic variables, temperature, laboratory results (e.g., electrolytes, hemoglobin, hematocrit), and personal concerns of the patient. Although the nurse makes the report, the FA and the surgeon ensure the inclusion of all necessary information. Just as the nurse reporting to the receiving caregiver uses active communication, so too should the FA clearly articulate any special patient needs that should be passed on to the receiving unit. Both the reporting nurse and the FA should receive confirmation of the information received (Chard, 2008).

In some institutions, the surgical team engages in a postprocedure debriefing immediately after the end of the procedure and before the patient is physically transported to the receiving unit (this process will vary among institutions). Components of the briefing can include confirmation of the exact procedure performed, correct counts (sponges, needles, instruments, other countable objects), information about specimens (how they were labeled), whether there were any problems with equipment or supplies, and a review of critical factors for patient recovery (WHO, 2008). Makary et al. (2006) describe their own briefing and debriefing sessions which promote communication and allow staff members to address potential problems before they become actual problems.

At the end of the surgical procedure and after confirming that the patient is hemodynamically stable and that there is no excessive bleeding, the FA assists in dressing the incision(s) and removing the drapes. All monitoring cables and intravenous lines should be secured and the transfer to the transport vehicle performed as a coordinated effort. It is common for the FA to accompany the patient to the postoperative unit and assist with the connection of monitoring lines and suction (for drainage tubes as necessary). By accompanying the patient, the FA has an opportunity to evaluate the patient's status and tolerance of position changes, transport, and other stimuli.

Postoperative Considerations
Postoperative Orders Postoperative orders (Table 8-8) are typically written after completion of the procedure and transfer to the receiving unit by the surgeon, PA, or an advanced practice nurse (APN). State regulatory agencies and individual facility credentialing by-laws determine who is permitted to write orders, which may be handwritten or entered into an electronic medical record. Utilizing

Table 8-8   Basic Postoperative Surgery Orders

- Date and time
- Admission note
- Medical record number
- Diagnosis
- Condition on admission
- Vital signs: When? How often?
- Activity: ambulate, out-of-bed (OOB) ad lib, bed rest, OOB bath room privileges with assistance only
- Deep vein thrombosis (DVT) prophylaxis
- Laboratory tests, special procedures, x-rays, electrocardiogram (ECG)
- Pain management
- Medications
- Diet
- Oxygen
- Comfort measures
- Wound care
- Drains and catheters: e.g., chest tube, drainage catheter, nasogastric tube, urinary drainage catheter (post-op)
- Consults: e.g., physical therapy, respiratory therapy, dietician, home health consult, discharge planning, social work

Source: Courtesy of Robert Blumm.

standing orders may save time and help prevent omissions in care but should not be substituted for individualized orders based on a patient's specific needs related to postoperative recovery.

Orders generally include indications for postoperative pain management, diet, activity, comfort measures, wound care, and lab work. Additional consultations with staff members from other disciplines (e.g., physical therapy, social work, discharge planning, dietary, respiratory) may also be ordered at this time. Many facilities have a medication reconciliation process that outlines the procedure for resuming medications after surgery.

Postoperative Complications   Postoperative complications are often related to the original surgery. Antonacci et al. (2008) reviewed unplanned returns to the OR and found that hemorrhage was the most common clinical incident (27.8%).

Wound and infectious complications that required reexploration comprised 24.3% of unplanned returns. Other unplanned returns to the OR were the results of technical difficulties or error (19.3%), device-related failures or mishaps (13.3%), and retained foreign bodies (1.3%).

Planned returns to the OR may occur when newly diagnosed conditions (unrelated to the admitting diagnosis) are identified during hospitalization. For example, a patient admitted for a renal transplant may fall and sustain a fracture that requires treatment. Another category of complications involves the conversion of patients from ambulatory to inpatient status. Reasons for this may be related to the need for antibiotic therapy, more aggressive pain management, or insertion of a drain. Complications may be specific to the procedure (e.g., a pacemaker fails to capture); general categories of complications include hemorrhage, infection, retained foreign bodies, airway/breathing problems, or device failures (Antonacci et al., 2009) (Table 8-9).

Table 8-9   General Postoperative Complications

Complication	Possible Preventive Measures
Infection, sepsis	Surgical sterile technique
	Prophylactic antibiotics
	Maintenance of normothermia; for cardiac surgery patients undergoing induced hypothermia, maintain normothermia before and after cardiopulmonary bypass
Hemorrhage, bleeding, hematoma	Effective surgical hemostasis
	Clotting factors infused as indicated
Metabolic derangements	Monitor/treat electrolyte, acid-base, other metabolic derangements
Cardiac complications: myocardial infarction, dysrhythmias; vascular graft failure	Preoperative assessment
	Intraoperative monitoring
	Beta blocker therapy; cardiac medications
	Pacing
	Careful excision and manipulation of grafts/conduits
Atelectasis, pneumonia	Postoperative coughing and deep breathing
	Nasotracheal suction
	Early ambulation
	Pain control
Pneumothorax (iatrogenic)	Chest tube insertion technique

(continued)

Table 8-9   *(Continued)*

Complication	Possible Preventive Measures
Respiratory failure	Ventilator support
Deep vein thrombosis (DVT), pulmonary embolus (PE)	Sequential compression devices
	Early ambulation
	DVT prophylaxis/treatment
	Adequate hydration
Urinary infection, retention	Ambulation
	Avoid bladder overdistension
	Early removal of urinary drainage catheter
	Adequate fluid status
Acute renal failure	Treat preexisting renal insufficiency
	Diuretics
	Electrolyte, acid-base balance maintained
	Maintain effective circulating blood volume
	Avoid nephrotoxic agents (e.g., amphotericin)
	Minimize use of intravascular contrast agents
Neurologic deficits: transient ischemic attack, stroke	Avoid ischemia, hypotension, hypertension
	Careful tissue handling, especially endovascular tissue
Mental status changes	Remove free tissue, fat, other particulate matter, or potential emboli from intravascular surgical sites
Pressure ulcers	Assessment, padding, treatment
	Avoid shearing forces
Wound dehiscence	Secure wound closure; reinforce as needed

Sources: Adapted from: Antonacci, A.C., Lam, S., Lavarias, V., Homel, P., & Eavey, R.D. (2008). Benchmarking surgical incident reports using a database and a triage system to reduce adverse outcomes. *Archives of Surgery, 143,* 1192–1197; Bilimoria, K.Y., Kmiecik, T.E., DaRosa, D.A., Halverson, A., Eskandari, M.K., et al. (2009). Development of an online morbidity, mortality, and near-miss reporting system to identify patterns of adverse events in surgical patients. *Archives of Surgery, 144,* 302–311; Doherty, G.M. (2006). *Current surgical diagnosis and treatment* (12th ed., Chapter 1). New York: Lange Medical Books/McGraw-Hill; Friedman, B., Encinosa, W., Jiang, H.J., & Mutter, R. (2009). Do patient safety events increase readmissions? *Medical Care, 47,* 583–590; Mann, B.D. (2009). *Surgery: A competency-based companion.* Philadelphia: Elsevier Saunders.

Rounding The current trend towards performing more procedures on an outpatient basis has made the practice of visiting patients on postoperative days almost obsolete. When possible, however, an effort should be made to visit patients from previous days even if this is not part of the usual job description. The FA can visit outpatients in the postoperative care unit before discharge; the visit can provide a preliminary indication of the course of recovery. Besides being an important patient satisfier, rounding provides an opportunity to determine postoperative progress and to assess and treat initial signs and symptoms of impending complications. The progress note (Table 8-10) can include a SOAP (subjective, objective, assessment, plan) note to direct care. A quick review of the medical record can provide information on vital sign trends, pain medication dosage, and results of any lab or pathology reports. Areas to focus on include:

- Vital signs (have they returned to baseline, or normal?)
- Pain control (is the current regimen meeting the patient's definition of acceptable management?)
- Status of dressing, amount of drainage, condition of surrounding skin
- Presence of nausea and vomiting, and treatment measures taken
- Ability to tolerate changes in position
- Respiratory status, including pulse oximetry readings
- Ability to take fluids and nourishment by mouth
- Status of IV and central lines, nasogastric (NG) tubes, urinary drainage catheters, chest tubes, and other tubes, lines and drains

Table 8-10   Daily Progress Note

- Date/time/attending
- Vital signs
- Lab or pathology reports
- Intravenous (IV) infusion lines
- Medications
- Complications
- Dressing change and drainage
- S.O.A.P. note:

    S (subjective)—How does the patient describe the condition in his/her own words?

    O (objective data)—Lab, radiology, or pathology results; summarize brief physical exam

    A (assessment)—Includes a summary of the patient's condition, progress, and problems. If multiple problems are present (e.g., COPD, PE, infection), number the problems.

    P (plan)—Based upon your findings and returned studies, what is your plan for this patient (e.g., diet, IVs, ambulation, sleep medications, pain control)? Will you alter, change, or eliminate medications? Will you need additional consultations? Should this patient remain on this unit or be transferred?

Source: Courtesy of Robert Blumm.

Patients should be encouraged to ask questions about their care, and patient teaching should be reinforced (see Chapter 9). Although a patient may have seemed lucid in the immediate postoperative period, medications are given that often have an amnesiac quality so that the patient may remember very little about the actual procedure. The FA should be prepared to answer the same questions multiple times, and enlist the assistance of family members to reinforce information.

Newer trends in the postoperative assessment of hospitalized patients include robotic telerounding, remote electronic intensive care units ("e-ICUs"), telewound care management, and other forms of telecommunication. Although these technologies may not yet be widely available, their use is growing steadily (Stokowski, 2008; Thacker, 2005).

Wound Healing Surgical wound management is based on knowledge of the physiology of wound healing and the factors that promote or interfere with the body's natural self-repair mechanisms. Healing tissue is subject to a process that progresses from injury through a variety of steps before creating tissue repair by primary or secondary intention (Figure 8-2). A number of factors can result in

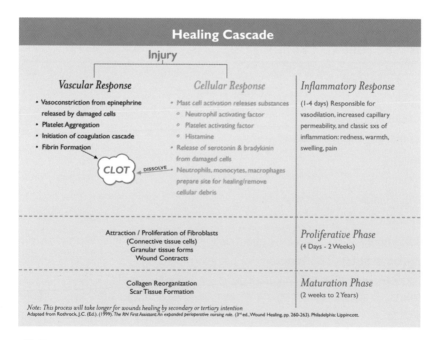

Figure 8-2

Wound healing cascade.

Source: Designed by Julie Mower.

Table 8-11   Factors That Delay Wound Healing

Age: both very young and very old

AIDS (acquried immunodeficiency syndrome)

Anemia

Autoimmune disorders
- Lupus erythematosus
- Multiple Sclerosis
- Crohn's disease
- Rheumatoid arthritis

Cancer

Chronic inflammatory disease

Endocrine disorders
- Diabetes mellitus
- Cushing's syndrome

Excessive activity

HIV (human immunodeficiency virus)

Hypertension

Altered nutritional status
- Increased body surface area (obesity)
- Malabsorption syndromes
- Excessive alcohol intake

Inadequate oxygenation

Smoking

Peripheral vascular disease

Peripheral neuropathy

Proximal nerve injury

Poor hygiene

Radiation
- Suppressed cell replication
- Endarteritis destroys blood supply

Source: Adapted from Rothrock, J.C. (1999c). Wound healing. In J. Rothrock (Ed.), *The RN First Assistant: An expanded perioperative nursing role* (3rd ed., pp. 259–286). Philadelphia: Lippincott; Singhal, H., Kaur, K., & Zammit, C. (2008). Wound infection. *emedicine specialties.* Retrieved May 6, 2009 from http://emedicine.medscape.com/article/188988-print

delayed wound healing (Table 8-11). An overview of wound classifications and healing is included in Chapter 3, Tissue Handling. This section will focus on techniques employed to enhance the wound healing process.

Classification   Wounds may be classified by etiology as either surgical or traumatic, and further subdivided as closed or open, based on the amount of tissue lost. A closed wound is always the preferred surgical technique because it reapproximates within hours of incision and heals with minimal scarring; this process is referred to as healing by primary intention.

Healing by secondary intention occurs in an open wound in which reapproximation of skin edges is impossible due to the amount of tissue lost. The body heals by filling in the defect with granulation tissue. The main mechanism of healing with secondary intention is contraction and movement of tissue towards the center of the wound. Although the goal is to heal the wound, the increased amount of scar tissue associated with healing from secondary intention can inhibit normal physiologic function in that area.

Healing by tertiary intention (also referred to as "delayed primary closure") occurs when a large wound cannot be closed by suturing due to the presence (or high suspicion) of infection. Examples include an infected sternal wound or infection of the mediastinum (mediastinitis). The wound may be left open to resolve the infectious process, after which the wound edges can be approximated. In this situation there is increased granulation and greater inflammation and scarring compared to healing by secondary intention (Diegelmann & Evans, 2004; Rothrock, 1999c). **Figure 8-3** illustrates the three stages of wound healing.

Special Wound Healing Applications   In areas where secondary closure is not possible, a skin graft or flap may be needed. A skin graft is a segment of dermis and epidermis that has been separated from its blood supply and site of origin (donor site) and transplanted to another area of the body (recipient site). The graft may consist of the epidermis with a portion (split-thickness) or all of the dermis (full-thickness). It is usually used as a permanent wound covering; infection, excessive swelling, or lack of blood flow to the graft will result in loss of graft and possibly loss of the tissue underneath. Frequently, the temperature of the OR will be increased to enhance the vasodilatory effect. Careful attention to wound dressings is very important to immobilize the site and decrease the formation of seromas or hematomas until the graft can "take."

Another special application relates to harvesting the greater saphenous vein for CABG surgery. A study examining saphenous vein harvesting by registered nurse first assistants (RNFAs) demonstrated fewer SSI compared to harvesting by surgical residents (Pear and Williamson, 2009). Although the study group consisted of RNFAs, the authors hypothesized that the RNFAs' results were due to their ability

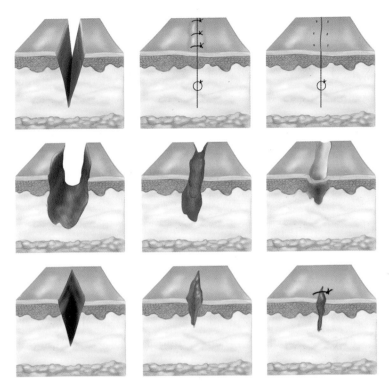

Figure 8-3

Types of wound healing. A [top]: Healing by primary intention. Wound is clean, in a straight line, with little loss of tissue. All wound edges are well approximated with sutures. Healing is usually rapid, with minimal scarring. B [middle]: Healing by secondary intention. Large wound with considerable loss of tissue. Natural healing occurs by formation of granulation tissue. Healing takes longer and results in more scarring. C [bottom]: Healing by tertiary intention. Time delay before wound is sutured. Greater granulation, greater risk of infection, greater inflammatory reaction than with healing by primary intention. Late suturing and development of more scar tissue.

Source: Adapted by M. Borman from Rothrock, J.C. (1999c). Wound healing. In J. Rothrock (Ed.), *The RN First Assistant: An expanded perioperative nursing role* (3rd ed., p. 260). Philadelphia: Lippincott.

to standardize and expedite the vein-harvesting process, a practice which nonphysician FAs may want to follow.

Preoperative Assessment   The FA will develop a plan of care based in part on a preoperative assessment of the patient's skin. The purposes for this include:

- Obtaining a baseline to compare any changes in skin integrity that may occur intraoperatively.

- Rescheduling procedures. Certain procedures, typically those that involve implants, are at increased risk for infection; thus, a patient with a presenting wound, elevated temperature, or other sign of an infectious process may need to be rescheduled. This is a discussion that is best conducted before the patient enters the OR.
- Making additional drapes and transparent adhesive barriers available prior to the start of the procedure. If the surgery is urgent or emergent, the FA will assist in draping off wounds not associated with the surgery to isolate them from the incision site. Intestinal or urinary stomas not involved in the procedure should also be isolated from the surgical field.

The single most important act the FA can perform to encourage wound healing is to avoid breaks in technique that predispose towards infection. The most frequent source of an SSI is the patient's own endogenous flora (Singhal et al., 2008). The amount of tissue traumatized during the surgical procedure will have a direct influence on the amount of time needed to heal, as well as the effectiveness of the body's natural ability to repair itself. Excessive handling of tissue and improper retracting techniques will cause additional damage. It is important when choosing an absorbable suture to match its absorption properties to the tissue being repaired. If the rate of absorption is quicker than the rate of healing, wound dehiscence, possible infection, and prolonged healing with an unsightly scar may result. Suture types and their concurrent absorption rates and tissue applications are discussed in Chapter 6.

A foreign body left in the wound will initiate a chronic inflammatory process, causing pain and excessive scar tissue to form around the object as the body attempts to break it down and remove it. Although counting sponges and instruments may become routine, it should be taken seriously because this is the last chance to account for items that will have disastrous consequences if retained.

Adequate blood flow to the site is a requisite to provide the oxygen and cellular components necessary to heal and fight infection. Hypoxia may be noted initially at the surgical site and is associated with bleeding of a darker red hue. The anesthesia care provider should be notified so that additional oxygenation measures may be initiated. The results of a meta-analysis by Qadan et al. (2009) revealed that an increased intraoperative oxygen concentration (80% as opposed to 30%) exerted a statistically significant beneficial effect on SSIs. The authors recommended that increased oxygen be used in conjunction with appropriate preoperative antibiotic administration, maintenance of normothermia, blood glucose control, and preservation of blood volume to reduce the incidence of wound infections. The benefits were greatest in patients undergoing colorectal surgery.

High-Risk Populations Certain patient populations and wound types are predisposed to delayed wound healing (see Table 8-11). Knowledge of this predisposition enables the FA to initiate actions to decrease the magnitude of this risk.

Weight Challenges According to the 2003–2004 National Health and Nutrition Examination Survey (National Center for Health Statistics, 2006), approximately 66% of adults 20 to 74 years old in the United States are considered obese or overweight. Because adipose tissue contains less vasculature, there is lower circulation to the injured area. The preponderance of comorbid conditions (diabetes, atherosclerosis, cardiovascular disease) typically associated with this population further increases the risk of delayed wound healing. These patients also challenge traditional wound closing and dressing techniques.

Although the prevalence of anorexia nervosa is much lower (0.3%–1%), this population poses its own unique set of challenges, including increased risk for poor wound healing and decreased skin turgor due to chronic dehydration (Denner & Townley, 2009).

Diabetes Mellitus This disease impairs the inflammatory response and is a primary cause of peripheral neuropathy (McCance & Huether, 2006). Concurrent vascular insufficiency reduces oxygen delivery to the tissues and decreases the ability of white blood cells to reach the area of injury. In addition, some pathogens are able to proliferate more rapidly in a sugar-rich environment. Diabetes is frequently associated with cardiovascular disease, which further compromises circulation to the injured area. The intraoperative management and treatment of elevated blood sugar has become the standard in many ORs. Close regulation of blood sugar may be a major determinant of wound morbidity (Singhal et al., 2008).

Trauma Multisystem trauma, along with the accompanying vasoactive drugs, massive transfusions, multiple surgeries, high risk for sepsis, and insertion of invasive monitoring devices, drains, and catheters, may overwhelm the body's innate ability to heal. All patients undergoing this level of stress become hyperglycemic as a result of the steroids given to reduce inflammation and the adrenocorticoid response to sympathetic nervous system stimulation (flight or fight) (see Diabetes discussion above).

Table 8-12 **Drugs That Impair Wound Healing**

Drug	Effect
Anticoagulants	Hematoma formation
Aspirin	Inhibits platelet activation
Warfarin (Coumadin®)	Impairs blood clotting
Anti-inflammatory including steroids	Suppresses inflammation
Ibuprofen	Suppresses protein synthesis
Naproxen	Suppresses epithelialization
	Increases incidence of bleeding
Chemotherapy	Arrests cell replication
	Suppresses inflammation
	Suppresses protein synthesis
	Decreases white blood cell count
Colchicine	Arrests cell replication
	Suppresses collagen transport
Diphenylhydantoin	Causes hypertrophic scars
Guarana (diet pill, contains caffeine, theobromine, theophylline)	Decreases platelet aggregation
Methysergide (Sansert®)	Causes excessive scarring
Penicillin	Liberates penicillamine
Pentazocine (Talwin®)	May cause extreme fibrosis

Sources: Adapted from Diegelmann, R.F., & Evans, M.C. (2004). Wound healing: An overview of acute, fibrotic, and delayed healing. *Frontiers in Bioscience, 9*, 283–289; Qadan, M., Akca, O., Mahid, S.S., Hornung, C. A., & Polk, H.C. (2009). Perioperative supplemental oxygen therapy and surgical site infection. *Archives of Surgery, 144*, 359–368; Rothrock, J.C. (1999c). Wound healing. In J. Rothrock (Ed.), *The RN First Assistant: An expanded perioperative nursing role* (3rd ed., pp. 259–286). Philadelphia: Lippincott.

Drugs Impaired wound healing is a side effect of many drugs (Table 8-12). Any drug that interacts with the healing cascade will affect healing. Patients taking these medications should be identified preoperatively so that action may be taken to mitigate the effect. In some cases, surgery may be postponed until the surgeon or anesthesia provider has judged that sufficient time has passed to allow the drug to clear the system.

Herbal medications (Table 8-13) should be investigated because certain herbs can inhibit platelet activity, increase blood pressure, or exacerbate the effects of anticoagulant medications. Many patients do not consider their herbal supplements to be "medications" or "drugs," so it is important for the FA

Table 8-13   **Herbal Medicines**

Agent	Pharmacologic Action	Concerns and Considerations
Echinacea (purple coneflower root)	Activates cell-mediated immunity	Decreases effectiveness of immunosuppressants; should not be taken by organ transplant patients
Ephedra	Increases heart rate and blood pressure through sympathomimetic effects	Increases risk of stroke and myocardial ischemia; may cause intraoperative hemodynamic instability
Feverfew	Inhibits platelet activity	Increases risk of bleeding
Garlic	Inhibits platelet aggregation; increases fibrinolysis	Increases risk of bleeding, especially in combination with other platelet inhibitors
Gingko	Inhibits platelet activation	Increases risk of bleeding, especially in combination with other platelet inhibitors
Ginseng	Inhibits platelet activation; lowers blood glucose; has many diverse effects	Increases risk of bleeding; has potential to decrease anticoagulant effect of warfarin; may cause hypoglycemia
St. John's wort	Inhibits neurotransmitter reuptake	Induces enzymes that affect warfarin and many other drugs; may affect calcium channel blockers and decrease serum digoxin levels

Source: American Society of Anesthesiologists. (2003). What you should know about your patient's use of herbal medicines and other dietary supplements. Retrieved May 7, 2009 from http://www.asahq.org/patientEducation/herbPatient.pdf; Association of periOperative Registered Nurses (AORN). (2005). *Safe medication administration tool kit.* Denver: AORN. Retrieved April 27, 2009, from www.aorn.org; Drain, C.B., & Odom-Forren, J. (2009). *Perianesthesia nursing: A critical care approach.* St. Louis: Saunders Elsevier.

to address these drugs specifically when talking with the patient (ASA, 2003; Barclay et al., 2008).

Nicotine is worth a special mention because cigarette smoking impairs oxygen delivery and pulmonary function, as well as causing vascular spasm and endovascular damage. Smoking cessation classes should be recommended to patients who smoke.

Application of Dressings   Dressings are initially applied under sterile conditions in the operating room to prevent wound and suture line contamination, protect wounds from additional trauma, and immobilize surrounding skin. A wound's

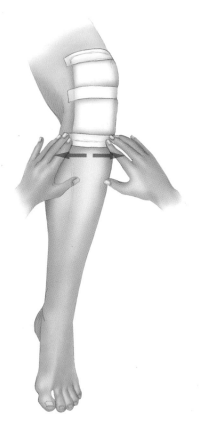

Figure 8-4

Application of dressing tape.

Source: Drawing by M. Borman

susceptibility to surface contamination is greatest during the first postoperative day. Because many surgeries are outpatient procedures, these dressings must withstand home and work activities in addition to the immediate postoperative period. Figure 8-4 illustrates the appropriate application of adhesive tape. Tape should be placed perpendicular to the incision; too much tension on the tape will cause shearing of the tissue. Use paper or hypoallergenic tape for patients with fragile skin (e.g., patients taking steroids, the elderly, and infants). Depending on the type of dressing, the patient may be instructed to remove dressings at home or leave them in place until the next office visit.

The FA promotes optimal healing by conducting a thorough preoperative assessment of risk factors for healing (e.g., diabetes, poor nutritional status) and careful postoperative observation of the wound. Interventions by the FA include monitoring the wound, obtaining cultures in the event of purulent drainage, and educating patients about wound care. Table 8-14 lists observations and interventions related to wound care.

Table 8-14 **Wound Assessments and Interventions**

Inspect wound to verify hemostasis

Assess wound for classic signs of inflammation

- Erythema
- Warmth
- Edema
- Pain/tenderness

Note any exudates; document color, consistency, odor; obtain/review culture results as appropriate

Monitor vital signs/pain

Elevate affected area as appropriate

Utilize proper technique for dressing changes

Monitor drainage system for amount and characteristics of drainage collection (as applicable)

Keep wound edges approximated

Provide written instructions for home care of incision, dressings, drains; clarify and verify patient's understanding

Maintain moist environment (use appropriate dressings to promote formation of granulation tissue and reepithelialization)

Protect wound from trauma (chemical/mechanical)

Review nutritional instructions prior to discharge; make referrals if indicated

Source: From Rothrock, J.C. (1999). Wound healing. In J. Rothrock (Ed.), *The RN First Assistant: An expanded perioperative nursing role* (3rd ed., p. 269). Philadelphia: Lippincott.

A high-risk patient may require complex wound care postoperatively. A consultation with a wound specialist nurse, who can be present during the surgical procedure to assess the wound, develop a postoperative plan of care, and suggest wound dressing techniques, is an excellent use of multidisciplinary resources.

Application of compressive wraps and pressure garments, although useful to control swelling, must not be applied so tightly as to impair blood flow to the area. Prolonged blanching, cyanosis, lack of pulses, and delayed capillary refill are signs of inadequate blood flow to the area and require immediate attention to correct the problem. The FA, along with other members of the health care team, must identify the physiological processes unique to each surgical patient and anticipate, prevent, and treat wound healing problems.

THE FAs ROLE IN PAIN CONTROL

Pain has a different meaning for different people at different times. A baseline assessment of preoperative pain is vital for effective postoperative pain management. Although the FAs may feel they have limited responsibility for control of pain, the actions taken in the OR have a direct effect on postoperative pain. The operative procedure produces acute pain as an unavoidable result of tissue damage at the site; however, another, possibly preventable source of pain is cutting or compressing nerve fibers, or damage to tissue not related to the surgical procedure.

Anesthetics and analgesics that allow the patient to tolerate the pain associated with the procedure have allowed advances in surgery. A thorough discussion of anesthesia is found in Chapter 10; this section will provide a brief discussion of the pathophysiology of pain and the FAs role in pain management.

TYPES OF PAIN

The most common types of pain associated with surgery are somatic pain, which results from damage to connective tissue, muscle, bone, or skin; and visceral pain, which refers to pain in the internal organs and the abdomen. Neuropathic pain may result from injury to nerves during surgery (McCance & Huether, 2006). Phantom pain, which may follow amputation of a limb, occurs in up to 80% of amputees (Flor et al., 2000). As the number of persons who survive land mines and other disasters grows, further research is warranted on the disruption of the "pain memory" associated with this phenomenon.

Even with emphasis on pain management and well-publicized regulatory standards, more than 50% of postoperative patients report moderate to severe pain; the elderly are especially vulnerable (Sauaia et al., 2005). Unrelieved postoperative pain results in:

- Delayed discharge
- Inability to perform activities of daily living
- Slower rate of healing
- Higher complication rates
- Unscheduled readmissions
- Diminished ability to cough and deep breathe, which increases the risk for respiratory complications
- Decreased activity, which puts the patient at risk for constipation, deep vein thrombosis, and ileus (Banks, 2007)

Undertreated acute postoperative pain may develop into chronic pain. In fact, 10% to 50% of patients undergoing such common procedures as inguinal hernia repairs, mastectomies, and coronary artery bypass grafting develop persistent chronic pain (Phippen et al., 2009).

Pathophysiology

The perception of pain arises from specialized nerve endings called nociceptors. Painful stimuli are then transmitted through two different types of nerve fibers: A delta fibers, which carry well-localized sharp pain sensations and are responsible for initiating reactions to acute pain; and smaller, C fibers, which are responsible for the diffuse burning or aching sensations that typically follow the initial onset of pain. The transmission of painful stimuli is modulated by three different types of neurotransmitters:

- Pain excitatory—facilitate the rapid transmission of the pain stimuli
- Pain inhibitory—substances such as endorphins and opioids that interrupt the transmission of painful stimuli
- Inflammatory—chemicals released by damaged cells which irritate the nociceptors (McCance & Huether, 2006)

The action of pain medications is based on blocking or enhancing these neurotransmitters.

All nerve fibers associated with pain eventually terminate in the dorsal horn of the gray matter in the spinal cord. From there, the painful stimuli travel to various areas of the brain. The thalamus is responsible for initiating the "fight or flight" response; the parietal lobe determines the cognitive or "meaning" aspect of pain; and the frontal lobe of the cerebral cortex allows expression of the pain, or what is observed (McCance & Huether, 2006).

The signs and symptoms of acute pain are predictable, and are directly related to the event (McCance & Huether, 2006). Vital sign changes include tachycardia, hypertension, fever, diaphoresis, and dilated pupils, which can all be attributed to activation of the sympathetic nervous system and the "fight or flight" response. Behavioral changes such as moaning or rocking may also be observed. However, the absence of any of these "normal" signs and symptoms of pain does not mean the patient is not experiencing discomfort. Age, gender, culture, ethnicity, other disease processes, past experience with other painful stimuli, and medications may all alter the presentation of pain. In addition, anxiety intensifies the response to pain (Symreng & Fishman, 2004). Because pain and anxiety have very similar signs and symptoms, interventions that address both are the most effective. Providing reassurance and education are two important ways the FA can contribute perioperatively towards the management of pain. For example, the FA can suggest two diversionary techniques—concentrating on breathing and muscle relaxation—to assist with pain control. Presence and touch are also powerful tools, and remaining with the patient and holding a hand, when appropriate, can do much to assuage the anxiety associated with the surgical experience.

Preoperative

In addition to the acute pain that follows surgery, many patients present with varying degrees of chronic pain preoperatively. This will need to be taken into account when planning an effective pain management program. Various tools for assessing pain are included in Chapter 7. The FA should be familiar with the pain assessment tool used by the facility, taking into account that not all patients understand how to use the popular 1–10 pain rating guide. The Wong-Baker FACES pain rating scale may be more appropriate for use in children or for those patients who do not understand English.

Patients should receive preoperative education focusing on ways in which pain will be treated, methods for assessing pain, and how and when to request analgesia (Joint Commission, 2009; Phippen, 2009). This information may also be utilized intraoperatively if the patient is receiving a local anesthetic.

Intraoperative

Virtually every surgical or invasive procedure involves some sort of pain intervention. The FA should be familiar with the anesthetic chosen for the procedure as well as the normal doses and side effects of any local anesthetics used on the field. All syringes must be labeled prior to administration of the drug (AORN, 2009a). The FA should never accept an unlabeled syringe.

Positioning (discussed in detail in Chapter 1) can be a major cause of both acute and chronic pain postoperatively. Gentle handling of the patient and adequate, appropriate padding are crucial. Extremities should never be forced past their usual range of motion. Nerve and tissue damage can occur from carelessly leaning on a patient's abdomen or arm. Permanent nerve damage can occur from a mayo stand resting on a patient's legs, or feet left crossed at the ankles. It is the FAs responsibility to help monitor the surgical field and check for alignment and pressure points after every change in patient position.

The length of time the patient is left in one position directly influences the degree of tissue and nerve damage and subsequent pain. The FA can significantly decrease the operative time with adequate wound exposure and rapid attention to bleeding vessels, by communicating needs to the circulating nurse in advance, and by thoroughly and efficiently completing such tasks as suturing and applying dressings. Beginning Oct. 1, 2008, Medicare/Medicaid no longer reimburses for charges associated with hospital-acquired pressure ulcers and deep vein thromboses; this should further encourage the exquisite attention to detail needed to prevent potential complications.

Due to improvements in surgical techniques, patients are now able to be discharged the same day for procedures that would have required several days' hospitalization only a few years ago. Laminectomies, anterior cruciate repairs, and laparoscopic cholecystectomies are just a few of the minimally invasive procedures for which patients are able to go home within 23 hours of surgery. Pain management techniques that traditionally included patient-controlled analgesia (PCA) or IV opioids are no longer an option for these procedures.

General Anesthesia   Although the FA is not personally involved in the administration of general anesthetic agents, remaining by the side of the patient and being prepared to assist the anesthesia care provider in the event of an emergency is an integral part of the FAs role. The FA should know the location of emergency carts (including code, difficult airway, malignant hyperthermia, and latex allergy carts) for every facility for which he or she holds practice privileges.

Regional Anesthesia
Epidural/Spinal Anesthesia   If the patient is scheduled for an epidural or spinal anesthesia, the FA may assist with opening kits, dispensing medications to the anesthesia care provider, and helping to position the patient. Two common positions for initiating spinal or epidural anesthesia are the sitting and the lateral decubitus (Miller, 2005).

Hypotension is the most common side effect for both these procedures; in addition to supporting the patient and returning him to a safe position, the FA may also be asked to assist the anesthesia care provider in obtaining fluids and other supplies.

Peripheral Nerve Blocks   The FA must anticipate the use of peripheral blocks for surgeries on extremities, especially for patients with cardiac and respiratory impairment. Peripheral nerve blocks can provide superior pain control compared to opioids, and may be administered as a single injection or continuous infusion of local anesthetics (Banks, 2007; Miller, 2005; Sargent & Dunfee, 2005). Depending on the medication used, a single intraoperative injection may provide hours of pain relief. Continuous infusion pumps typically provide pain medications for 72 hours, after which time they are discontinued, often by the patient or family member (Banks, 2007). These methods allow the patient to make the initial transition from hospital to home with minimal discomfort. Additional advantages are decreases in surgery and recovery time, decrease in opioid side effects, and the ability of the patient to move him/herself after the procedure (Sargent & Dunfee, 2005). FAs should be familiar with the location and technique for performing peripheral nerve blocks because they often assist the surgeon or anesthesia care provider with placement of the block.

Local and Moderate Sedation   This technique involves injecting the anesthetic medication directly into the wound site. Local anesthetics have an opioid-sparing effect (reducing the amount of opioid needed), thus decreasing the risk of their side effects (Banks, 2007). This type of anesthetic is frequently chosen for patients with cardiac and/or pulmonary dysfunction, who may not be able to tolerate a general anesthetic. These patients may be awake and alert through part of the intraoperative period and will require additional reassurance and emotional comfort (Phillips, 2007). The FA can assist by communicating the actions of the team to the patient before they occur and by keeping conversation brief, appropriate, and centered on the patient. Words that may have an anxiety-provoking meaning, such as "knife," "cut" or "burn," should be avoided.

The most frequently used medications for local infiltration are Xylocaine (lidocaine) and Marcaine (bupivacaine). Ropivacaine may be used in continuous local anesthetic infusion pumps. Table 8-15 outlines the drugs most commonly used for local anesthesia. Epinephrine may be added for its vasoconstrictive properties and to prolong the analgesic action of the drug. It should never be used in areas of compromised circulation, terminal digits (fingers and toes), or the penis due to the risk of tissue ischemia and necrosis. Furthermore, the incision should never be made before the area is tested for lack of sensation.

Postoperative

The choice of postoperative pain medication is based on:

- the type of surgery
- the age of the patient
- presence of hepatic or renal dysfunction
- comorbid conditions and their concurrent medications with the potential for drug interactions
- allergies and sensitivities
- cultural beliefs
- previous experiences with pain and surgery (AORN, 2009b)

Patient-controlled analgesia (PCA) is typically initiated in the Post Anesthesia Care Unit (PACU). This method allows the patient to administer IV pain medications

Table 8-15   Local Anesthetics

Amides

- Lidocaine (intermediate duration)
- Prilocaine (intermediate duration)
- Bupivacane (long duration)
- Etidocaine (long duration)
- Mepivacaine (intermediate duration)
- Ropivacaine (long duration)
- Levobupivacaine (long duration)

Esters

- Cocaine (intermediate duration)
- Chloroprocaine (short duration)
- Tetracaine (long duration)
- Procaine (short duration)

Local anesthetics block the generation and propagation of nerve impulses. The choice of a local anesthetic (short-acting, long-acting) depends on the duration of the surgery, the regional anesthetic technique used (e.g., subcutaneous infiltration, peripheral nerve block, central neural blockade), and the potential for local or systemic toxicity (e.g., the ester-type local anesthetics are hydrolyzed by cholinesterase enzyme and have a more rapid clearance than most amides).

Sources: Adapted from Davis, T.C. (2009). Local Anesthetics. In Drain, C., & Odom-Forren, J. (Eds.), *Perianesthesia nursing: A critical care approach.* St. Louis: Saunders Elsevier; Rothrock, J.C. (1999). *The RN First Assistant: An expanded perioperative nursing role.* Philadelphia: Lippincott.

via a button connected to a programmable pump (ASPN, 2008).The FA may assist in the pain management program by helping to identify patients who are appropriate for this type of pain control. Children, those patients who cannot physically manipulate a dispensing button, and confused patients are not good candidates for this type of analgesia management.

The patient should be an active partner in selecting his pain management program, and the FA can serve as an advocate in communicating patient preferences to the rest of the health care team. Nonpharmacologic comfort measures (e.g., ice, elevation, positioning) are part of everyone's scope of practice. Inquiries about the intensity of the pain, its location, quality, and measures to alleviate it should be part of every postoperative encounter.

Documenting progress

The daily progress note (see Table 8-10) summarizes the patient's condition and alerts caregivers, consultants, and other staff members to special needs. Referrals for physical therapy or cardiac rehabilitation are also documented in the progress notes. Reviewing documentation by all members of the multidisciplinary team, including the nurses' notes, may alert the FA and the attending physician to include pertinent information in the discharge orders.

Discharge Planning Information obtained from the admission assessment provides baseline information for discharge planning (Hinshaw, 2006; Rothrock, 1999b). The patient's functional status and ability to perform activities of daily living (bathing, self-feeding, dressing, toileting, dressing, and grooming) should be considered in the discharge order (Table 8-16).

The patient's prognosis, functional status, and support system are among the factors that influence the decision to refer the patient to the home, an extended-care facility, or to a hospice. Discharge orders should include a complete list of medications (including directions for use and possible side effects), dietary recommendations, follow-up appointments, and information about emergency contacts.

Patient education (see Chapter 9) should provide information about postoperative wound care (including reportable signs and symptoms of complications) as well as medications, diet, and activity. Patients and their significant others should be encouraged to ask questions before and after discharge. Keeping a diary (which includes written questions for the caregiver) facilitates effective communication during follow-up visits (or telephone calls). Clarifying misconceptions is important to promote optimal patient outcomes.

Table 8-16   Discharge Orders

Discharge Orders
• Date/time
• Discharge to: home, nursing home, extended care facility, hospice
• Medications
• Diet
• Activities
• Self-care
• Follow-up appointments with appropriate services or physicians
• In emergency: return to hospital via Emergency Department or call physician

Source: Discharge orders courtesy of Robert Blumm, MA, PA-C, DFAAPA.

In preparation for discharge, the FA can identify learning needs that can enhance or impede recuperation (Rothrock, 1999b). Factors to address include:

- Potential problems that can endanger the patient's safety (e.g., unstable gait)
- Knowledge of the problem that necessitated surgery (e.g., possible long-term effects of coronary artery disease on future coronary-related events)
- Concerns about potential complications (e.g., risk for bleeding in a patient taking anticoagulant medications)
- Skills and equipment required for management of the problem (e.g., need for a walker or special braces)

The FA's role in achieving quality outcomes affects all aspects of the patient's experience—whether the care is provided in an ambulatory or tertiary care setting—and reflects both independent critical thinking and interdependent multidisciplinary collaboration. The FA plays a significant role throughout the continuum of care.

GLOSSARY

EARLY WOUND COMPLICATIONS

Infections

Please note: Additional treatment for many of these conditions will include antibiotic therapy and prolonged hospitalization with the potential need for additional surgery. These complications result in additional pain, suffering, loss of wages, and possible permanent changes in quality of life. After October 1, 2008, Medicare/Medicaid no longer reimburses for health care-associated infections.

Cellulitis: bacterial infection that spreads in tissue planes; usually causes intense inflammation manifested locally as tenderness, pain, swelling, erythema, and warmth.

Abscess: localized bacterial infection marked by a circumscribed area of pus (necrotic tissue, bacteria, and white blood cells). Abscesses tend to develop point tenderness and fluctuate on palpation. They are often under high pressure and tend to seed bacteria, causing bacteremia or sepsis by invasion of vascular spaces, or cellulitis from involvement of adjacent tissues.

Gas gangrene: rapidly progressive infection arising from injuries associated with devitalized muscle and decreased local oxygen tension. Swelling and pain occur early (within 24 hours) after injury and may be associated with crepitus from gas formation in the muscles. Often, the wound produces a thin, watery, brown, foul-smelling discharge that may contain gas bubbles and bacteria. Skin overlying the affected area may appear bronze-colored and dusky; dark red muscle may protrude through the wound. Such a patient faces impending septic shock. Treatment consists of immediate surgical exploration of the wound with decompression of the involved muscle compartment, wide excision, and muscle debridement.

Dehiscence: breakdown and separation of tissue layers in a wound, usually occurring five to eight days postoperatively. Although half of all cases are associated with infection, dehiscence may also occur in many patients who did not demonstrate a cutaneous "healing ridge" of tissue in their incisions. Poorly managed ischemic wounds and wound closure under extreme tension are other common causes of dehiscence. If dehiscence is noted within six hours and is caused by premature suture removal, the wound is immediately resutured. Otherwise, the wound is usually managed with open packing and secondary or delayed primary closure. When there is serosanguinous drainage from an abdominal wound five to eight days after surgery and the healing ridge is absent, the wound should be explored to define the extent of fascial dehiscence; significant fascial dehiscence may lead to evisceration. If immediate operative reclosure is not possible, then evisceration may be prevented with abdominal binders and bed rest.

Seroma or Blood Collections
Seroma: collection of serum that frequently complicates wounds involving undermined tissues, such as mastectomy flaps or large incisions in obese patients. Although these collections are initially sterile and resistant to infection, they quickly become susceptible to contamination and should be drained. Hemorrhage within a wound may be related to hypertension, coagulopathy, or excessive postoperative motion; however, most wound hematomas are the result of surgically controllable bleeding, such as an unligated vessel. These should be evacuated under sterile conditions, because they predispose wounds to infection and may take months to organize and resorb. They can be resutured unless infection or ongoing bleeding is present.

LATE WOUND COMPLICATIONS
Incisional hernia: considered to be a hospital-acquired failure in healing. It usually occurs after abdominal wounds and is rare in chest or flank incisions. The most common cause of incisional hernia is wound infection, but technical errors in closing wounds, severe obesity, and prior dehiscence all predispose to this complication.

Epithelial cyst: membranous sac occasionally seen along suture lines, which may be prevented by properly timed skin suture removal (usually within five days).

Fibrosis: excessive accumulation of scar tissue typically found in Crohn's disease and other chronic inflammatory conditions, esophageal and urethral strictures, and breast capsules following implant surgery.

Suture sinus: small abscesses in or near a wound associated with localized infection around a suture; they persist as long as the suture remains in the tissue and may resolve spontaneously after several weeks as the suture is ejected from the wound. Suture sinuses occur most frequently with silk, cotton, or heavy multifilament sutures.

Hypertrophic scars and keloids: large, firm masses of fibrotic, collagenous tissue that arise in healing wounds for unknown reasons. Certain ethnic types (African Americans and Asians) and younger patients may be more susceptible to these lesions, which tend to occur around joints where areas of varying motion and tension exist.

Contracture: shortening of skin and soft tissues adjacent to an area of injury. Motion around joints may be severely limited, and distortion of adjoining tissue structures may result.

Source: From Rothrock, J.C. (Ed.). (1999). *The RN First Assistant: An expanded perioperative nursing role.* (3rd ed., pp. 273–277). Philadelphia: Lippincott.

REFERENCES

1. Agency for Healthcare Research and Quality (AHRQ). (2006). TeamSTEPPS™. Retrieved May 10, 2009 from http://teamstepps.ahrq.gov
2. Agency for Healthcare Research & Quality (AHRQ). (2009). Health care-associated infections (Safety Primer). Retrieved February 26, 2009 from http://psnet.ahrq.gov/primer.aspx?primerID=7
3. American Society of Anesthesiologists. (2003). What you should know about your patient's use of herbal medicines and other dietary supplements. Retrieved May 7, 2009 from http://www.asahq.org/patientEducation/herbPatient.pdf
4. American Society of Anesthesiologists. (2008). ASA physical status classification system. Retrieved December 27, 2008 from http://www.asahq.org/clinical/physicalstatus.htm
5. American Society of Perianesthesia Nurses (ASPAN).(2008). ASPAN patient information. Retrieved May 13, 2009 from http://aspan.org
6. Antonacci, A.C., Lam, S., Lavarias, V., Homel, P., & Eavey, R.D. (2008). Benchmarking surgical incident reports using a database and a triage system to reduce adverse outcomes. *Archives of Surgery, 143,* 192–197.
7. AORN. (2009a). *Perioperative standards and recommended practices: Safe medication practices.* Denver, CO: AORN.
8. AORN. (2009b). *Perioperative standards and recommended practices: Patient outcomes* (p. 29). Denver, CO: AORN.

9. Banks, A. (2007). Innovations in postoperative pain management: Continuous infusion of local anesthetics. *AORN Journal, 85,* 904–914.

10. Barclay, L., & Murata, P. (2008). AAP addresses use of complementary and alternative medicine. *Medscape medical news.* Retrieved December 17, 2008 from http:///www.medscape.com/viewarticle/584824

11. Bilimoria, K.Y., Kmiecik, T.E., DaRosa, D.A., Halverson, A., Eskandari, M.K., et al. (2009). Development of an online morbidity, mortality, and near-miss reporting system to identify patterns of adverse events in surgical patients. *Archives of Surgery, 144,* 302–311.

12. Catalano, K. (2008). Knowledge is power: Averting safety-compromising events in the OR. *AORN Journal, 88,* 987–995.

13. Centers for Medicare and Medicaid Services (CMS). (2009). Hospital acquired conditions. Retrieved April 26, 2009 from http://www.cms.hhs.gov/HospitalAcqCond

14. Chard, R. (2008). Clinical issues: Implementing a process for hand-off communications. *AORN Journal, 88,* 1005–1006.

15. Clancy, C.M. (2007). Teamwork in the perioperative setting. *AORN Journal, 86,* 18–22.

16. Culver, D.H., Horan, T.C., Gaynes, R.P., et al. (1991). Surgical wound infection rates by wound class, operative procedure, and patient risk index. National nosocomial infections surveillance system. *American Journal of Medicine, 91,* 152S–157S.

17. Denner, A. M., & Townley, S.A. (2009). Anorexia nervosa: Perioperative implications. *Continuing Education in Anaesthesia, Critical Care, and Pain, 9,* 61–64.

18. Diegelmann, R.F., & Evans, M.C. (2004). Wound healing: An overview of acute, fibrotic, and delayed healing. *Frontiers in Bioscience, 9,* 283–289.

19. Dorsey, C. (2009). Handle specimens and cultures. In M.L. Phippen, B.C. Ulmer, & M.P. Wells (Eds.) *Competency for safe patient care during operative and invasive procedures* (pp. 447–464). Denver: Competency & Credentialing Institute.

20. Epstein, R.M., Mauksch, L., Carroll, J., & Jaén, C.R. (2008). Have you really addressed your patient's concerns? *Family Practice Management, 15,* 35–40. Retrieved May 11, 2009 from http://www.medscape.com/viewarticle/578921

21. Feuchtinger, J., Halfens, R.J., & Dassen, T. (2005). Pressure ulcer risk factors in cardiac surgery: A review of the research literature. *Heart Lung, 34,* 375–385.

22. Flor, H., Birbaumer, N., & Sherman, R. (2000). Phantom limb pain. *Pain Clinical Updates, 13*(3). Retrieved May 13, 2009 from www.iasp-pain.org

23. Friedman, B., Encinosa, W., Jiang, H.J., & Mutter, R. (2009). Do patient safety events increase readmissions? *Medical Care, 47,* 583–590.

24. Gawande, A.A., Studdert, D.M., Orav, E.J., Brennan, T.A., & Zinner, M.J. (2003). Risk factors for retained instruments and sponges after surgery. *New England Journal of Medicine, 348,* 229–235.

25. Geerts, W.H., Bergqvist, D., Pineo, G.F., Heit, J.A., Samama, C.M., et al. (2008). Prevention of venous thromboembolism. *Chest, 136 Suppl,* 3815–4535.

26. Hall, M.C. (2007). Surgical Care Improvement Project (SCIP) Module 1: Infection prevention update. Retrieved April 26, 2009 from http://cme.medscape.com/viewarticle/557689

27. Haridas, M., & Malangoni, M.A. (2008). Predictive factors for surgical site infection in general surgery. *Surgery, 144,* 496–503.

28. Haynes, A.B., Weiser, T.G., Berry, W.R., et al. (2009). A surgical safety checklist to reduce morbidity and mortality in a global population. *New England Journal of Medicine, 360,* 491–499.

29. Hegarty, J., Walsh, E., Burton, A., Murphy, S., O'Gorman, F., & McPolin, G. (2009). Nurses' knowledge of inadvertent hypothermia. *AORN Journal, 89*, 701–713.

30. Hinshaw, D.B. (2006). Management of the older surgical patient. In G. Doherty (Ed.), *Current surgical diagnosis and treatment* (12th ed., pp. 69–74). New York: Lange Medical Books/McGraw-Hill.

31. The Joint Commission. (2009). *Hospital accreditation standards: PC.01.02.07* (p 263). Oakbrook Terrace, IL: The Joint Commission.

32. The Joint Commission. (2008a). SCIP core measures Retrieved April 26, 2009 from http://www.jointcommission.org/ PerformanceMeasurement/ PerformanceMeasurement/ SCIP+Core+Measure+Set.htm

33. The Joint Commission.(2008b). Universal protocol for preventing wrong site, wrong procedure, wrong person surgery. Accreditation program: Hospital. National patient safety goals. Retrieved April 26, 2009 from http://www.jointcommission. org/NR/rdonlyres/AEA17A06-BB67-4-C4E-B0FC-DD195FE6BF2A/0/UP_HAP_20080616.pdf

34. The Joint Commission. (October 2008c). 2009 national patient safety goals. Retrieved May 9, 2009 from http://www. jointcommission.org/NR/rdonlyres/ D619D05C-A682-47CB-874A-8-DE16D21CE24/0/HAP_NPSG_Outline.pdf

35. The Joint Commission. (2008d). Anticoagulation therapy. Retrieved May 9, 2009 from http://www.jointcommission.org/AccreditationPrograms/ LongTermCare/Standards/09_FAQs/ NPSG/Medication_safety/ NPSG.03.05.01/Anticoagulation+ therapy.htm

36. Kaye, K.S., Anderson, D.J., Sloane, R., Chen, L.F., Choi, Y., Link, K., et al. (2009). The effect of surgical site infection on older operative patients.

Journal American Geriatric Society, 57, 46–54.

37. Kiekkas, P., Poulopoulou, M., Papahatzi, A., & Panagiotis, S. (2005). Effects of hypothermia and shivering on standard PACU monitoring of patients. *AANA Journal, 73*, 47–53.

38. King, C. (1999). Infection control. In J. Rothrock (Ed.), The RN First Assistant: An expanded perioperative nursing role (3rd ed.). Philadelphia: Lippincott.

39. Kurz, A., Sessler, D.I., & Lenhardt, R. (1996). Perioperative normothermia to reduce the incidence of surgical-wound infection and shorten hospitalization.

40. Makary, M.A., Sexton, J.B., Freischlag, J.A., Millman, E.A., Pryor, D., Holzmueller, C., et al. (2006). Patient safety in surgery. *Annals of Surgery, 243,* 628–635.

41. Mann, B.D. (2009). *Surgery: A competency-based companion.* Philadelphia: Elsevier Saunders.

42. McCance, K.L., & Huether, S.E. (2006). *Pathophysiology: The biologic basis for disease in adults and children* (5th ed.). St. Louis, MO: Elsevier.

43. MedQIC. Home site for Surgical Care Improvement Project (SCIP). Retrieved April 26, 2009, from http://www. qualitynet.org/dcs/ContentServer?c=MQ Parents&pagename=Medqic/Content/Pa rentShellTemplate&cid=1122904930422 &parentName=Topic

44. Mews, P. (2009). Establish and maintain a sterile field. In M.L. Phippen, B.C. Ulmer, & M.P. Wells (Eds.), *Competency for safe patient care during operative and invasive procedures*(pp. 215–282). Denver: Competency & Credentialing Institute.

45. Miller, R.D. (Ed.). (2005). *Miller's Anesthesia* (6th ed.). Philadelphia, PA: Elsevier.

46. Mundy, L.M., Doherty, G.M., & Cobb, J.P. (2006). Inflammation, infection, & antimicrobial therapy. In G. Doherty & L. Way (Eds.), *Current surgical diagnosis*

& treatment (12th ed., pp. 97–126). New York: Lange Medical Books/ McGraw-Hill.

47. National Center for Health Statistics. (2006). *Prevalence of overweight and obesity among adults: United States, 2003–2004.* U.S. Department of Health and Human Services, Centers for Disease Control and Prevention, National Center for Health Statistics. Hyattsville, MD: Author. Retrieved May 14, 2009, from http://www.cdc.gov/nchs/products/pubs/ pubd/hestats/overweight/overwght_ adult_03.htm

48. NICE-SUGAR Study Investigators. (2009). Intensive versus conventional glucose control in critically ill patients. *New England Journal of Medicine, 360,* 1283–1297.

49. Oram, D.H. (2006). Basic surgical skills. *Clinical Obstetrics and Gynaecology, 20,* 61–71.

50. Paige, J.T., Aaron, D.L., Yang, T., Howell, D.S., Hilton, C.W., et al. (2008). Implementation of a preoperative briefing protocol improves accuracy of teamwork assessment in the operating room. *The American Surgeon, 74,* 817–823.

51. Pear, S.M., Williamson, T.H. (2009). The RN First Assistant: An expert resource for surgical site infection prevention. *AORN Journal, 89,* 1093–1097.

52. Phillips, N. (2007). *Berry and Kohn's operating room technique* (11th ed.). St. Louis, MO: Mosby.

53. Phippen, M.L., Ulmer, B.C., & Wells, M.P. (2009). *Competency for safe patient care during operative and invasive procedures.* Denver, CO: Competency and Credentialing Institute.

54. Pronovost, P.J., Holzmueller, C.G., Young, J., Whitney, P., Wu, A.W., et al. (2007). Using incident reporting to improve patient safety: A conceptual model. *Journal of Patient Safety, 3,* 27–33.

55. Qadan, M., Akca, O., Mahid, S.S., Hornung, C.A., & Polk, H.C. (2009).

Perioperative supplemental oxygen therapy and surgical site infection. *Archives of Surgery, 144,* 359–368.

56. Ranji, S.R., Shetty, K., Posley, K.A., et al. (2007). Prevention of healthcare-associated infections. In K. Shojania, K. McDonald, R. Wachter, & D. Owens (Eds.), Closing the quality gap: A critical analysis of quality improvement strategies. Technical Review 9. Rockville, MD: Agency for Healthcare Research and Quality. Retrieved April 26, 2009 from http://psnet.ahrq.gov/primer. aspx?primerID=7

57. Rathbun, S. (2009). The Surgeon General's call to action to prevent deep vein thrombosis and pulmonary embolism. Cardiology patient page. *Circulation, 119,* e480–e482.

58. Reines, H.D., & Seifert, P.C. (2005). Patient safety: Latex allergy. *Surgical Clinics of North America, 85,* 1329–1340.

59. Rothrock, J.C. (1999a). The diagnostic process. In J. Rothrock (Ed.), *The RN First Assistant: An expanded perioperative nursing role* (3rd ed., pp. 105–126). Philadelphia: Lippincott.

60. Rothrock, J.C. (1999b). Perioperative patient preparation. In J. Rothrock (Ed.), *The RN First Assistant: An expanded perioperative nursing role* (3rd ed., pp. 1127–1152). Philadelphia: Lippincott.

61. Rothrock, J.C. (1999c). Wound healing. In J. Rothrock (Ed.), *The RN First Assistant: An expanded perioperative nursing role* (3rd ed., pp. 259–286). Philadelphia: Lippincott.

62. Sargent, C.A., & Dunfee, M.T. (2005). Knee block anesthesia for arthroscopic procedures. *AORN Journal, 82,* 20–36.

63. Sauaia, A., Min, S., Leber, C., Erbacher, K., Abrams, F., & Fink, R. (2005). Postoperative pain management in elderly patients: Correlation between adherence to treatment guidelines and patient satisfaction. *Journal of the American Geriatrics Society, 53,* 274–282.

64. Sewchuk, D., Padula, C., & Osborne, E. (2006). Prevention and early detection of pressure ulcers. *AORN Journal, 84*, 75–96.

65. Singhal, H., Kaur, K., & Zammit, C. (2008). Wound infection. *emedicine specialties.* Retrieved May 6, 2009 from http://emedicine.medscape.com/article/188988-print

66. Stokowski, L.A. (2008). Healthcare anywhere: The pledge of telehealth. *Medscape Nurses.* Retrieved November 5, 2008 from http://www.medscape.com/viewarticle/581800

67. Symreng, I., & Fishman, S.M. (2004). Pain and anxiety. *Pain Clinical Updates,* *12*(7). Retrieved May 13, 2009 from www.iasp-pain.org

68. Thacker, P.D. (2005). Physician-robot makes the rounds. *Journal of the American Medical Association, 293,* 150.

69. Woolever, D.R. (2008). The art and science of clinical decision making. *Family Practice Management, 15,* 31–36.

70. World Health Organization (WHO). (2008). Surgical safety checklist. Retrieved May 9, 2009 from http://www.who.int/patientsafety/safesurgery/tools_resources/SSSL_Checklist_finalJun08.pdf

9

Patient Education

Denise O'Brien

Preparing patients for surgical, diagnostic, and interventional procedures requires assessment of patient educational needs, knowledge of teaching/learning principles, the information needed by the patient, and educational resources. Quality care includes providing patients and families with appropriate information for decision making. When patients are adequately prepared for procedures, benefits to the patient include shorter stays, less anxiety, fewer complications, as well as improved knowledge, compliance, satisfaction, and discharge preparation (Stern & Lockwood, 2005). Patient education is a multidisciplinary effort that uses the knowledge and expertise of FAs, physicians, nurses, and other health care providers to improve outcomes for surgical patients.

GOALS, PURPOSE, AND BENEFITS OF PATIENT EDUCATION IN THE PERIOPERATIVE SETTING

Increasing the patient's sense of self-worth, decreasing anxiety, and reducing facility and provider liability are all goals of patient education (O'Brien, 2008). Patients and their families/caregivers need information provided in a form that they can understand and use. In addition, they are empowered when the focus is on the patient instead of on the provider or facility. Patient-centered care views the patient as a partner, engages the patient in interactions that identify and alleviate vulnerabilities, and allows shared authority over care decisions (Hobbs, 2009). The intended result is an educated surgical patient who understands and complies with preoperative regimens, discharge instructions, and overall health management.

The Joint Commission (TJC) in its 2008 report on Healthcare at the Crossroads (TJC 2008b) aptly notes that the patient has an enormous stake in his or her care and should be respected as an equal partner. The notion of "patient as partner" has significant implications for the quality and safety of patient care. Family members or others to whom the patient is emotionally tied are also part of this health care partnership. According to the report, adopting patient-centered care values is essential for improving patient safety and patient and staff satisfaction. When patient-centered care values are adopted, barriers to patient and family engagement, such as low health literacy and personal and cultural preferences, are identified and addressed.

Positive effects of preoperative patient education include less anxiety and fear, shorter recovery time, decreased length of stay (LOS) by 1.5 days, fewer postoperative complications, less analgesia use, increased patient satisfaction, and improved compliance with treatment regimens (Joanna Briggs Institute, 2000; Kiyohara et al., 2004; Roach, Tremblay, & Bowers, 1995; Shuldman, 1999; Sjöling et al., 2003). Other positive effects are lower levels of psychological distress and physical pain. Various patient outcomes measures have been studied; they include knowledge of preoperative, intraoperative, and postoperative procedures, compliance, satisfaction, skills, physical coping, mobility, independence, and discharge preparedness (Joanna Briggs Institute, 2000).

By definition, patient education focuses on patients and their families/caregivers. They need adequate information and support for successful navigation of the perioperative experience. Johansson et al. (2007) promote a model of empowering patient education within a patient-centered model of care. Consisting of an individually tailored amount of knowledge, their model of empowering education includes biophysiological (signs, symptoms), functional (activities of daily living), experiential (feeling, experiences), social (social network), ethical (individual rights), and financial (payments, benefits) issues. Their research with orthopedic patients suggests that preadmission counseling that focuses on empowering patients with knowledge and uses appropriate methods to achieve empowerment were highly effective in patient education. Another example of a patient-centered care model empowers elderly patients through choice, again focusing care on the patient instead of the usual provider or system (Merriman, 2008). Patient-centered models such as these promote discharge readiness that is grounded in both patient knowledge and preferences.

Compliance—The Joint Commission Requirements

TJC accreditation standards underscore the requirement that patients receive both oral and written information about their care, treatment, and services in a comprehensible form. Understanding information through effective communication improves patient safety and reduces risk for surgical patients. Rationales and elements that specify performance criteria accompany each TJC standard. Standards that address patient education fully expect that such education will assess learning requirements specific to the patient's needs, identify any barriers, and develop plans to address those needs. It is also important to take into account religious and cultural beliefs, emotional barriers, desire and motivation to learn, learning preferences, physical or cognitive abilities and limitations, and barriers to communication as appropriate (TJC, 2008a). Appendix 9-1 identifies sample materials available from TJC for providing and measuring patient education.

Educational and Developmental Considerations

Before patient education content and programs can be developed, information about patient characteristics is required. Patient characteristics that influence educational planning and development include age; primary language; reading level; sensory limitations; physical condition; developmental level; mental, emotional, or educational limitations; and motivation and attitude (O'Brien, 2008). Knowing the patient's learning preferences helps to individualize learning materials. Awareness of adult learning principles is also helpful when one is preparing educational programs and materials.

Pediatric education depends in part on the developmental stage of the child. Various theories of developmental stages exist and are useful when FAs are involved in planning educational programs and materials. Children feel less anxiety and show less postoperative negative behavior when they take part in educational programs, but these programs may require significant financial investment (Rice et al., 2008). Because higher parental anxiety can lead to increased distress in children, parents should be included in all pediatric teaching.

Choosing a teaching method for a child requires evaluation of the child's age and developmental level, the family's available resources, and the cognitive abilities of both child and parent (O'Brien, 2008). Four- to twelve-year-olds may enjoy taking a facility tour and playing with puppets or models. The three- to seven-year-old may want to draw, act out events, or describe them; play therapy with puppets or dolls may also be effective as a learning method. Films or videos are most effective in the seven- to twelve-year-old age group and can be viewed anywhere. Models allowing visualization and manipulation of equipment are most effective with three- to six-year-olds but are useful with all ages. Breathing masks, circuits, splints, IV tubing, and models of anatomical parts are just some of the educational tools available to the FA.

INFLUENCES ON LEARNING

Physiological, emotional, cultural, and environmental barriers challenge the learning process for all ages and developmental levels (O'Brien, 2008). Language barriers significantly interfere with comprehension. Individual health beliefs, attitudes, levels of stress, coping skills, anxiety, and social support also need to be considered. Evaluating present knowledge, previous experience, prior education, perceptions and expectations, as well as potential misinformation about the procedure will allow FAs to provide more effective educational materials for the patient.

The personal knowledge and experience of the FA also influence preoperative education (Fitzpatrick & Hyde, 2006). Depending on previous involvement with patient education, some FAs will benefit by attending patient education workshops. Learning how to teach effectively is a necessity.

GENERAL EDUCATIONAL PRINCIPLES

Patient education may occur every time the FA has an encounter with the patient. Preoperative education begins when surgery is scheduled and when the FA provides new information, reinforces previously learned information, and assesses new learning needs. Rankinen et al. (2007) found that patients do not receive as much knowledge as they expect and that not all patients need the same amount or level of information. Individualized patient education, based in part on what the patient specifically wants to know, provides the greatest benefit.

In his early work a half century ago, Miller (1956) established that the average individual recalls at best about seven bits or "chunks" of new information. However, even today, clinicians often disregard Miller's early work and overload patients with information and fail to use any memory-enhancing techniques (Sandberg et al., 2008). For example, reinforcing information and using multimodal approaches to provide information help patients improve retention. Structuring information with a statement such as "now I will tell you what will happen when you arrive in the operating room," and then following it with a review of information helps patients remember what they were told.

LEARNER ASSESSMENT

FAs, as well as other health care providers, need to ask, "What is it that the patient wants to know?" Many health care providers believe they already know what that information is. However, Keulers et al. (2008) found that surgeons underestimated patient desire for preoperative information. In their study, patients wanted to know about all aspects of the hospital admission process, postoperative period, and self-care. In contrast, surgeons in the study reportedly—and erroneously—believed patients wanted to focus specifically on aspects of their disease, examination results, and the operation.

Another aspect of learner assessment is patient health literacy and its impact on the ability to learn and comprehend information. Comprehending health information is not a simple, straightforward task (Box 9-1). The Institute of Medicine defines health literacy as "the degree to which individuals have the capacity to obtain, process, and understand basic health information and services needed to make appropriate health decisions" (IOM, 2004, p. 34). Literacy itself is an issue for a large proportion of the population of the United States (National Assessment of Adult Literacy, 2003). English literacy is lacking in 5% of the population; nearly a third of the population has only basic understanding

---

Box 9-1	**Provider-Patient Communication Regarding Total Knee Replacement**

A recent study confirmed that health care providers and patients often have different ideas about the need for total knee replacement (TKR). The study was based on questionnaire responses from providers and patients at baseline and after office consultation on the need for TKR. Coded audiotranscripts of communication behaviors in the provider/patient encounter were also reviewed. The final sample consisted of responses from 27 health care providers (5 physicians, 17 medical residents, and 5 physician assistants) and 74 patients.

Analysis showed that provider-patient agreement was modest to poor on the following issues: whether the patient should have TKR; the severity of the patients' osteoarthritis; and the expected benefits and risks for TKR. About 20% of the time, providers' and patients' responses differed on whether TKR was even recommended. Moreover, providers generally viewed the severity of osteoarthritis as less severe and expressed less concern about surgical complications than patients did.

Differences between provider and patient concerns about surgery were significant when patients were less participatory. Aspects of communication that could improve provider-patient concordance include more active patient participation, provider partnership building, and patient perceptions about the provider's ability to impart information. The authors suggest that although providers and patients in this study may have discussed the nature of surgery and its expected benefits, they may not have had adequate conversations about the patients' need for TKR.

The study authors note that future research is needed on how providers can be both comprehensive and comprehensible in the provision of clinical information and in discovering patients' beliefs and concerns. They also suggest examining the role of companions in consultations because they often serve as surrogates or advocates.

Source: Adapted from Street, Jr., R., Richardson, M.N., Cox, V., & Suarez-Almazor, M.E. (2009). (Mis) Understanding in patient-health care provider communication about total knee replacement. *Arthritis Care and Research, 61,* 100–107.

of English; and up to 22% possess reading and math skills that are below basic levels. About 50% of Americans have difficulty using text to accomplish routine tasks. Health literacy also encompasses educational, social, and cultural factors; these influence individual expectations. Health literacy (and basic literacy) considerations are essential when developing content, materials, and programs for patient education if that education is to assist patients in effectively obtaining, processing, and understanding basic health information (Rothrock, Zulick, & Zulick, 2009).

TOOLS/METHODS

Tools and methods to deliver patient education vary widely. Options include printed information, learning packages, audiovisual presentations, and individual or group teaching. The FA shares responsibility with other members of the health care team to identify the most appropriate educational tools and methods to teach and communicate particular health information.

Pamphlets and written materials are effective tools to provide preoperative information. Pamphlets and other written materials improve knowledge of the condition requiring surgery, the surgical procedure, exercise or skills necessary for self-care, and time taken to learn the exercises or skills (Joanna Briggs Institute, 2000). Pamphlets are more effective when given before admission and focus specifically on the intended surgical procedure (Joanna Briggs Institute, 2000; Stern & Lockwood, 2005). Pamphlets are available in a variety of languages. Any pamphlet or other written material should be provided in the patient's language of choice. The patient and family/caregiver also need sufficient time to read the materials and should be encouraged to ask questions about them. When indicated, interpreters must be part of the process. If necessary, a cultural "broker" should be used when the patient's cultural beliefs are likely to affect the proposed care (Wilson-Stronks & Galvez, 2007). This is critical if the FA helps to secure informed consent (Box 9-2).

Giving the patient and the family/caregiver only written information is likely to lead to inadequate education (Johansson et al., 2005). The FA should supplement written information with verbal explanations and clarification. Sufficient time should be provided for questions and further clarification. Patients should be asked to "repeat back" or "teach back" key information in their own words and demonstrate skills requisite for proper home care during surgical recovery. It may also help to suggest that patients or their families write down questions. That way, when the FA makes rounds, the questions will be ready, and clarification or repetition can proceed according to what the patient needs and wants to know.

Box 9-2	Informed Consent

Informed consent is a central element of safe surgical patient care. The National Quality Forum's Safe Practices for Better Healthcare–2009 Update is a list of 34 evidence-based measures for use in applicable clinical care settings to reduce the risk of harm to patients. Among these is Safe Practice 5—specifying the need for improved communication during the informed consent process. Well-informed patients are more likely to receive care that reflects their own values, are better prepared for requisite self-care, are more satisfied with the care they receive, and are more likely to have increased trust in their caregivers.

Safe Practice 5: Ask each patient or legal surrogate to "teach back," in his or her own words, key information about the proposed treatments or procedures for which he or she is being asked to provide informed consent.

To engage in this safe practice for informed consent, the FA can:

- Ask each patient or his or her legal surrogate to recount what he or she has been told during the informed consent discussion.
- Use informed consent forms written in simple sentences and in the primary language of the patient or legal surrogate.
- Engage the patient in a discussion about the nature and scope of the procedure covered by the consent form.
- Provide an interpreter or reader to assist non–English-speaking patients or legal surrogates, vision-impaired or hearing-impaired patients, and low-literacy patients.
- Verify that patient and or family member/legal surrogate can state the name of the procedure and, using their own words, describe it.

In its Speak-Up™ Campaign, The Joint Commission (TJC) further encourages patients as follows:

- At the surgery facility, the staff will ask you to sign an Informed Consent form. Read it carefully. It lists:
  - Your name
  - The kind of surgery you will have
  - The risks of your surgery
  - That you talked to your doctor about the surgery and asked questions
  - Your agreement to have the surgery
- Make sure everything on the form is correct.
- Make sure all of your questions have been answered. If you do not understand something on the form—speak up.

Sources: Modified from TJC: Speak Up™: *Help avoid mistakes in your surgery.* www.jointcommission.org/GeneralPublic/Speak+Up/wss_tips.htm. Retrieved April 17, 2009 from www. jointcommission ect; National Quality Forum. (2009). *Safe practices for better healthcare-2009 update.* Washington, DC: National Quality Forum. Retrieved April 17, 2009 from http://www.qualityforum.org/Search.aspx?keyword=safe+practices

Educational materials should most often be written at the fifth- or sixth-grade reading level (Seifert, 2008). The Rapid Estimate of Adult Literacy in Medicine (REALM) (Box 9-3) is a tool to screen an adult patient's reading ability. Readability tests such as the Flesch-Kincaid Readability Test, Gunning-Fog Index, Fry formula, and SMOG (Simple Measure of Gobbledygook) are available to ensure that materials are written at an appropriate level. These provide analyses of the difficulty of the material, are easy to use, and offer a simple method to evaluate readability during development of patient education materials. Simply analyzing the reading level, however, is not sufficient to ensure that educational materials will be valuable to the patient or understood.

All educational materials should be reviewed for accuracy, clarity, and ease of comprehension. Considering the population for whom the materials are intended, ask yourself, "What are the average educational level, literacy level, primary language, and age range of the audience?" Summarizing key information and focusing on main points help patients to identify important information more easily (Johansson et al., 2004).

Video formats offer additional visual information and can supplement written and verbal information, potentially lessening patient anxiety (Bondy et al., 1999; Ruffinengo et al., 2009). Although computer-assisted instruction has not been

Box 9-3	Measuring Health Literacy: The Rapid Estimate of Adult Literacy in Medicine (REALM) Tool

Among several approaches to measuring health literacy is the Rapid Estimate of Adult Literacy in Medicine or REALM. This tool uses a simple medical word recognition and pronunciation test to screen the adult patient's reading ability in medical settings. FAs can administer and score the test in less than 3 minutes. Patients read from a list of 66 common medical terms that they may encounter. The medical terms are arranged in three columns according to the number of syllables and pronunciation difficulty. Thus, column one (single syllable, easy to pronounce) may contain the word "pill." The second column contains words with more syllables that are more difficult to pronounce; this list may contain words such as "notify," "prescription," or "exercise." The final column contains the most difficult words; here one would find words such as "anemia," "diagnosis," or "osteoporosis." Each correctly read and pronounced word increases the patient's score by one word or point. Scores can then be translated into four reading levels, based on grade level: grades 0–3 (0–18 words), grades 4–6 (19–44 words), grades 7–8 (45–60 words), and grade 9 and above (61–66 words).

Source: Modified from Rothrock, J.C., Zulick, K.M., & Zulick, P.A. (2009). Patient education and health literacy. *Perioperative Nursing Clinics 4*, 131–139.

as well reviewed as other instructional methods, data related to its use are available (Stern & Lockwood, 2005). In studies examining informed consent knowledge, for example, interactive computer programs improved knowledge retention and perceived understanding (Bollschweiler, 2008). In another study comparing physician-provided information and an interactive computer program, patients achieved higher knowledge levels with the interactive computer program, and satisfaction equaled that of seeing the physician in person (Keulers et al., 2007). Although the use of videos or computer instruction may be useful in providing standardized and initial information for surgical patients, the FA must still answer questions or discuss treatment options in person.

Downloadable podcasts using portable video technology for viewing are a newer option used in some health care centers for patient education (Abreu et al., 2008). The podcasts are available from the hospital's website for download to view on the patient's home computer or portable media player. Similarly, many institutions provide patient learning channels and intranet access to in-house education programs via satellite. These are additional options for providing educational materials.

Internet-based education is also being evaluated for patient education. Heikkinen et al. (2008) found that internet-based education was as effective as face-to-face education by a nurse in increasing cognitive empowerment. Benefits of this method include its flexibility; it allows the patient to choose when and where the education is completed, and the patient is able to return to it as needed. Box 9-4 presents sample criteria the FA might use to evaluate websites and direct patients to them.

Group teaching has also been found to be as effective as individual teaching (Joanna Briggs Institute, 2000). Organizing groups before procedures may be

---

Box 9-4   **Sample Criteria for Evaluating Patient Education Websites**

- Accuracy: Is the information accurate? Is the information source clearly stated? Does the information have a date?
- Authority: Whose Website is it? If an author is identified, what credentials are offered to establish credibility? Is contact information provided so you can reach the author or publisher?
- Currency: Is the information up-to-date? When was it first posted and how recently was it updated? To gauge currency, compare the information with that available through other sources and check out hyperlinks.
- Coverage: What topics are covered and how complete is the coverage? Do hyperlinks connect to other reliable sites? Is the information well presented, with a balance of text and graphics? Do the graphics teach something or are they just decorative? Is the information written at a level that a patient could understand?

challenging, but they can offer another method to deliver educational programming. Providing education to a group requires less teaching time and offers a more cost-effective alternative to individual sessions. Group teaching also allows patients and their families to interact with others undergoing surgery. This may be comforting to both patient and family.

SPECIFIC PREOPERATIVE EDUCATION

Preoperative teaching is more effective if provided before admission. Recommended preparational content describes the planned procedure on the day of surgery including expected behaviors, possible alterations in comfort after the procedure, and strategies to reduce and manage pain (O'Brien, 2008). Patients and caregivers need clear instructions, reinforced verbally and in writing, about fasting from solids and liquids (see Chapter 10). Current medications should be reviewed with the patient and specific instructions given regarding medications that are to be stopped before the day of surgery and those that should be continued. Medications requiring special instructions include anticoagulants, insulin, and antihypertensive medications. Patients should bring medicine inhalers to the hospital, as applicable. All valuables and jewelry (including body jewelry) are to be left at home or with an adult companion/family member. To reduce risks for surgical site infection, patients bathe or shower with an antibacterial cleanser the evening before and morning of the procedure per hospital policy (AORN, 2009).

The FA must reinforce the requirement for a responsible adult companion, and if needed, a ride home when the ambulatory surgery patient is ready for discharge. Facility policies vary regarding transportation requirements and the need for companions to stay in the facility during the procedure. Knowing facility policy about these issues and having ready access to resources such as risk management or legal counsel will be beneficial to the FA when questions arise, as they often do (O'Brien, 2008).

SPECIFIC POSTOPERATIVE EDUCATION

Before surgery, anticipated postoperative behaviors are also discussed with the patient and caregiver. These may include passive exercises or the correct use of compression stockings/sequential compression devices (SCDs) (to reduce venous thromboembolism [VTE] risk); ambulation; effective deep breathing/coughing (to reduce respiratory complications); dressings, drain, or cast care; and diet/fluid needs or restrictions. Patients should also receive information about the signs and symptoms that indicate complications that should be reported to the unit nurse, physician, or FA; plans for follow-up care; pain management strategies; and who to contact in an emergency after leaving the facility.

Patient Education for Pain Management

Patient and family education is central to effective pain management. Pain management may be first discussed when the patient agrees to surgery (Figure 9-1). General information includes what to expect about pain management, method

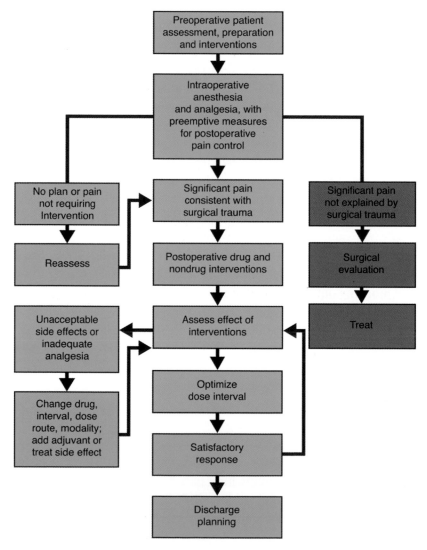

Figure 9-1

Flow chart for the management of postprocedure pain.

Source: Courtesy of Phippen, M.L., Ulmer, B.C., & Wells, M.P. (2009). *Competency for safe patient care during operative and invasive procedures* (Fig. 18.1, pp. 559). Denver: CCI.

of pain assessment, use of a pain rating scale, methods for administration of postoperative analgesia, possible combined anesthesia techniques to promote pain relief, and postdischarge pain management.

Pain rating scales are an important tool to help patients identify their pain intensity; the goal is to provide sufficient pain relief so the patient can perform activities related to satisfactory recovery or improved function. When discussing pain, it is helpful for the FA to identify patient attitudes about pain and previous experiences with pain. Ask about previous surgery and the prior effectiveness of previous pain management strategies. Using a pain scale as an example, ask the patient what an acceptable level of pain is. Acceptable pain levels differ, but the goal should be comfort and function. Ask simple questions, allow time for responses, and repeat or rephrase your questions as necessary. Pay attention to anxiety about pain. Confirm patient preferences and acceptable pain levels. This helps to uncover possible unrealistic expectations that the FA can address before surgery. This information may become part of a comprehensive postoperative pain management plan, collaboratively designed by health care providers (physician, FA, nursing staff, and others), the patient, and his or her family/caregiver. For examples of pain intensity rating scales, please refer to **Figure 7-3** in Chapter 7, Assessment.

Both pharmacological and nonpharmacological measures to manage pain should be reviewed. Relaxation techniques such as slow rhythmic breathing, listening to music of the patient's choice, distraction, guided imagery, aromatherapy, and massage can all help with mild to moderate pain. These rarely, however, can substitute for pharmacological control of severe postoperative pain.

The focus of pharmacological relief should be on managing pain and relieving severe discomfort so that the patient can rest and recover. Whether this is via nurse-administered analgesics or patient-controlled analgesia (PCA) therapy, the goal of pain management is to reduce the peaks and valleys in the pharmacologic agent's blood level concentrations. Thus, the suggestion that pain relief be administered as needed or "prn" is an outdated concept; by the time it is needed, the pain has already become higher on the intensity scale and the analgesic is at a subtherapeutic level. Thus, around-the-clock or set-interval pain relief schedules are more likely to provide effective pain control (Wells, McCaffery, & Pasero, 2008). Balanced analgesia is a multimodal approach to postoperative pain relief, combining opioids, nonsteroidal anti-inflammatory drugs (NSAIDs), and local anesthetics. Each of these agents acts through a different mechanism to interfere with the physiological pain sequence: NSAIDs inhibit pain mediators at the injury site, opioids attach to receptor sites in the spinal cord and brain, and local anesthetics block sensory inflow.

DISCHARGE PLANNING AND INFORMATION

Before the FA discharges a patient, he or she informs and educates the patient about follow-up care, treatment, and services. When deciding when the patient will be ready for discharge, the FA should share this follow-up information with the patient and family. This is important so both patient and family can prepare for the needed postdischarge care, treatment, and services. In addition, the patient and family should understand the reason for discharge or transfer. If transfer is necessary, the FA should review information about any alternatives to the transfer.

The FA, often along with members of an interdisciplinary discharge-planning team, educates the patient and family about how to obtain any continuing care, treatment, and services that he or she will need. Then, the FA or another member of the discharge-planning team provides written discharge instructions in a manner that the patient, or the patient's family or caregiver, can understand. One recent study found that patients participating in a hospital program that provided detailed, personalized instructions at discharge had 30% fewer subsequent emergency visits and hospital readmissions than patients who received usual care at discharge (AMA Care Transitions, 2009). These personalized instructions were designed to be appropriate for the patient's age, language, and ability to understand, and included a review of medication routines and assistance with arranging follow-up appointments.

Discharge information enhances the patient's active participation in recovery and rehabilitation (Table 9-1), boosts confidence in managing postoperative concerns (Henderson, 2001), and prevents adverse events after discharge (Box 9-5). Follow-up telephone calls by nurses help identify any patient concerns

Table 9-1 **Discharge Planning**

The patient and family are compliant with the rehabilitation process and the therapeutic regimen after the procedure		
Outcome	**Risk Factors**	**Outcome Indicators**
Patient and family participate in rehabilitation process	• Demonstrate less than adequate recall of information about past procedure experiences or demonstrate misunderstanding, misinterpretation, or misconceptions • Inaccurately follow through with previous instructions • Inadequately perform a self-care skill	• Can the patient and/or family describe in their own words the anticipated physical and psychological effects of the operative or invasive procedure? • Do the patient and/or family express their feelings regarding the operative or invasive procedure and its expected outcomes?

- Demonstrate inappropriate or exaggerated behaviors such as hysteria, hostility, or apathy
- Low readiness for reception of information (anxiety)
- Lack of interest or motivation to learn
- Cognitive limitations
- Uncompensated short-term memory loss
- Inability to use materials or information resources owing to factors such as cultural or language differences
- Unfamiliarity with information

- Does the patient verbalize expectations about pain relief?
- Can the patient and/or family member state the measures that can be taken to alleviate pain?
- Can the patient and family members identify family and community support systems?
- Is the patient able to demonstrate turning, coughing, deep breathing, incision splinting, passive leg exercising, and ambulating?
- Can the patient and or family describe anticipated steps in postprocedure activity resumption?
- Do the patient and/or family indicate that they understand verbal and written discharge instructions? Can they describe these instructions in their own words?
- Are the patient and/or family able to demonstrate implementation of therapeutic treatments such as dressing change and administration of medication?
- Activity intolerance: Decreased strength and endurance related to age, the presence of disease, or the effect of surgery/invasive procedure
- Chronic pain or discomfort
- Acute pain or discomfort after surgery/invasive procedure
- Uncompensated perceptual-cognitive impairment
- Is the patient performing the activities of daily living (eating, bathing, toileting, dressing, and grooming)?
- Is the patient able to implement prescribed therapeutic regimens such as dressing changes and administration of medication?

Source: Adapted from Phippen, M.L., Ulmer, B.C., & Wells, M.P. (2009). *Competency for safe patient care during operative and invasive procedures* (Fig. 18.11, pp. 539–540). Denver: CCI.

or information needs and provide reassurance (**Box 9-6**). Considerations when evaluating discharge instructions include language, health literacy, cultural beliefs, access, and family/other caregiver support. All instructions must be evaluated for accuracy. Asking patients questions and using teach-back processes (e.g.,

Box 9-5	Adverse Events after Hospital Discharge

The posthospital discharge period can be perilous for patients and their families. A surprisingly large number of patients experience possibly preventable adverse events within 3 weeks of discharge. Of these, adverse drug events are the most common postdischarge complication, followed by hospital-associated infections and procedure-related complications.

These patient safety threats can be ascribed to problems in discharge planning and postdischarge care. In particular, adverse drug events can be attributed to the frequency of new medications or changes in medications during hospitalization. Problems with accurate medication reconciliation can result in the potential for inadvertent medication discrepancies and adverse drug events—particularly for patients with low health literacy or those prescribed high-risk medications or complex medication regimens.

Even if appropriate steps are taken to ensure medication safety, patients and their families still assume a large responsibility for care after discharge. Accurately assessing patients' abilities to care for themselves after discharge sometimes is a coordinated multidisciplinary effort. Failure to enlist appropriate resources to help with the transition from hospital to home (or another health care setting) may leave patients vulnerable. Alleviating vulnerabilities is part of patient-centered care.

Ensuring safe care transitions requires a systematic approach. AHRQ recommends three key areas to be addressed prior to discharge:

- *Medication reconciliation:* The patient's medications are cross-checked to ensure that no chronic medications were discontinued that should not be stopped and to ensure the safety of new prescriptions.
- *Structured discharge communication:* Information on medication changes, any pending tests and studies, and any other follow-up needs are accurately and promptly communicated to outpatient physicians or other care providers (such as the primary care physician or NP/PA).
- *Patient education:* Patients (and their families) understand their diagnosis, can state it in their own words, can repeat their follow-up needs, and can name whom to contact with questions or problems after discharge.

Discharge checklists, structured postdischarge phone calls, and generic standardized discharge instructions for patients may all be considered in achieving the above goals. During patient satisfaction surveys, satisfaction with the care transition process should be considered as a patient survey measure to assess and improve the process of discharge education.

Source: Adapted from Agency for Healthcare Research and Quality (AHRQ): *Patient safety primer: Adverse events after hospital discharge*, Retrieved April 26, 2009 from http://psnet.ahrq.gov/primer. aspx?primerID=11

Note: Chapter 13 lists resources FAs may find helpful regarding discharge instructions and other information regarding preventing adverse events postdischarge.

Box 9-6	Sample Questions That Might Be Asked During Postdischarge Follow-Up Phone Calls

Research by Flanagan (2009) suggests that postdischarge follow-up phone calls may be most helpful to patients when they are made at 12 and 24 hours after surgery. Early phone calls (12 hours postsurgery) may focus primarily on symptoms of nausea, vomiting, and a sore throat (for patients who were intubated). The 24-hour post-discharge follow-up call is probably most significant in terms of discovering self-reports of problems and concerns.

- How are you feeling?
- Is your pain adequately controlled?
- What level of pain are you experiencing (on a scale of 0 to 10)?
- Have you taken pain medication?
- Do you have any particular problems related to your procedure?
- Did you receive verbal and written instructions?
- Do you have someone helping you? Have they reviewed the instructions? How long will they plan to help you?
- Do you have any questions regarding your instructions?
- Have you been following the instructions?
- Is there anything else you would like to ask me?

Sources: Modified from Flanagan, J. (2009). Postoperative telephone calls: Timing is everything. *AORN Journal, 90*(1), 41–51; Phippen, M.L., Ulmer, B.C., & Wells, M.P. (2009). *Competency for safe patient care during operative and invasive procedures* (p. 577). Denver: Competency & Credentialing Institute.

return demonstration or repeating instructions in their own words) help to assess comprehension.

Potential complications need to be identified for patients and caregivers. Common postoperative concerns include fatigue, pain management, and resuming activities of daily life (Gilmartin, 2007). Gilmartin (2007) also found that patients have significant concerns about resumption of sexual activity, skin discoloration, and swelling and bruising, as well as a need for written information that supports verbal discharge information. Ambulatory surgery patients and their families/caregivers need to be aware of potential symptoms, management strategies, and postdischarge emergency contact information.

FAs should not depend solely on verbal instructions to adequately prepare patients and their families/caregivers for discharge (McMurray et al., 2007). Written materials support the patient preparing for discharge. Individualized instructions are more useful to the patient and caregiver. Additionally, telephone follow-up not only assists patient and caregiver but can also validate the extent of retention and usefulness of discharge information (Hodgins et al., 2008; McMurray et al., 2007).

Patient discharge information includes diet recommendations (when and what to eat); medication reconciliation and instructions (Box 9-7) (new prescriptions, when to resume regular medications, and precautions regarding operating machinery, including driving); and pain management (Box 9-8) (when to take medications, when to call if pain not relieved). Also discussed with the patient and

---

Box 9-7	Medication Reconciliation

Errors are common when patients are discharged from the hospital. Up to 66% of patients experience a medication error on discharge. Significantly, unintended discontinuation of chronic medications occurs in 11.4% of patients admitted for short surgical procedures. These errors of omission are most common at discharge. Erroneous medication lists prompted the Joint Commission to establish medication reconciliation in 2005 as a National Patient Safety Goal (NPSG). Medication reconciliation is also on the National Quality Forum (NQF) Safe Practices for Better Healthcare list.

Steps to follow for medication reconciliation on admission are:

1. Obtain and record a complete medication history (both prescription and over-the-counter drugs and an allergy history).
2. Assure that admitting orders are written.
3. Compare the orders and the medication history and identify possible discrepancies (performed by another provider, such as the nurse or a pharmacist).
4. Contact the prescriber to resolve the discrepancy, if one exists (performed by another provider, such as the nurse or a pharmacist).

On discharge, follow a similar process. In contrast to admission, however, the FA, nurse, or pharmacist also uses the most recent medication administration record as a source of information and follows these steps:

1. Review any medication changes that were based on the institution's drug formulary (such as name of medication). Reconcile whether the patient will resume the drug they were taking on admission or whether they will continue with the formulary version.
2. Determine which medications will be continued and which will be discontinued.
3. Write or secure prescriptions for the patient (if within scope of practice).
4. Clearly communicate the discharge medication list to the patient. A simple, printed discharge list that includes names of medications, dose, indication, and directions can reduce postdischarge medication errors. This list can also be copied for the next provider of care.

Source: Adapted from Meisel, S., Hasan, A., & Scudder, L.E. (2009). Falling through the cracks: Medication reconciliation at admission and discharge. Retrieved April 21, 2009 from online at http://cme.medscape.com/viewprogram/19223

Box 9-8	Suggested Steps in Educating Patients About Managing Their Pain

- Explain the purpose of a pain rating scale. The patient should understand that it is his or her right and responsibility to communicate when pain levels are personally unacceptable.
- Review the specific pain rating scale that will be used. There are many scales available, and if the patient cannot use one scale, alternative scales should be reviewed.
- Discuss the concept of pain so that the patient understands pain is an experience that can range from mild to moderate to severe. It is helpful to have the patient give examples of kinds of pain experienced in the past, and then use one of those examples as practice in using the pain rating scale.
- Have the patient set goals for comfort and his or her personal recovery.

Source: Adapted from Wells, N., McCaffery, M., & Pasero, C. (2008). Improving the quality of care through pain assessment and management. In R.G. Hughes (Ed.), *Patient safety and quality: An evidence-based handbook for nurses* (Ch. 17, pp. 469–521). Rockville, MD: Agency for Healthcare Research and Quality.

caregiver are potential medication side effects (i.e., dizziness, constipation); bowel habits (increase dietary fiber and fluids, use stool softener); and wound, dressing, or drain care (when to change, required supplies, signs/symptoms of infection, when to call physician). The patient and family/caregiver also need to know follow-up plans including return visit to the physician, when to resume activities of daily living and return to work, and what to do in case of emergency (who to call, where to go). Checklists are useful discharge planning tools; a sample checklist is presented in Table 9-2.

FUTURE ISSUES

Additional data are needed to support evidence-based patient education practices and demonstrate the value of patient education. Research is needed on use of teaching materials for patients with limited English proficiency and limited literacy skills. Studies are also recommended to evaluate the potential benefits of various learning modalities (e.g., pamphlets, videos, computer-assisted instruction) on larger populations of preoperative patients undergoing different surgical procedures. Results of these studies can help determine the most effective format (or combination of formats) and timing of instruction, as well as measure changes in the ability of patient and caregiver to comprehend and retain information.

Table 9-2 Sample Discharge-Planning Checklist

SOCIAL SUPPORT

- Does the patient live alone?
- Who will stay with the patient? For how long?
- What is the ability of the caregiver?
- Who will drive the patient home?
- Is the patient the primary care provider for another family member?
- Does the patient drive?
- Who is the emergency contact when the patient is alone?

HOME ENVIRONMENT

- Does the home have stairs?
- Is an elevator available?
- How far is the walk from the car to inside the home?
- What is the relationship of the bedroom, bathroom, and kitchen?
- Where is the telephone located?
- Is there a list of emergency contacts available by the telephone?
- Has someone removed safety hazards, e.g., throw rugs and small objects?
- Has someone moved cooking utensils to the countertop as needed?
- Is there adequate food in the home?
- Are there entertainment sources, e.g., books, puzzles, television, movies, radio, crafts?

MEDICAL AND SURGERY–RELATED NEEDS

- Supply of prescription medications: ongoing and surgery-specific.
- Equipment needed for recovery, e.g., wheelchair, crutches, braces, cold packs, etc.
- Wound-care supplies.
- Follow up physician appointment: Date? Transportation?

Source: Courtesy of Phippen, M.L., Ulmer, B.C., & Wells, M.P. (2009). *Competency for safe patient care during operative and invasive procedures* (Fig. 18.11, p. 574). Denver: CCI.

REFERENCES

1. Abreu, D.V., Tamura, T.K., Sipp, J.A., Keamy, D.G., Jr., & Eavey, R.D. (2008). Podcasting: Contemporary patient education. *Ear Nose Throat Journal, 87,* 210–211.
2. American Medical Association (AMA). (2009, February). *Care transitions: Performance measurement set (Phase I: Inpatient discharges and emergency department discharges).* Status: For Public Comment. Retrieved June 24, 2009, from http://www.mhakeystonecenter.org/documents/March%202009/Tab%20XIa%20PCPI%20Care%20Transition%20Measures.pdf

3. Association of periOperative Registered Nurses: Recommended practices for preoperative patient skin antisepsis. (2009). In *AORN perioperative standards and recommended practices* (pp. 549–567). Denver, CO: AORN.

4. Bollschweiler, E., Apitzsch, J., Apitsch, J., et al. (2008). Improving informed consent of surgical patients using a multimedia-based program? Results of a prospective randomized multicenter study of patients before cholecystectomy. *Annals of Surgery, 248*, 205–211.

5. Bondy, L.R., Sims, N., Schroeder, D.R., Offord, K.P., & Narr, B.J. (1999). The effect of anesthetic patient education on preoperative patient anxiety. *Regional Anesthesia and Pain Medicine, 24*, 158–164.

6. Fitzpatrick, E., & Hyde, A. (2006). Nurse-related factors in the delivery of preoperative patient education. *Journal of Clinical Nursing,15*, 671–677.

7. Gilmartin, J. (2007). Contemporary day surgery: Patients' experience of discharge and recovery. *Journal of Clinical Nursing, 16*, 1109–1117.

8. Heikkinen, K., Helena, L-K., Taina, N., Anne, K., & Sanna, S. (2008). A comparison of two educational interventions for the cognitive empowerment of ambulatory orthopaedic surgery patients. *Patient Education and Counseling, 73*, 272–279.

9. Henderson, A., & Zernike, W. (2001). A study of the impact of discharge information for surgical patients. *Journal of Advanced Nursing, 35*, 435–441.

10. Hobbs, J.L. (2009). A dimensional analysis of patient-centered care. *Nursing Research, 58*, 52–62.

11. Hodgins, M.J., Ouellet, L.L., Pond, S., Knorr, S., & Geldart, G. (2008). Effect of telephone follow-up on surgical orthopedic recovery. *Applied Nursing Research, 21*, 218–226.

12. Institute of Medicine. (2004). Health literacy: A prescription to end confusion. *Institute of Medicine of the National Academies.* Washington, DC: National Academies Press.

13. Joanna Briggs Institute (2000). Knowledge retention from pre-operative patient information. *The Joanna Briggs Institute: Best practice–evidence based practice information sheets for health professionals (4*, pp. 1–6). Adelaide, South Australia: Joanna Briggs Institute.

14. Johansson, K., Salanterä, S., Katajisto, J., & Leino-Kilpi, H. (2004). Written orthopedic patient education materials from the point of view of empowerment by education. *Patient Education and Counseling, 52*, 175–181.

15. Johansson, K., Nuutila, L., Virtanen, H., Katajisto, J., & Salanterä, S. (2005). Preoperative education for orthopaedic patients: Systematic review. *Journal of Advanced Nursing, 50*, 212–223.

16. Johansson, K., Salanterä, S., & Katajisto, J. (2007). Empowering orthopaedic patients through preadmission education: Results from a clinical study. *Patient Education and Counseling, 66*, 84–91.

17. Keulers, B.J., Welters, C.F.M., Spauwen, P.H.M., & Houpt, P. (2007). Can face-to-face patient education be replaced by computer-based patient education? A randomised trial. *Patient Education and Counseling, 67*, 176–182.

18. Keulers, B.J., Scheltinga, M.R.M., Houterman, S., Van Der Wilt. G,J., & Spauwen, P.H.M. (2008). Surgeons underestimate their patients' desire for preoperative information. *World Journal of Surgery, 32*, 964–970.

19. Kiyohara, L.Y., Kayano, L.K., Oliveira, L.M., et al. (2004). Surgery information reduces anxiety in the pre-operative period. *Revista do Hospital das Clínicas, 59*, 51–56.

20. McMurray, A., Johnson, P., Wallis, M., Patterson, E., & Griffiths, S. (2007). General surgical patients' perspectives of the adequacy and appropriateness of discharge planning to facilitate health

decision-making at home. *Journal of Clinical Nursing, 16*, 1602–1609.

21. Merriman, M.L. (2008). Pre-hospital discharge planning: Empowering elderly patients through choice. *Critical Care Nursing Quarterly, 31*, 52–58.

22. Miller, G.A. (1956). The magical number seven, plus or minus two: Some limits on our capacity for processing information. *Psychological Review, 63*, 81–97.

23. National Center for Education Statistics (2003). *The 2003 National assessment of adult literacy (NAAL).* (NCES 2003-495 REVISED) Jessup, MD: U.S. Department of Education Institute of Education Sciences. Retrieved June 19, 2009, from http://nces.ed.gov/pubs2003/2003495rev.pdf

24. O'Brien, D. (2008). Patient education and care of perianesthesia patient. In C.B. Drain & J. Odom-Forren (Eds.), *PeriAnesthesia nursing: A critical care approach* (5th ed.). St. Louis, MO: Saunders Elsevier.

25. Rankinen, S., Salanterä, S., Heikkinen, K., et al. (2007). Expectations and received knowledge by surgical patients. *International Journal for Quality in Health Care, 19*, 113–119.

26. Rice, M., Glasper, A., Keeton, D., & Spargo, P. (2008). The effect of a preoperative education programme on perioperative anxiety in children: An observational study. *Paediatric Anaesthesia, 18*, 426–430.

27. Roach, J.A., Tremblay, L.M., & Bowers, D.L. (1995). A preoperative assessment and education program: Implementation and outcomes. *Patient Education and Counseling, 25*, 83–88.

28. Rothrock, J.C., Zulick, K.M., & Zulick, P.A. (2009). Patient education and health literacy. *Perioperative Nursing Clinics, 4*, 131–139.

29. Ruffinengo, C., Versino, E., & Renga, G. (2009). Effectiveness of an informative video on reducing anxiety levels in patients undergoing elective coronarography: A RCT. *European Journal of Cardiovascular Nursing, 8(1)*, 57–61.

30. Sandberg, E.H., Sharma, R., Wiklund, R., & Sandberg, W.S. (2008). Clinicians consistently exceed a typical person's short-term memory during preoperative teaching. *Anesthesia & Analgesia, 107*, 972–978.

31. Seifert, P.C. (2008). Summer reading. *AORN Journal, 88*, 177–178.

32. Shuldham, C. (1999). A review of the impact of pre-operative education on recovery from surgery. *International Journal of Nursing Studies, 36*, 171–177.

33. Sjöling, M., Nordahl, G., Olofsson, N., & Asplund, K. (2003). The impact of preoperative information on state anxiety, postoperative pain and satisfaction with pain management. *Patient Education and Counseling, 51*, 169–176.

34. Stern, C., & Lockwood, C. (2005). Knowledge retention from preoperative patient information. *International Journal of Evidence-Based Healthcare, 3*, 45–63.

35. The Joint Commission. (2008a). Comprehensive accreditation manual for hospitals: The official handbook. Oakbrook Terrace, IL: The Joint Commission.

36. The Joint Commission. (2008b). *Health care at the crossroads: Guiding principles for the development of the hospital of the future.* Retrieved June 20, 2009, from www.jointcommission.org

37. Wells, N., McCaffery, M., & Pasero, C. (2008). Improving the quality of care through pain assessment and management. In R.G. Hughes (Ed.), *Patient safety and quality: An evidence-based handbook for nurses* (pp. 469–521). Rockville, MD: Agency for Healthcare Research and Quality.

38. Wilson-Stronks, A., & Galvez, E. (2007). *Hospitals, language, and culture: A snapshot of the nation.* Oakbrook Terrace, IL: The Joint Commission and the California Endowment. Retrieved June 19, 2009, from http://www.yvcc.edu/coe/pdf/hlc_paper.pdf

APPENDIX 9-1   SAMPLE JOINT COMMISSION RESOURCES FOR PATIENT EDUCATION

Stewart, M. (2008, March). *A Prescription for Patient Education: Assessing Patient Needs.* A Joint Commission Resource Audioconference. Information available at /www.jcrinc.com/Audio-Conferences/Prescription-for-Patient-Education/1401/.

Program overview: Focus on the Five Rights of Patient Education:

- Have the right patient.
- Know how to identify the right time for patient education.
- Recognize how the right place/setting can affect learning.
- Understand the importance of delivering the right information.
- Match learning styles with the right route of educational material delivery.

Stewart, M. (2008, November). *A Prescription for Patient Education: Outcome Measurements.* A Joint Commission Resource Audioconference. Information available at /www.jcrinc.com/Audio-Conferences/Prescription-for-Patient-Education/1401/.

Program overview: Patients who understand are able to actively participate in their treatment process to reach their goals. However, how do we assess what patients need and how effectively they comprehend the information we provide them? What tools and techniques have we used to ensure that our patients understand and apply information to participate actively in their health care plan? This program identified specific strategies to determine outcome measurements for patient education and further explored the benefits to both the patient and provider when a foundation of compliance and cooperation has been established.

SPEAK UP™ INITIATIVES

Health care organizations have reported printing Speak Up™ materials for patient rooms; sponsoring local public service announcements; including Speak Up™ content in patient information materials, websites and community newsletters; distributing material at health fairs; sharing content on closed-circuit patient education television; using materials for staff education and orientation; and distributing it on bedside tent cards. Since its launch in 2002, the Speak Up™ program has grown to include 11 campaign brochures and four posters, as well as Spanish language versions of all brochures.

SPEAK UP™ MATERIALS

All Speak Up™ materials are available at http://www.jointcommission.org/
PatientSafety/SpeakUp. The brochures are in Macintosh file format to enable
designers or printers to easily download and print as many copies as a health care
organization needs to distribute to its patients, staff, and community members.
Note: These files are not PC-compatible—they were created for designers or
commercial printers. The brochures include a blank panel for organizations to
insert their own patient safety information, logo, and contact information.

10 Anesthesia

Russell R. Lynn

Many patients feel vulnerable about undergoing anesthesia, which can be described as a state in which one experiences a loss of sensation and awareness. Patient-centered care can alleviate patient vulnerabilities (Hobbs, 2009). Generally, the state of anesthesia is achieved by pharmacologic agents that provide amnesia, analgesia, and muscle relaxation. The delivery of anesthetic agents requires the anesthesia provider to formulate a patient-specific anesthetic plan, to monitor and assess the patient's physiologic response to the anesthetic and surgical procedure, and to manipulate the administration of anesthetic as needed. The safety of present-day anesthetic practice can be directly attributed to the ability to safely monitor critical parameters of a patient's ventilation, oxygenation, perfusion, and temperature (Bankert, 2000) (Table 10-1).

HISTORY OF MODERN ANESTHESIA

Considered one of the three most significant advances in health care in the 19th century, the discovery of ether's anesthetic property 150 years ago dramatically changed the practice of surgery (Garde, 1996). Before the development of anesthesia, only procedures deemed life-saving, such as amputations of gangrenous limbs or drainage of an abscess, were performed, and often speed mattered more than did the surgeon's skill. Patients were prepared for surgery using ice, whiskey, hashish, opioids, a blow to the head, and even strangulation. Often surgeons used "muscle men" to restrain and gag the patient during a procedure (Kaul, 2006). As one can imagine, mortality was quite high before the advent of anesthesia.

Table 10-1 Monitors Used to Assess the Anesthetized Patient

Oxygenation

- Pulse oximetry
- Direct observation of patient's skin color
- Oxygen monitors within anesthesia equipment
- Arterial blood gas sampling

Ventilation

- Auscultation of breath sounds
- Precordial stethoscope
- Esophageal stethoscope
- Capnography (identification of expired carbon dioxide)
- Direct observation of the patient's chest
- Arterial blood gas sampling
- Ventilation pressure and spirometry monitoring

Perfusion

- Electrocardiogram tracing
- Esophageal stethoscope
- Auscultation of heart sounds
- Pulse oximetry
- Blood pressure (noninvasive or arterial line)
- Urine output
- Central venous pressure monitoring
- Evaluation of surgical blood loss (suction and sponges)

Temperature

- Esophageal stethoscope
- Skin temperature monitoring
- Central core temperature

Neuromuscular Function

- Nerve stimulation (when neuromuscular blocking drugs [NMBDs] have been administered)

Positioning

- Continued monitoring and assessment

Note: This document mandates continued clinical observation and vigilance throughout anesthesia care that applies to all patients. The standards also dictate that the means for monitoring shall be immediately available and, if omitted, must be documented by the anesthesia provider.

Source: Adapted from The American Association of Nurse Anesthetists. (2005). *The scope and standards for nurse anesthesia practice.* Park Ridge, IL: Author.

PREANESTHESIA EVALUATION

Before the administration of any anesthetic agent, a thorough preanesthesia assessment takes place. While a routine in-hospital evaluation is usually conducted by an anesthesia provider on the day before or the morning of surgery, preoperative anesthesia consultation typically takes place days to weeks before surgery, often scheduled in conjunction with preadmission testing. It provides an opportunity for the anesthesia provider to meet and interview the patient, identify and document comorbid diseases, selectively order other diagnostic tests, optimize management of preexisting medical conditions, and discuss aspects of perioperative care, such as postoperative pain management (ASA, 2002). Studies show that these preoperative anesthesia consultations reduce patient anxiety, cancellations on the day of surgery, and length of hospital stay (Wijeysundera et al., 2009). Elements of this assessment include:

- Preoperative fasting status
- Airway assessment
- Focused systematic physical assessment with particular attention to respiratory, cardiac, hepatic, and renal function
- Review of past medical and surgical history
- List of all current medications, including dosages
- Notation of reactions to previous anesthetics
- Identification of any allergies
- Documentation of use of tobacco, alcohol, illicit drugs, alternative or complementary medications, and homeopathic drugs and treatments (ASA, 2003)

Another evaluation must be completed and documented by an individual qualified to administer anesthesia within 48 hours of surgery or anesthesia (Joint Commission, 2009).

An American Society of Anesthesiologists (ASA) physical status classification is then assigned to the patient based on the preanesthesia assessment (Table 10-2) and informed consent for both the surgical procedure and anesthesia is verified

Table 10-2   ASA Physical Classification System

P1	A normal healthy patient
P2	A patient with mild systemic disease
P3	A patient with severe systemic disease
P4	A patient with severe systemic disease that is a constant threat to life
P5	A moribund patient who is not expected to survive without the operation
P6	A declared brain-dead patient whose organs are being removed for donor purposes

Source: American Society of Anesthesiologists. *ASA physical status classification system.* Retrieved June 3, 2009 from http://www.asahq.org/clinical/physicalstatus.htm

before administration of any sedatives. The ASA has established an algorithm to follow for patients with recognized or unrecognized difficult airways (ASA, 2003) (Figure 10-1; Table 10-3). If this airway assessment reveals findings consistent

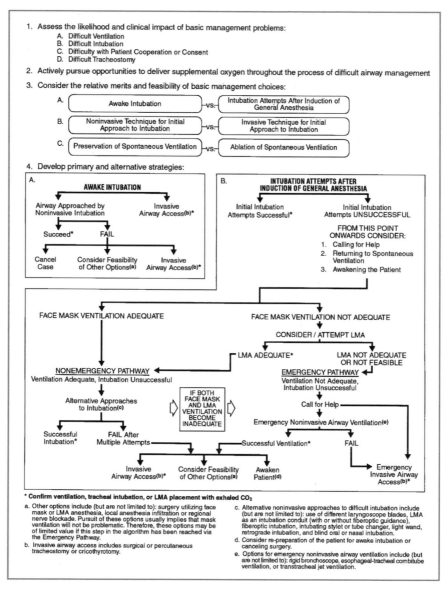

Figure 10-1

ASA difficult airway algorithm.

Source: From "Practice guidelines for management of the difficult airway," American Society of Anesthesiologists, 2003, *Anesthesiology, 98* (5), p. 1273. Copyright © 2003 by the American Society of Anesthesiologists. Reprinted with permission of Lippincott Williams & Wilkins, Publishers, and ASA. Reprinted with permission of ASA.

Table 10-3   Airway Assessment Using the Mallampati Score

Airway management decision making includes prospective determination of the potential for a difficult airway. The Mallampati score is one evaluation method used to determine if a patient requires alternative airway management. The anesthesia provider performs direct oral pharyngeal visualization, looking for the tongue, soft and hard palate, uvula, and tonsillar pillars. Patients with a higher Mallampati grade tend to have poorer visualization during direct laryngoscopy; in patients with a Mallampati score of 4, no posterior structures can be seen (see scoring below).

Class 1: able to visualize soft palate, entire uvula, and tonsillar pillars

Class 2: able to visualize soft palate, partial uvula

Class 3: able to visualize hard and soft palate only

Class 4: able to visualize hard palate only

Sources: Modified from Birnbaumer, D.M., & Pollack, C.V. (2002). The difficult airway: Evaluation of the difficult airway. Retrieved May 7, 2009 from www.medscape.com/viewarticle/430201_2; Downing, J.W., & Baysinger, C.L. (2008). Lost in translation: The Mallampati score? *Anesthesiology, 109,* 931–932.

with an anticipated "easy" airway, then intubation of the patient generally proceeds after induction of general anesthesia. However, based on airway assessment and type of surgery, the anesthesia provider may choose to secure the patient's airway while awake, using fiberoptic equipment to ensure a patent airway before induction of anesthesia and loss of spontaneous ventilation.

Preoperative fasting (Table 10-4) is required to reduce the risk of regurgitation and aspiration of gastric contents. During induction of general anesthesia, protective reflexes in the airway are diminished. The goal of preoperative fasting is to decrease both volume and acidity of gastric contents. When urgent and emergency surgical procedures are required, the patient is presumed to have a "full stomach" regardless of fasting status. Several other conditions (Table 10-5) in which gastric emptying is slowed or gastric acidity is increased also require the presumption of a "full stomach." The anesthesia provider may order or administer an antacid, histamine-2 (H_2) blocker, or Reglan® to the patient presumed to have a "full stomach."

RAPID SEQUENCE INDUCTION FOR GENERAL ANESTHESIA

In the OR, the anesthesia provider induces general anesthesia using a rapid sequence technique and the Sellick maneuver for patients identified as having a "full stomach." Rapid sequence induction (RSI) (Box 10-1) refers to the administration of a hypnotic agent immediately followed by a rapid-acting muscle relaxant (succinylcholine); the airway is then quickly secured by inserting an endotracheal

Table 10-4 **Preoperative Fasting Guidelines**

The FA needs to be familiar with fasting guidelines to be able to monitor the patient and reinforce instructions for patients and families about preoperative fasting. FAs can use the "2-4-6-8" mnemonic as a way to remember the guidelines.

Summary of Fasting Recommendations to Reduce the Risk of Pulmonary Aspiration*

Ingested Material	Minimum Fasting Period (hours)**
Clear liquids***	2
Breast milk****	4
Infant formula	6
Nonhuman milk	6
Light meal*****	6
Regular meal	8

*These recommendations apply to healthy patients who are undergoing elective procedures. They are not intended for women in labor. Following the guidelines does not guarantee complete gastric emptying.
**The fasting periods noted above apply to all ages.
***Examples of clear liquids include water, fruit juices without pulp, carbonated beverages, clear tea, and black coffee.
****Nonhuman milk is similar to solids in gastric emptying time, and therefore the amount ingested must be considered when determining an appropriate fasting period.
*****A light meal typically consists of toast and clear liquids. Meals that include fried or fatty foods or meat tend to prolong gastric emptying time. Both the amount and type of foods ingested must be considered when determining an appropriate fasting period.

Sources: Adapted from ASA (1999). Practice guidelines for preoperative fasting and the use of pharmacologic agents to reduce the risk of pulmonary aspiration: Application to healthy patients undergoing elective procedures: A report by the American Society of Anesthesiologists Task Force on Preoperative Fasting. (1999). *Anesthesiology, 90,* 896–905; Crenshaw, J.T., & Winslow, E.H. (2008). Preoperative fasting duration and medication instruction: Are we improving? *AORN Journal, 88,* 963–976.

Table 10-5 **Conditions Which Slow Gastric Emptying or Increase Gastric Acidity**

1. Trauma
2. Bowel obstruction
3. Pregnancy
4. Obesity
5. Diabetes mellitus
6. Renal failure

tube (ETT) (**Figure 10-2**) and inflating the cuff on the ETT. The Sellick maneuver (**Figure 10-3**) refers to manual pressure applied on the cricoid cartilage, the only tracheal cartilage that forms a complete ring. Downward pressure on the cricoid

---

Box 10-1   Sample Rapid Sequence Induction

- All equipment is available and functional—this includes laryngoscopes, endotracheal tubes (ETTs), suction, No. 11 blade, pulse oximeter/end tidal CO_2 monitor, electrocardiogram (ECG), and blood pressure (BP) monitors.
- IV access is established.
- Preoxygenation with nonrebreather mask or Ambu bag—valve-assisted ventilations with the application of cricoid pressure.
- Premedications, if any, are administered.
- The induction agent is administered.
- The paralytic agent is given immediately following induction.
- Laryngoscopy and intubation is performed.
- ETT placement is confirmed (listening for bilateral equal breath sounds, absence of breath sounds over the stomach, esophageal detector, presence of end-tidal CO_2, observing symmetrical chest expansion).
- Cricoid pressure is then released.
- ETT is secured.
- Patient is ventilated with additional paralysis and sedation as needed.

Source: From Pousman, R.M. (2008). Rapid sequence induction for prehospital providers. Retrieved June 3, 2009 from http://www.uam.es/departamentos/medicina/anesnet/journals/ijeicm/vol4n1/rapid.htm#V.%20 Rapid%20Sequence%20Induction

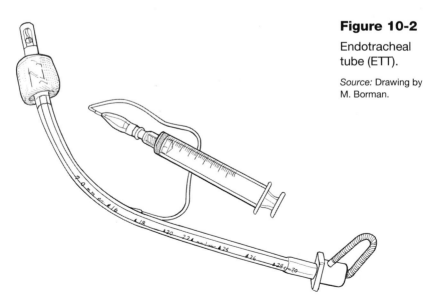

Figure 10-2

Endotracheal tube (ETT).

Source: Drawing by M. Borman.

cartilage seals the esophagus and thereby prevents regurgitation of gastric contents into the oropharynx and subsequent aspiration into the lungs. Atelectasis and chemical pneumonitis, potential sequelae of aspiration, are associated with

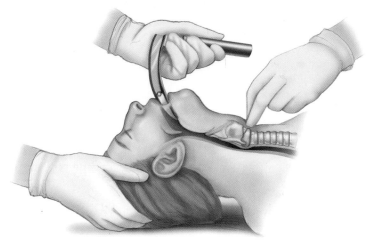

Figure 10-3

Cricoid pressure. Anesthetic induction agents result in the loss of esophageal tone and protective laryngeal reflexes. Cricoid pressure achieves occlusion of the upper esophagus between the cricoid and sixth cervical vertebra.

Source: Drawing by M. Borman.

increased morbidity and mortality (ASA, 1999; ASA, 2003; Nagelhout & Zaglanic-zny, 2005). Prevention of regurgitation and possible pulmonary aspiration of gastric contents depends on proper technique in applying cricoid pressure. The FA, if she or he is assisting the anesthesia provider, uses the following recommended technique (Beavers, Moos, & Cuddeford, 2009):

- If you are right-handed, stand facing the patient's head, on the patient's right side.
- With your right hand (use of the dominant hand is best for achieving the correct amount of pressure), identify the anatomy.
- Using the three-finger technique, place your thumb on the right side of the patient's trachea, your first finger directly on the cricoid cartilage, and your second finger on the left side of the trachea.
- Using the thumb and index finger technique, place the thumb and index finger over the cricoid cartilage, as if you are picking up a small item.
- With either technique, at the direction of the anesthesia provider, apply about 2 kg of pressure on the cricoid ring directly backwards towards the vertebral column if the patient is awake.
- Increase the pressure to about 4 kg in the unconscious patient, still applying pressure directly backwards towards the vertebral column.

- Only reduce or terminate cricoid pressure at the direction of the anesthesia provider.

The anesthesia provider develops an anesthetic plan guided by the preoperative patient assessment and the type and expected duration of the planned surgical procedure. Anesthesia can be achieved by many means, including moderate sedation, monitored anesthesia care (MAC), administration of local anesthetic agents (infiltrated into the surgical site by the surgeon or FA), regional anesthesia (a local anesthetic used to achieve a central or peripheral nerve block), and general anesthesia (the administration of intravenous [IV] or inhalational anesthetics).

Moderate Sedation Sedative agents provide a dose-dependent alteration in consciousness. This is achieved by the use of one or a combination of several agents (Table 10-6). Patients who receive moderate sedation require monitoring, as noted earlier in Table 10-1. Emergency airway equipment is available should the patient's spontaneous ventilations become inadequate. Because a non-anesthesia provider may be monitoring the patient, personnel with the ability to convert to general anesthesia must be immediately available.

Table 10-6   **Anesthetic Agents**

Benzodiazepines

Midazolam, Diazepam, Lorazepam

Opioids

Codeine, Hydromorphone, Morphine, Fentanyl, Alfentanil, Sufentanil, Remifentanil

Barbiturates

Thiopental, Methohexital

Nonbarbiturate Hypnotics

Etomidate, Propofol, Ketamine

Inhalational Agents

Isoflurane, Sevoflurane, Desflurane, Halothane, Nitrous Oxide

Depolarizing Muscle Relaxant

Succinylcholine

Nondepolarizing Muscle Relaxants

Vecuronium, Rocuronium, Cisatracurium, Pancuronium

Local Anesthetics

Chloroprocaine, Procaine, Tetracaine, Prilocaine, Lidocaine, Mepivacaine, Bupivacaine, Levobupivacaine, Ropivacaine, Etidocaine

Local Anesthesia   Local anesthetics disrupt afferent nerve impulses along the nerve fiber (Nagelhout & Zaglaniczny, 2005). Such agents are divided into two groups, based on the method by which they are metabolized. Agents dependent on hepatic metabolism (primarily microsomal cytochrome P 450) are referred to as "amide locals." Agents metabolized by ester hydrolysis are referred to as "ester locals" (Table 10-7). Ester hydrolysis occurs rapidly through the action of esterase found in the plasma, red blood cells, and the liver (Nagelhout & Zaglaniczny, 2005). Although the duration of action of local anesthetic agents depends on their chemical structure, the site of injection also contributes to the duration of the agent. Local anesthetic agents injected into areas with higher perfusion have shorter duration. They have greater exposure to hepatic degradation or plasma esterases compared to agents injected into areas with lower perfusion.

Epinephrine is often added to a local anesthetic to cause vasoconstriction. This vasoconstriction decreases blood flow to the area, thereby prolonging the duration of the agent and simultaneously decreasing surgical blood loss. The FA should communicate the use of vasoconstrictors with local anesthetics to the anesthesia provider because such use may cause severe hemodynamic alterations. It should also be noted that vasoconstrictors should never be injected into an area of terminal circulation such as the ear, finger tip, or toes. Local anesthetic agents can be infiltrated into the surgical site by the FA or surgeon.

If plasma concentration of a local anesthetic agent becomes significantly elevated, cardiovascular and central nervous system (CNS) involvement may be dramatic. The patient may complain of a metallic taste, circumoral numbness or a numb tongue, tinnitus, lightheadedness, and visual disturbances. Speech may become slurred, and muscle twitching may occur. Seizures, unconsciousness, respiratory arrest, and

Table 10-7   Ester and Amide Local Anesthetics

Ester Locals	Amide Locals
Procaine	Lidocaine
Chloroprocaine	Mepivacaine
Tetracaine	Prilocaine
Cocaine	Bupivacaine
	Levobupivacaine
	Ropivacaine
	Etidocaine
	Articaine

cardiovascular collapse may also ensue. The most common cause of local anesthetic toxicity is accidental intravascular injection. Careful aspiration before injection of a local anesthetic by the FA prevents this situation (Nagelhout & Zaglaniczny, 2005).

Regional Blocks   Local anesthetics can be injected into specific areas of the body (central or peripheral) to "block" large bundles of nerve fibers so as to render a loss of sensation to a specific region. Examples of peripheral blocks include an interscalene or axillary block for an upper extremity procedure or a femoral nerve block for a lower extremity procedure. Examples of a central block include a subarachnoid or epidural block for procedures in the lower abdomen, perineal area, or lower extremities.

Injection of local anesthetics to achieve a central block (e.g., subarachnoid or epidural block) causes relaxation of vascular tone as nerve fibers known as *B* fibers become blocked by the local anesthetic. This results in a sympathectomy, which obstructs sympathetic activity below the level of the block. A sympathectomy may lead to profound hypotension. Nerve fibers that control the heart rate arise from the thoracic spinal nerves located between T1 and T4. When the level of the block rises to this area, profound bradycardia occurs. The diaphragm is innervated by spinal nerves which originate from C3–C5. If the level of the block rises to this area, ventilatory effort may be inhibited and support required (Nagelhout & Zaglaniczny, 2005).

Absolute and relative contraindications for regional anesthesia are noted in Table 10-8 (Nagelhout & Zaglaniczny, 2005). Anesthesia emergencies require the

Table 10-8   Contraindications to Regional Anesthesia

Absolute Contraindications	Relative Contraindications
Patient refusal	Uncooperative patient
Infection at injection site	Infection peripheral to injection site
Abnormal coagulation studies (See Appendix I for normal values)	Patient on anticoagulant therapy
Severe hypovolemia	Hypovolemia
Sepsis	Patient with back pain or prior lumbar surgery
Increased intracranial pressure	
Critical aortic stenosis (an aortic valve orifice reduced to 0.5–0.7 cm^2) (Morgan et al., 2006)	

assistance of all members of the surgical team. The FA must be skilled in resuscitation techniques and competent in the use of resuscitative equipment.

GENERAL ANESTHESIA

General anesthesia has three phases: induction, maintenance, and emergence. Before administering anesthesia, airway management supplies are readied (oxygen, oral suction, equipment needed for ventilation and intubation, and resuscitative medications). During induction the patient is preoxygenated with 100% oxygen. This allows for a period of apnea before securing the airway without the patient experiencing an episode of desaturation. Once the patient is preoxygenated and standard monitors are placed (see Table 10-1), an IV hypnotic agent is given to render the patient unconscious. At this point the anesthesia provider may insert a supraglottic airway device such as a laryngeal mask airway (LMA) (Figure 10-4). If positive pressure ventilation or muscle relaxation is required for the procedure, a muscle relaxant is administered, an ETT is placed (see Figure 10-2), and positive ventilation initiated. The intubating dose of the muscle relaxant (neuromuscular blocking drug, or NMBD) is followed by a maintenance dose when continued muscle relaxation is desired.

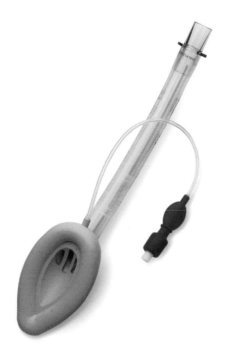

Figure 10-4

Laryngeal Mask Airway (LMA)

Source: Courtesy of Phippen, M.L., Ulmer, B.C., & Wells, M.P. (2009). *Competency for safe patient care during operative and invasive procedures* (Fig. 7.1, p. 157). Denver: CCI.

During maintenance, amnesia is achieved using a potent inhalation agent or infusion of a hypnotic agent (see Table 10-6). Analgesia is achieved by the administration of narcotics. Additional muscle relaxant, if required, is given intravenously. During this phase, the anesthesia provider monitors all bodily functions and provides support to maintain hemodynamic stability. It is critical that the anesthesia provider be aware of continuing developments in the surgical field as they occur. Ongoing communication with the surgical team helps guide the anesthesia provider with additional monitoring and management of the patient in terms of fluid and blood replacement, hemodynamic support, placement of invasive monitoring devices, and special modifications and considerations in laparoscopic procedures (Box 10-2).

Box 10-2	Anesthesia Considerations During Laparoscopic Robotic-Assisted Surgical Procedures

Precautions with Steep (45°) Trendelenburg and Lithotomy Positions

Rationale: To maintain positive air exchange and cardiac function intraoperatively and postoperatively, especially in patients who have cardiopulmonary conditions; to prevent postoperative nerve damage.

Special Considerations:

- Maintain Trendelenburg and lithotomy position precautions, such as protecting/padding the ulnar, peroneal, and popliteal nerves. Assess for any previous nerve damage prior to the surgical procedure, and document thoroughly.
- If patient has a history of cardiopulmonary conditions, begin by placing the patient in steep Trendelenburg using small adjustments once general anesthesia is induced and endotracheal tube (ETT) is secured. Continue with small adjustments until the steepest (45°) Trendelenburg is obtained prior to "docking." This will assist the patient with tolerating the steep (45°) intraoperative Trendelenburg position. It will further allow the operative team and anesthesia care provider to assess changes in hemodynamic and cardiopulmonary function.
- If partial CO_2 (PCO_2) begins to rise intraoperatively, consider lowering the CO_2 abdominal insufflation pressure from the usual setting of 15 mm Hg to 10–12 mm Hg. Reducing the CO_2 insufflation may assist with decreasing end-tidal CO_2 ($ETCO_2$).
- The anesthesia provider may adjust the ventilation settings by increasing the rate of ventilation to "blow off" excess CO_2 and adjust the inspiratory pressure to allow delivery of the desired tidal volume. These adjustments help prevent barotrauma to the lung.
- Steep Trendelenburg (45°) places added stress on the patient's ventilation. The anesthesia provider may use pressure-controlled ventilation versus volume-controlled ventilation to help to maintain optimum saturation and normocarbia.

(continued)

Box 10-2	Anesthesia Considerations During Laparoscopic Robotic-Assisted Surgical Procedures (*Continued*)

Pad and Protect Eyes and Face

Rationale: Prevent corneal abrasions and facial injury.
   Special Considerations:

- Tape eyes closed. Use eye ointment per normal practice. If eye ointment is used, inform patient preoperatively that eyes may be blurred upon awakening.
- Pad eyes with eye pads and place foam pillow over face and secure.
- After endotracheal extubation, protective eye wear is kept in place until the patient is fully awake. Eyes may become drier than usual due to decreased intraoperative fluid maintenance. This can cause patients to rub their eyes more often, increasing the possibility of corneal abrasion especially during the awakening from general anesthesia.

IV Fluid Management

Rationale: Prevent or minimize pharyngeal, laryngeal, and periorbital or facial edema. Maintain safe airway management intraoperatively and postoperatively. Decrease venous congestion which can be exacerbated with intraoperative IV fluid hydration maintenance.
   Special Considerations:

- Place second IV access (18-gauge or 20-gauge) when patient is under general anesthesia. This allows dual IV access to replenish IV fluid volume postoperatively and provides an emergent IV access if needed. Placing the extra IV access when patient is under general anesthesia diminishes patient discomfort and anxiety associated with IV access placement. The anesthesia provider may use the same arm for both IV accesses if there are contradictions or limitations to using the other arm, such as when a patient has previously had a lymph node dissection or mastectomy. This prevents lymphedema postoperatively.
- Limit IV fluids to less than 2 liters (2,000 ml) intraoperatively. Monitor and titrate urine output according to safe fluid management protocol of facility.
- Once procedure is complete, the anesthesia provider begins rehydration utilizing both IV access sites.

Modifying Surgical Draping Intraoperatively

Rationale: Prevent contamination of extra long robotic camera/scope and cords when placing them in and out of robotic camera arm holder. Maintain sterile surgical field.
   Special Considerations:

- After draping and unfolding abdominal drape over patient's head, use an extra 3/4 sheet (instead of the abdominal drape) as the barrier screen between anesthesia and the surgical field. Secure it high on two IV poles (which are on either side of the head of the bed). Position the IV poles at least 2 feet from the head of OR bed.

Pain Management & Other Medication Considerations

Rationale: Maintain pain control, minimize postoperative nausea and vomiting (PONV), and promote healing.

Special Considerations:

- The anesthesia provider may titrate pain medication intraoperatively.
- The anesthesia provider may need to administer additional muscle relaxant intraoperatively to decrease intra-abdominal movement caused by ventilation or intra-abdominal breathing movements. This provides for safe dissection in a stable/nonmoving field.
- Surgeon or FA may inject trocar sites prior to incisions. They may choose to use local anesthetic without epinephrine if the patient has hypertension.
- The anesthesia provider and surgeon may agree on patient administration of ketorolac when beginning to close the trocar sites. This will depend on the patient's renal function and any other contradictions for administering ketorolac.
- The anesthesia care provider may administer preoperative antiemetics or other medications to prevent PONV per antiemetic protocol of facility.

Source: Adapted from Danic, M., Chow, M., Alexander, G., Bhandari, A., Menon, M., et al. (2007). Anesthesia considerations for robotic-assisted laparoscopic prostatectomy: Review of 1,500 cases. *Journal of Robotic Surgery, 1,* 119–123.

Emergence occurs at the end of the surgical procedure. Muscle relaxants are antagonized with a cholinesterase-inhibiting agent, the anesthetic agent is discontinued, and spontaneous ventilation resumes. The patient is assessed to determine adequacy of spontaneous ventilation, return of muscle tone, and level of consciousness. Once it is determined that the patient has emerged from anesthesia and is ready for extubation, the oropharynx is suctioned and the ETT removed. The patient is closely observed immediately after extubation to assure adequate respiratory effort. Once stable, the patient is readied for transport and transfer to the Post Anesthesia Care Unit (PACU) or other discharge unit, such as the Intensive Care Unit (ICU) or ambulatory recovery.

The transport vehicle is brought into the OR. The armboard (if used) is removed from the OR bed and the transport vehicle is moved next to the OR bed and all wheels locked. The transport vehicle should be at the same height or slightly lower than the OR bed (Nelson, Motacki, & Menzel, 2009). If the patient is alert and can move him- or herself, the anesthesia provider moves the IV solution (as applicable) to an IV pole on the transport vehicle. The safety strap is removed, and the anesthesia provider asks the patient to move slowly to the transport vehicle. The FA or another person stands at the side of the transport vehicle (this may be referred to as "stand by for safety"), leans against it, and assists the patient. After the patient is positioned on the transport vehicle, any residual skin prep solution is wiped off, the skin dried and assessed, the patient covered with a warm blanket, and the side rails raised on the transport vehicle.

If the patient is unable to move himself or herself, four people normally must assist in the move, using an ergonomically safe handling protocol. Lateral transfer is done, often with a roller/slide technique or a bed-tilt technique. Mechanical devices such as a mechanical lift with supine sling, mechanical lateral transfer device, or an air-assisted device are necessary for large, unconscious patients (AORN, 2007). The anesthesia provider leads a planned count and gives the "OK to move" call. The FA should not attempt to move the patient without clearance from the anesthesia provider. Personnel assisting with the transfer should maintain the patient's body alignment, support the extremities, and maintain the airway. As with an alert patient, after the patient is moved to the transport vehicle, any residual skin prep solution is wiped off, the skin dried and assessed, the patient covered with a warm blanket, and the side rails raised on the transport vehicle. The patient is now ready for transfer. The FA often accompanies the anesthesia provider to PACU or other discharge recovery unit and participates in the handoff report.

HANDOFF REPORT

When the patient is transferred to the PACU, ICU, or another recovery area, the anesthesia provider, FA, and perioperative nurse may be involved in transport and a handoff report. It is recommended that a standardized approach be used for handoff communication. Patient-specific information such as the following is communicated (DeJohn, 2009):

- The surgical procedure performed
- Type of anesthesia and medications administered and the patient's response
- Current condition
- Drains
- Physiological problems encountered or that may be anticipated; if a surgical Apgar score is used, the blood loss, lowest recorded heart rate, and lowest recorded mean arterial pressure are reported (Regenbogen, 2009)
- Baseline temperature
- Fluids administered
- Urinary output
- Estimated blood loss (EBL)
- Relevant medical history
- Allergies
- Specific orders for postoperative problems
  - Pain medications
  - Nausea medications
  - Sedatives
- Other pertinent information
- Any special needs

Opportunity is given for the receiving nurse to ask questions and receive answers (Mascioli et al., 2009). Interruptions during handoffs are limited to minimize the possibility that information fails to be conveyed or is forgotten.

POSTANESTHESIA EVALUATION

Within 48 hours after surgery or anesthesia, an individual qualified to administer anesthesia must complete a postanesthesia evaluation. This evaluation is guided by policies and procedures established by the medical staff.

POTENTIAL ANESTHESIA EMERGENCIES

Anesthesia providers must be able to recognize and manage a variety of intra-operative emergencies, including:

Laryngospasm   Following extubation, residual oral secretions may stimulate the vocal cords, causing them to spasm and close in what is known as a laryngospasm. In this situation the patient cannot breathe. When laryngospasm occurs, positive-pressure mask ventilation is attempted first in an effort to push the cords apart. If unsuccessful, the muscle relaxant succinylcholine is administered to relax the vocal cords into the open position and restore ventilation.

Malignant Hyperthermia   Malignant hyperthermia (MH) is a rare but life-threatening genetic condition, with an incidence estimated at 1:50,000 adults and 1:15,000 children (Rosenberg et al., 1996; Rosenberg et al., 2001) (Box 10-3). MH is triggered by exposure to succinylcholine or one of the potent inhalation agents, such as Isoflurane, Sevoflurane, or Desflurane. MH susceptibility has an

Box 10-3	Malignant Hyperthermia Trends and Outcomes in the U.S.

Malignant hyperthermia (MH) is a potentially fatal, complex genetic disorder. In this study, researchers used a national database representing hospital discharges from 2000 through 2005 to determine incidence of MH and its risk-adjusted in-hospital mortality. During this six-year period, the number of MH cases increased from 372 to 521 per year, with an estimated incidence rate of MH episodes of 13.3 per million hospital discharges in 2005. On the other hand, mortality rates significantly declined from 12.5% in 2000 to 6.5% in 2005. Regression analysis established that in-hospital mortality was associated with increasing age (the mean age of MH patients was 39), female gender, co-morbidity, source of admission to hospital, and geographic region of the US (mortality was more than three times greater in the southern U.S.).

Source: Adapted from Rosero, E. B., Adesanya, A. O., Timaran, C. H., et al. (2009). Trends and outcomes of malignant hyperthermia in the United States, 2000 to 2005. *Anesthesiology, 110,* 89–94.

autosomal inheritance and is characterized as a calcium regulation disorder of skeletal muscle cells. When exposed to a triggering agent, increased levels of calcium accumulate within the skeletal muscle cell. This is accompanied by muscle rigidity, elevated end-tidal carbon dioxide, tachycardia or arrhythmias, acidosis, rapid elevation in temperature, cola-colored urine (from myoglobinuria) and cyanosis (Nagelhout & Zaglaniczny, 2005). If this occurs in the OR, it is imperative that the entire perioperative team communicate and work collaboratively to employ the interventions noted in Table 10-9.

Table 10-9   Emergency Therapy for Malignant Hyperthermia

Acute Phase Treatment

1. Get Help. Get Dantrolene. Notify surgeon.
   a. Discontinue volatile agents and succinylcholine.
   b. Hyperventilate with 100% oxygen at 10 L/min flow rate.
   c. Halt procedure as soon as possible.

2. Infuse dantrolene sodium (2.5 mg/kg) rapidly IV via large-bore IV if possible.
   a. Dissolve the 20 mg in each vial with at least 60 ml of preservative-free sterile water for injection. Reconstitution requires vigorous shaking until the mixture is clear. Reconstituted dantrolene must be used within 6 hours.
   b. Repeat until signs of MH are reversed.
   c. Sometimes more than 10 mg/kg dantrolene sodium is necessary.

3. Bicarbonate for metabolic acidosis.
   a. Administer 1–2 mEq/kg if blood gas values are not yet available.

4. Cool patient's core temperature.
   a. If temperature > 39 $^\circ$C, lavage open body cavities, stomach, bladder, or rectum.
   b. Apply ice to body surface.
   c. Infuse cold saline IV.
   d. Stop cooling if temperature < 38 $^\circ$C.

5. Dysrhythmias usually respond to treatment of acidosis and hyperkalemia.
   a. Use standard drug therapy, except for calcium channel blockers, which may cause hyperkalemia or cardiac arrest in the presence of dantrolene.

6. Hyperkalemia—treat with hyperventilation, sodium bicarbonate, glucose, insulin, and calcium chloride.

7. Follow end-tidal CO_2, electrolytes, blood gases, Creatine kinase, core temperature, urine output and color, coagulation studies.

Sources: Modified from Malignant Hyperthermia Association of the United States (MHAUS). (2009). Emergency therapy for malignant hyperthermia. Retrieved September 25, 2009 from http://www.mhaus.org/index.cfm/fuseaction; AORN malignant hyperthermia guide. In *Perioperative standards and recommended practices* (p. 127–163). (2009). Denver, CO: AORN.

During the preanesthesia evaluation interview, the anesthesia provider queries the patient about past experiences with anesthesia. Specific questions relate to past anesthetic problems for either the patient or a family member. If there is reason to suspect a past MH event, a diagnostic muscle biopsy (the Caffeine-Halothane Contracture Test [CHCT]) is performed to determine MH susceptibility (Hernandez et al., 2009). If MH susceptibility is confirmed, this information is communicated during the pre-op briefing (sometimes called a "huddle") and/or during the time out (Paige et al., 2008). The anesthesia provider avoids triggering agents as part of the anesthetic plan and ensures that the needed equipment, along with dantrolene sodium, is available in the event an episode is triggered. In some institutions, an MH cart is brought to the room. The cart has essential medications, but the code cart may also be needed for its additional medications (e.g., to treat any arrhythmias).

PATIENT SAFETY

Use of Checklists   The World Health Organization (WHO) developed a Surgical Safety Checklist which was piloted worldwide (WHO launches safe surgery saves lives, 2008). The 19-item checklist is organized around the sign-in, time out, and sign-out (Haynes et al., 2009) (**Box 10-4**). During the pilot research, use of the

---

Box 10-4	**Participation by the Anesthesia Provider in the WHO Recommended Checklist for Surgical Patient Safety**

During the sign-in, specific items in the checklist for the anesthesia provider are:

- Confirmation of patient identity
- Confirmation of surgical procedure, surgical site, and consent
- Completion of an anesthesia safety checklist
- Application of pulse oximeter
- Review of any allergies
- Evaluation of airway for possible difficult airway or aspiration risk
- Establishment of adequate IV access and plans for fluid replacement if significant blood loss is expected

During the time out, the anesthesia provider:

- Fully participates in the institution's time out protocol
- Discusses anticipated patient-specific concerns
- Confirms, as appropriate, administration of prophylactic antibiotics

At the conclusion of the procedure, during the sign-out, the anesthesia provider reviews with the surgeon and perioperative nurse key concerns and plans for the patient's recovery and postoperative management.

Source: Modified from World Health Organization. *Implementation manual WHO surgical safety checklist (first edition).* Retrieved May 7, 2009 from http://www.who.int/patientsafety

checklist reduced death rates and complications from surgery. The Association of periOperative Registered Nurses (AORN), the Anesthesia Patient Safety Foundation, the Council on Perioperative and Surgical Safety (CSPS), along with numerous other professional societies, have endorsed this initiative (Surgical safety council endorses WHO checklist, 2009). In addition to use of a checklist, the initiative encourages more open communication and discussion of anticipated perioperative critical events among all perioperative staff. The use of the checklist is not a substitute for the implementation of the Joint Commission's Universal Protocol, which mandates a time out. At a minimum, the time out includes that the surgical procedure has been verified with the surgical consent; the patient has been correctly identified; the surgical team agrees with the surgical procedure to be done; the patient is in the correct surgical position; special equipment or implants are available; and the preoperative antibiotic has been administered (if applicable) (Dillon, 2008). If the surgical team agrees with the time out information, the procedure begins. If any discrepancy exists, the procedure does not begin until the discrepancy is resolved.

Temperature Management   The anesthesia provider and surgical team implement many interventions to prevent unplanned hypothermia. In the OR, heat may be transferred from the anterior surfaces of the patient's body to the environment by four primary mechanisms—radiation, convection, conduction, and evaporation (Figure 10-5). Compounding the potential for inadvertent hypothermia from the cold OR environment are the effects of anesthesia itself. In an effort to keep warm, the body initially responds to the cold OR environment with vasoconstriction. This transfers heat to the core to protect vital organs. Following the induction of general anesthesia, there is corresponding vasodilatation. The heat is now transferred from the core to the cold periphery. Hypothermia, defined as a core temperature of less than 36 °C (Odem-Forren, 2007), increases risk of surgical site infection, length of stay, and morbidity and mortality. To prevent inadvertent, unplanned hypothermia, the following can be done (Paulikas, 2008):

- Recommend that the patient bring or that the institution provide the patient with socks and a head covering.
- Use forced-air, temperature regulating patient gowns in preop holding (if available); these allow the patient to regulate temperature to individual comfort.
- Verify with the perioperative nurse that the OR temperature is no less than 20 °C.
- Determine whether active patient warming is required. Upper-body or lower-body temperature-regulating devices are applied as indicated.

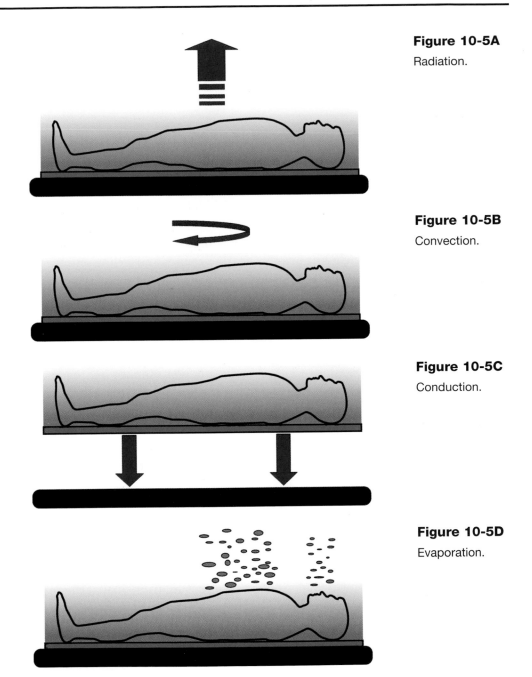

Figure 10-5A
Radiation.

Figure 10-5B
Convection.

Figure 10-5C
Conduction.

Figure 10-5D
Evaporation.

Figure 10-5

The four primary mechanisms for heat transfer from the patient to the environment.

Source: Courtesy of Phippen, M.L., Ulmer, B.C., & Wells, M.P. (2009). *Competency for safe patient care during operative and invasive procedures* (Figs. 7.2, 7.3, 7.4, 7.5, p. 167). Denver: CCI.

- Use appropriate temperature-monitoring device during the surgical procedure.
- Recommend that OR solutions be warmed to body temperature (near 37 °C).
- Consider adding a heated humidifier to the anesthesia circuit in general anesthesia.
- Use fluid warmers for IV fluids and blood products.

Awareness During Anesthesia   Although the actual incidence of awareness with recall (AWR) is unclear, it is a known anesthesia-related problem during general anesthesia, with a reported incidence of 0.1% to 0.2%. For patients, the possibility of awakening during the procedure is a cause of anxiety. Unintended awareness during general anesthesia involves the patient having some recollection of events during his or her surgery, including possibly hearing sounds and feeling sensations or even pain. While these episodes are often brief, they may be traumatic for the patient. In its Practice Advisory, the ASA makes several recommendations and statements related to monitoring of patients for intraoperative awareness (ASA, 2005). Multiple modalities are recommended, including clinical assessment of purposeful or reflex movement, combined with conventional monitoring systems as noted in Table 10-1. Decisions to use a brain function monitor are made on a case-by-case basis by the anesthesia provider for each patient. At-risk patients include patients who cannot tolerate a deep anesthetic. Providing a lighter-than-normal anesthetic to at-risk patients (Box 10-5) may be necessary. The anesthesia provider generally discusses this with the patient in advance of surgery, unless circumstances do not permit such a discussion. The ASA and American Association of Nurse Anesthetists (AANA) collaborated in the development of a patient information booklet on awareness under general anesthesia. Information on accessing this and other patient education materials developed for patients undergoing general anesthesia are listed in Chapter 13.

Prevention of OR Fires   In addition to the use of safety checklists and preop briefings, the ASA has issued a practice advisory for the prevention and management of OR fires. Estimates suggest there are between 50 and 200 fires annually in the U.S., with 20% resulting in severe injury or death. These estimates may be low because the U.S. lacks a national mandatory reporting system (ASA, 2008).

Understanding the way in which an OR fire occurs allows the perioperative team to focus on prevention. Three components, the well-known "fire triangle," must exist for a fire to occur: heat, fuel, and oxygen. It is incumbent upon the entire perioperative team to prevent situations in which an OR fire may occur. Care should be taken to minimize or avoid surgical fire risks, including safe

Box 10-5	Risk Factors, Causes, and Sequelae of Awareness During Anesthesia

Awareness during anesthesia, although uncommon, is of interest to anesthesia providers. It is a specific vulnerability in patient-centered care, and researchers continue to seek information on its incidence, risks, causes, and sequelae. This meta-analysis reviewed cases of awareness published in scientific journals from 1950 through 2005. The 271 cases of awareness discovered were compared with a control group of 19,504 patients who did not experience awareness during anesthesia. The most frequent cause of awareness was overly light anesthesia (87%). A history of awareness was present in 1.6% of cases. Patients who experienced awareness were more likely to be female, younger, and undergoing cardiac and obstetrical procedures. Aware patients received fewer anesthetic drugs and were more likely to experience episodes of tachycardia and hypertension during surgery. Fifty-two percent of aware patients voiced complaints, including an inability to move, feelings of helplessness, sensation of weakness, hearing noises and voices, sleep disturbances, and fear about future anesthesia. More than 20% of aware patients suffered psychological symptoms.

Based on this analysis, researchers suggest that the two most common risk factors are light anesthesia and a history of awareness.

Source: Ghoneim, M.M., Block, R.I., Haffaman, M., & Mathews, M.J. (2009). Awareness during anesthesia: Risk factors, causes and sequelae: A review of reported cases in the literature. *Anesthesia & Analgesia, 108,* 527–535.

management of ignition and fuel sources and proceeding with the use of electrosurgery only after flammable surgical prep solutions have completely dried and vapors have dissipated (ASA, 2008). The oxygen-enriched atmosphere (OEA) in the OR exacerbates surgical fire risk. In an OEA, the electrosurgery unit (ESU) active electrode can serve as an ignition source. The drapes, prep solution, and other supplies that come in contact with the patient can serve as fuels.

Perioperative team members have a combined responsibility to reduce the risk of surgical fires. In addition to participation in specific surgical fire drills and education sessions, the team should communicate with one another about surgical fire risks. The anesthesia provider and surgical team collaborate to minimize the accumulation of oxygen under drapes, decrease use of open oxygen sources, and keep open oxygen sources, such as oxygen delivered via nasal cannula, out of the surgical site. This is critical during head and neck surgery. When supplemental oxygen is being delivered during head and neck surgery, the FA should arrange the drapes to minimize oxygen buildup underneath, keep fenestration towels used in draping as far from the incision site as possible, and consider using an incise drape to isolate head and neck incisions from oxygen and vapors of alcohol-based prep solutions. When using the ESU, the FA should communicate with the anesthesia provider, requesting, if possible, that any supplemental oxygen greater than 30% concentration be stopped one minute before activation of the ESU (ECRI, 2006). In many ORs, a fire risk assessment is part of the time out. If it is determined that a high-risk situation exists, team members should agree on the methods for preventing and managing a fire. Each team member is assigned a specific fire management task to perform in the event of a fire (e.g., removing the tracheal tube, stopping the flow of airway gases). If a fire occurs, each team member then performs his or her preassigned task (ASA, 2008).

CONCLUSION

All members of the surgical team engage together in achieving safety goals and efficient, effective patient outcomes. Essential to the achievement of these common goals and desired patient outcomes is open communication and successful collaboration. Such collaboration, which fosters clinical staff involvement in mutual delivery of specific care processes, maximizes care efforts related to patient safety and optimal outcomes, and extends quality improvement efforts across the entire team is the topic of the next chapter.

GLOSSARY

Atelectasis: collapse of part or all of a lung.

Cholinesterase-inhibiting agent: prevents breakdown of the neurotransmitter acetylcholine (ACh) by acetylcholinesterase, thereby enhancing the activity of acetylcholine.

Circumoral numbness: numbness around the mouth.

Depolarizing muscle relaxant: ACh receptor agonist (e.g., succinylcholine); produces a visible response that includes muscle contraction or fasciculation.

Desaturation: the reduction of the oxygen saturation level below a specified amount.

Myoglobinuria: protein in the urine; typically a result of increased muscular activity or trauma.

Nondepolarizing muscle relaxant: binds to ACh receptor, preventing ACh from activating receptor sites; may be short-acting (SA), intermediate-acting (IA) or long-acting (LA), e.g., mivacurium (SA), rocuronium (IA), vecuronium (IA), atracurium (IA), pancuronium (LA).

Normocarbia: normal concentration of carbon dioxide in blood.

Pneumonitis: inflammation of lung tissue (e.g., pneumonia).

Rapid sequence induction (RSI): the preferred method of endotracheal intubation with patients suspected of having a full stomach or who have not adhered to fasting guidelines, and are therefore at greater risk for vomiting and aspiration. RSI results in rapid unconsciousness (induction) and neuromuscular blockade (paralysis), using weight-based doses of an induction agent immediately followed by a paralytic agent.

Sellick maneuver: application of pressure to the cricoid cartilage (also referred to as "cricoid pressure") to prevent gastric contents from leaking into the pharynx and causing potential aspiration.

Tinnitus: ringing in the ears.

REFERENCES

1. Association of periOperative Registered Nurses (AORN). (2007). *AORN guidance statement: Safe patient handling and movement in the perioperative setting.* Denver, CO: AORN.

2. American Society of Anesthesiologists (ASA). (2005). Practice advisory for intraoperative awareness and brain function monitoring. A report by the American Society of Anesthesiologists Task Force on intraoperative awareness. *Anesthesiology, 104,* 847–864.

3. American Society of Anesthesiologists (ASA). (2002). Practice advisory for preanesthesia evaluation. A report by the American Society of Anesthesiologists Task Force on preanesthesia evaluation. *Anesthesiology, 96,* 485–496.

4. American Society of Anesthesiologists (ASA). (2008). Practice advisory for the prevention and management of operating room fires: A report by the American Society of Anesthesiologists Task Force on operating room fires. *Anesthesiology, 108,* 786–801.

5. American Society of Anesthesiologists (ASA). (1999). Practice guidelines for preoperative fasting and the use of pharmacologic agents to reduce the risk of pulmonary aspiration: Application to healthy patients undergoing elective procedures: A report by the American Society of Anesthesiologists Task Force on preoperative fasting. *Anesthesiology, 90,* 896–905.

6. American Society of Anesthesiologists (ASA). (2003). Practice guidelines for management of the difficult airway: An updated report by the American Society of Anesthesiologists Task Force on management of the difficult airway. *Anesthesiology, 98,* 1269–1277.

7. Bankert, M. (2000). *Watchful care: A history of America's nurse anesthetists.* New York: Continuum Publishing Company.

8. Beavers, R.A., Moos, D.D., & Cuddeford, J.D. (2009). Analysis of the application of cricoid pressure: Implications for the clinician. *Journal of Perianesthesia Nursing, 24,* 92–102.

9. DeJohn, P. (2009). ASCs take steps to improve handoffs. *OR Manager, 25,* 26–27, 29.

10. Dillon, K.A. (2008). Time out: An analysis. *AORN Journal, 88,* 437–442.

11. ECRI. (2006). Guidance article: Surgical fires: A patient safety perspective. *Health Devices, 35,* 46–66.

12. Garde, J.F. (1996). The Nurse anesthesia profession. *Nursing Clinics of North America, 31,* 567–580.

13. Haynes, A.B., Weiser, T.G., Berry, W.R., Lipsitz, S.R., Breizat, A.H.S., et al. (2009). A surgical safety checklist to reduce morbidity and mortality in a global population. *New England Journal of Medicine, 360,* 491–499.

14. Hernandez, J.H., Secrest, J.A., Hill, L., & McClarty, S.J. (2009). Scientific advances in the genetic understanding and diagnosis of malignant hyperthermia. *Journal of Perianesthesia Nursing, 24,* 19–34.

15. Hobbs, J.L. (2009). A dimensional analysis of patient-centered care. *Nursing Research, 58,* 52–60.

16. The Joint Commission. (2009). Further changes for 2009 standards. *OR Manager, 25,* 10.

17. Kaul, T.K. (2006). Happy birthday–Anesthesia. *Journal of Anaesthesiology Clinical Pharmacology, 22,* 333–335.

18. Mascioli, S., Laskowski-Jones, L., Urban, S., & Moran, S. (2009). Improving handoff communication. *Nursing, 39,* 52–55.

19. Morgan, E.M., Mikhail, M.S., & Murray, M.J. (2005). *Clinical anesthesiology* (4th ed.). New York, NY: McGraw-Hill.

20. Nagelhout, J.J., & Zaglaniczny, K.L. (2005). *Nurse anesthesia.* St. Louis, MO: Elsevier Saunders.

21. Nelson, A.L., Motacki K., & Menzel, N.V. (2009). *The illustrated guide to safe patient handling and movement.* New York: Springer Publishing Company.

22. Odem-Forren, J. (2007). Postoperative patient care and pain management. In J.C. Rothrock (Ed.), *Alexander's care of the patient in surgery* (13th ed.). St. Louis: Elsevier.

23. Paige, J.T., Aaron, D.L., Yang, T., Howell, D.S., Hilton, C.W., et al. (2008). Implementation of a preoperative briefing protocol improves accuracy of teamwork assessment in the operating room. *The American Surgeon, 74,* 817–823.

24. Paulikas, C.A. (2008). Prevention of unplanned perioperative hypothermia. *AORN Journal, 88,* 358–364.

25. Regenbogen, S.E., Ehrenfeld, J.M., Lipsitz, S.R., Greenberg, C.C., Hutter, M.M., et al. (2009). Utility of the Surgical Apgar Score: Validation in 4,119 patients. *Archives of Surgery, 144,* 30–36.

26. Rosenberg, H., Fletcher, J.E., & Seitman, J. (2001). Malignant hyperthermia and other pharmacologic disorders. In P. Barsh, B. Cullen, & R. Stoelting (Eds.), *Clinical anesthesia* (4th ed.). Philadelphia: Lippincott Williams & Wilkins.

27. Rosenberg, R., Leith, P., & Hannallah, R. (1996). Evaluation of the difficult pediatric patient: Ambulatory anesthesia. *Anesthesia Clinics of North America, 14,* 753–767.

28. Surgical safety council endorses WHO checklist: OR manager e-mail bulletin. (2009). Retrieved May 7, 2009 from www.ormanager.com

29. Wijeysundera, D.N., Austin, P.C., Beattie., W.S., Hux, J.E., & Laupacis, A. (2009). A population-based study of anesthesia consultation before major noncardiac surgery. *Archives of Internal Medicine, 169,* 595–602.

30. WHO launches "safe surgery saves lives." (2008). *Journal of the Anesthesia Patient Safety Foundation Newsletter, 23,* 21–36.

11 The First Assistant and Collaborative Practice

Mary K. Weis

New strategies, policy initiatives, delivery models, and payment methods are changing the way health care is delivered. The successful transformation of the health care system depends, in part, on effective collaboration among members of the health care team. In today's health care system, delivery processes involve numerous interfaces and patient handoffs among multiple patient care providers who possess varying levels of education and occupational training. In addition, the patient care environment offers an ever-broadening range of treatment options and complex care strategies. Too often, however, care is fragmented, and there is evidence of overreliance on physicians directing care, lack of patient/family participation in setting health care goals, wasted resources, diminished effectiveness, and dissatisfaction among providers and patients (Markus et al., 1995; McEwen, 1994). Moreover, research on patient outcomes has demonstrated that physician behavior alone cannot produce quality patient care in hospitals: quality outcomes are more closely linked to teamwork (Fagin, 1992; Prescott, 1993; The Joint Commission, 2005).

OVERVIEW: DEVELOPMENT OF MULTIPLE PROVIDERS OF FIRST ASSISTING SERVICES

In 1894, an operating room (OR) team consisting of surgeons, nurses, and assistants was recommended and introduced at the Johns Hopkins Hospital in Baltimore (Kneedler, 1994). At about the same time, in Rochester, Minnesota, the Mayo brothers were among the first to provide an opportunity to expand the role of nurses in the OR and to include them in patient care by training them to provide anesthesia to their patients (Clapesattle, 1941). Although the operating room nurse's duties at that time centered mainly on maintaining instruments, supplies, and equipment; managing the sterilizing room; preparing dressings; and passing instruments, the team concept fostered shared responsibilities and a growing mutual respect.

By World War I, OR nursing had evolved into a distinct specialty with formal education programs and specialized training. The nurse's focus shifted from technical concerns to more patient-centered activities. Their additional responsibilities included maintaining an aseptic environment, supervising non-nursing personnel, and preparing the surgical patient for the procedure. First assisting services were performed and became increasingly more common as the war progressed. A shortage of qualified first assistants (FAs) influenced the decision to train nurses for this role.

First assisting by non-physicians was further promoted during World War II, when the demand for assistants became so great that even non-nursing technicians were trained to assist. After the war, the shortage of nurses forced hospitals to hire technicians trained in the armed forces. In 1962, former Navy hospital corpsmen were hired to assist with operative procedures and were classified as "physician assistants" (PA).

The role of the PA became established in the 1960s. In 1965, the first four PA students, all ex-Navy hospital corpsmen, began training in the first PA program at Duke University. In 1969, the American Hospital Association and Joint Commission on Hospital Accreditation released a report on the "Utilization of Physician's Assistants in the Hospital" (Physician Assistant History Center, 2004). In 1971, the American Medical Association (AMA) began work on national PA certification and delineated educational standards. A PA certification exam was developed in 1973, and in 1974, the American College of Surgeons published the "Essentials of an Approved Educational Program for the Surgeon's Assistant" (Physician Assistant History Center, 2004). The curriculum of PA programs includes a surgical rotation to prepare the PA student for the role. In addition to their broad medical care training, PAs may enhance their education through postgraduate surgical programs (see Chapter 13 for a list of resources for PAs).

Over the years, the Association of periOperative Registered Nurses (AORN) has issued position statements clarifying the role responsibilities of registered nurses as first assistant (RNFA) in surgery and defined standards for their educational programs (see Chapter 13 for a list of resources for RNFAs). The Association has also fostered the RNFA role by creating the RNFA Specialty Assembly to serve as a forum for the discussion of issues, to provide educational opportunities, and to act as a representative in regulatory and legislative arenas. Professional recognition has been enhanced by a rigorous certification process for RNFAs and by the development of a core curriculum which serves as the infrastructure for education programs. (see Chapter 13 for a list of resources for RNFA's).

The Association of Surgical Technologists (AST) has developed the role of the Certified First Assistant (CFA). In this role, a certified surgical technologist is educated and certified to assist the surgeon in surgery (see Chapter 13 for a list of resources for CFAs).

In 1990, the United States Congress granted reimbursement for Advanced Practice Nurses (APN) assisting in surgery. Since that time, faculty in programs that educate RNFAs have redesigned the curriculum to prepare the APN to be a qualified assistant in surgery. Using competency assessment and remediation for APNs with limited perioperative experience, RNFA programs prepare APNs with an expanded skill base in perioperative routines and the critical thinking needed to fulfill the role as a FA during surgery (see Chapter 13 for a list of resources for APNs).

COLLABORATION AND TEAMWORK

Well-coordinated, integrated care not only promotes staff satisfaction and enhances patient outcomes but also results in cost savings (Fagin, 1992) and fewer technical errors and problems during surgery (Catchpole et al., 2008). When health care professionals do not communicate effectively, patient safety is at risk for several reasons, including lack of critical information, misinterpretation of information, unclear orders, and overlooked changes in patient status (The Joint Commission, 2005). It is in this context of patient safety that collaboration as a practice model is essential in surgical patient care (**Box 11-1**). Accordingly, collaborative models are being advocated by professional organizations, accrediting bodies, regulatory reformers, and government agencies (Henneman et al., 2005). One such model, Transforming Care at the Bedside (TCAB), was begun by the Robert Wood Johnson Foundation and the Institute for Healthcare Improvement (Stefancyk, 2009). Two essential elements of this model are patient-centered care and teamwork.

DEFINITION OF COLLABORATIVE PRACTICE

According to Adler and colleagues (1995), collaboration is a process of many individuals working together toward a mutual goal. Disch and her colleagues (2001) describe collaboration as a process of joint decision making, joint ownership of decisions, and collective responsibility for the outcomes of those decisions. Lockhardt-Wood (2000) further notes the need for self-confidence and the ability to share information on an equal basis. Interprofessional collaboration in surgical patient care is exemplified as health care providers assume complementary

Box 11-1	NQF Safe Practices for Better Healthcare—2009

Teamwork and collaboration both improve the safety of health care delivery to surgical patients and their families. Safe care depends, in part, on clear and accurate communication, systematic teamwork, and universal implementation of best practices for effective team functioning. The National Quality Forum's Safe Practices for Better Healthcare were developed for all clinical care settings to reduce the risk of error and harm to patients. In the OR, factors such as pressure for room turnover, varying patient acuity, scheduling conflicts and issues, complex technology, and other competing demands can disrupt team-based care. Collaboration, sincerely executed and valued by each member of the surgical team, significantly contributes to positive outcomes for surgical patients in the face of these contrary pressures.

NQF Safe Practice 3: there should be organization-wide approaches in place that address team-based care through teamwork training, skill building, and team-led performance improvement strategies to reduce preventable harm to patients.

Sources: Adapted from National Quality Forum. (2009). *Safe practices for better healthcare—2009 update: A consensus report.* Washington, DC: National Quality Forum; Sterchi, L.S. (2007). Perceptions that affect physician-nurse collaboration in the perioperative setting. *AORN Journal, 86,* 45–57.

roles and work together cooperatively, sharing responsibility for problem solving and making decisions about plans for patients' surgical care. Such collaboration increases surgical team members' awareness of each others' unique knowledge and skills and leads to improved decision making for safe patient outcomes. Unlike more traditional employer/employee relationships, a valid collaboration has no rigid power structure. The surgical FAs contribution is his or her knowledge, expertise, and surgical skills. The scope of each provider's responsibility is defined by the relevant discipline's standards of practice, state practice acts, and institutional standards.

For the FA, a collaborative team effort may include perioperative staff, surgeons, anesthesia providers, social workers, pharmacists, physical and respiratory therapists, and nutritionists (Figure 11-1). It also includes the patient, whose well-being is the goal of the entire team. Full and effective relationships and partnerships require new behaviors and new ways of thinking.

COMPONENTS OF COLLABORATION

In a landmark study on collaboration, Knaus and colleagues identified 12 critical components: trust, knowledge, shared responsibility, mutual respect, communication, cooperation, coordination, conflict management, integrity, independence, optimism, and a sense of humor (Knaus et al., 1986).

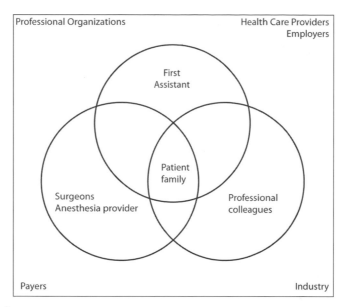

Figure 11-1

Collaborative model.

The patient and family are the focus of the multidisciplinary health care delivery team. The First Assistant also collaborates with health care providers, employers, industry representatives, payers, and members of professional organizations to improve patient care.

Source: Modified from Seifert, P.C. (1999). *The RN First Assistant and collaborative practice. In J.C. Rothrock (Ed.), (1999). The RN First Assistant: An expanded perioperative nursing role* (3rd ed., Fig. 14–1, p. 344). Philadelphia: Lippincott.

Trust

Trust develops over time as the surgical team works together and comes to know and appreciate each other's knowledge and skill level. Trust is the primary component of all relationships and is the building block of collaborative efforts. Thus, without trust, there can be no collaboration. Working in a climate of trust and respect fosters feelings of satisfaction and serves as a unifying force in collaborative endeavors (Alpert, 1992). As indicated by Norsen, Opladen, and Quinn (1995), communication is hampered, autonomy becomes suppressed, and coordination is haphazard without the element of trust. When trust is lacking, cooperation ceases to exist, assertiveness becomes threatening, and responsibility is avoided.

Knowledge

Knowledge empowers people to achieve and provides a basis for clinical competence. Knowledge requires a basic understanding of the surgical procedure, disease state, or problem. A collaborating FA is expected to possess basic knowledge about the surgical procedure or know where to obtain that knowledge. Knowledge and competence in practice are fundamental to the establishment of trust and respect among collaborating care providers. As a function of knowledge, competence is more than a demonstration of adequate clinical skills. To be competent as an FA, one must develop professional maturity, self-confidence, and the motivation necessary to effectively combine direct and indirect care responsibilities in a dynamic surgical environment (Sheely & McCarthy, 1998).

Shared Responsibility
In shared responsibility, there is joint decision making. Intertwined with the concept of shared responsibility is the element of equality. The FA and surgeon have joint responsibility to provide high-quality, safe patient care and to make clinical decisions that support optimal patient outcomes. Although the ultimate decision rests with the surgeon, shared responsibility balances accountability and promotes mutual respect.

Mutual Respect
Mutual respect embodies reciprocal esteem for each surgical team member's individual worth and excellence. This is communicated both verbally and nonverbally by acknowledging other team members' opinions and expertise. In the spirit of working together, mutual respect diminishes the competition that destroys relationships. With mutual respect comes shared responsibility to provide for a safe and optimal surgical outcome.

Communication
Effective communication skills are crucial to the success of any collaborative endeavor. Shared information must be relevant, accurate, complete, and timely. Collaboration is an interactive process; mere technical competence and a sufficient knowledge base are insufficient. All surgical team members need to exchange information and ideas directly and share in the discussions that integrate information and contribute to sound decisions.

Cooperation
Cooperation involves a joint effort from the entire surgical team on behalf of the patient, with identification of a common goal from all participants involved in the plan of care. The pooling of specialized services leads to integrated interventions.

Coordination
Coordination enhances productivity and requires a conscious, methodical effort. It is work performed by individuals towards a common goal, without duplication of efforts. The circulating nurse and the scrub person, often a surgical technologist, perform tasks independently while preparing for the surgical procedure but coordinate their

efforts to ensure a smooth safe delivery. The FA provides critical information for the preparation of requisite supplies and equipment, smoothing the flow of the surgical procedure. Communication must always be clear for effective coordination.

Conflict Management

Conflicts usually occur when people have different goals, different ways to reach shared goals, or different values. These issues need to be resolved, either before beginning a surgical procedure or after the conclusion of the procedure. The inability of a member of the surgical team to adapt to the collaborative environment may result in an impasse. Such a situation cannot be changed without great effort, using energy that is taken away from the surgical procedure. The best approach for moving beyond conflict is to accept that personality conflicts occur and that health professionals need to work collaboratively around conflicts when they arise in the OR. Conflict and conflict management are not necessarily negative—they can lead to discussion, spur action, and force the parties to address the causes of conflict and improve collaboration.

Integrity

Wikipedia suggests that "integrity" means "consistency of actions, values, methods, measures, and principles" (Wikipedia, 2009a). Although integrity is closely aligned to ethics, it is independent of ethical burden. It is the basic core value by which one decides right from wrong. Integrity forms the foundation of growth in a person so that, when an ethical dilemma arises, the FA has sound values on which to base decisions.

Independence

Independence is a characteristic that gives a person the freedom to act alone, without the influence and control of others, in matters of opinion without compromising one's knowledge, beliefs, or values (Birmingham, 2002). Independence and autonomy are virtually synonymous. An independent scope of practice includes self-governance and accountability for one's knowledge and actions. Autonomy is earned and articulated through certification within one's area of practice, delineations in scope of practice, state practice acts, and institutional standards, rules, and regulations. In practice, autonomy must be legitimized by members of the surgical team. Members of the collaborative team foster each other's autonomy by demonstrating confidence, respect, and trust, which enables the FA to function independently within delegated duties and defined scope of practice.

Optimism

Optimism allows an individual to see the world as a positive place (Wikipedia, 2009b). Optimism is the disposition or tendency to look on the favorable side of events. It is the ability to foresee a favorable result despite seemingly insurmountable problems (Birmingham, 2002). Pessimism has no place in the OR. The surgical effort needs to be focused on the patient's best interest, and the patient's rights need to be respected at all times. Optimism provides the support needed to look for effective alternatives in dire situations.

Sense of Humor

Humor can be a valuable social support to reduce stress. When recipients of humor view it as esteeming, humor enhances cohesion with others and increases morale. For humor to enhance work relationships and decrease work-related stresses, it must be thoughtfully chosen and timed (White, 1993).

BARRIERS TO COLLABORATION

Although different members of the surgical team work autonomously at times, they are still part of the surgical team. Efforts to provide a safe surgical experience are jeopardized by potential communication and collaboration barriers among team members. The Agency for Healthcare Research and Quality (AHRQ) has identified common barriers that can occur—between physicians and residents, surgeons and anesthesia providers, surgeons and FAs, and between FAs and other surgical team members (Hughes, 2008) (Box 11-2). Identified barriers include diversity and cultural differences; disruptive behavior; varying levels of preparation, qualifications, and status; and differences in norms, all of which are addressed below.

Diversity and Cultural Differences

The United States is one of the most ethnically and culturally diverse countries in the world. Given that diversity, different cultural backgrounds may pose barriers to collaboration. In all interactions, cultural differences may tend to worsen communication problems (Hughes, 2008). Individuals from some cultures are not normally assertive and will not challenge opinions openly. Such individuals may communicate in indirect ways. Indirect communication can affect the understanding of nonverbal messages. In some cultures, there are specific meanings for eye contact, facial expressions, nods of head, tone of voice, and manners of touching an individual. Awareness of such differences in communication behaviors is essential to effective FA practice.

Disruptive Behavior

Disruptive behavior has a significant effect on safe patient care. Research has shown that delays in patient care and recurring problems from unresolved disputes are often the unintended by-product of physician-nurse disagreements (Prescott, 1993). Staff who witness poor performance may be hesitant to speak up for fear of retaliation, or because they believe it will not improve the

Box 11-2	Common Barriers to Interprofessional Communication and Collaboration

Personal values and expectations

Personality differences

Hierarchy

Disruptive behavior

Culture and ethnicity

Generational differences

Gender

Historical interprofessional and intraprofessional rivalries

Differences in language and jargon

Differences in schedules and professional routines

Varying levels of preparation, qualifications, status

Differences in requirements, regulations, and norms of professional education

Fears of diluted professional identity

Differences in accountability, payment, and rewards

Concerns regarding clinical responsibility

Complexity of care

Emphasis on rapid decision making

Source: Adapted from Hughes, R.G. (2008). Agency for Health Care Research and Quality, Advancing excellence in healthcare. In *Patient safety and quality: An evidence-based handbook for nurses* (Vol. 2, pp. 2–272). Rockville, MD: Agency for Health Care Research and Quality.

situation (Patterson, 2009). Disruptive behavior and communication problems have a negative effect on patient safety and can lead to potentially preventable adverse events (Rosenstein et al., 2008). Zero tolerance policies, fully supported throughout the institution, are essential to ensuring respectful work environments (Dellasega, 2009) (Box 11-3).

In health care environments, physicians have historically been perceived to be at the top of the hierarchy (Hughes, 2008). Perceived hierarchy differences weaken the collaborative interactions that are needed to deliver safe patient care. When perceived hierarchical differences become overarching, care providers on the lower end of the hierarchy tend to be uncomfortable speaking up about problems or concerns. Consequently, physicians may feel that the environment is collaborative and that communication is open, while nurses and other care providers perceive communication problems. Intimidating behavior, especially by individuals at the top of the hierarchy, can hinder communication and give

Box 11-3	Recommendations to Address Disruptive Behavior

Recognition of the problem. Awareness of the problem of disruptive behavior is essential. Institutional commitment to champion professional standards of behavior must be established and clearly visible.

Clear definitions and examples of disruptive behaviors. These may include such behaviors as intimidation, threats, profane language, racial or ethnic jokes, physical attack, property damage, engaging in actions intended to frighten and coerce, bullying, the "silent treatment," spreading rumors, making fun of someone, using body language to convey an unfavorable opinion, sexual harassment, and failure to adhere to institutional policies.

Development and full enforcement of zero tolerance policy for disruptive behavior. Such a policy and its expectations should be communicated to all individuals providing and receiving services in the facility. Potential consequences of disruptive behavior should be clearly delineated.

Uniform approach to reporting complaints/incidents of disruptive behavior. This should include a clause verifying that an individual who reports an incident will experience no reprisal or retribution. Patients and their families who witness such behavior or believe they are victims of it should be able to report complaints. When this is the case, prompt investigation and apology are recommended and appropriate.

Code of conduct. This must address and define acceptable behaviors.

Education and training. This should focus on awareness, appropriate behavior, having difficult discussions, adhering to codes of conduct, respect, relationship building, conflict resolution, basic etiquette, and communication competence. Education and training programs should be conducted annually.

Intervention strategies. A process to manage disruptive and inappropriate behaviors is created and utilized by institutional leaders. Everyone is held accountable under the code of conduct. Intervention strategies include disciplinary processes when necessary. They should ensure access to support services for victims of incidents.

Sources: Adapted from Dellasega, C.A. (2009). Bullying among nurses. *American Journal of Nursing, 109,* 52–58; Goldberg, E. (2008). Reducing horizontal bullying in nursing. *The Pennsylvania Nurse, 63,* 10; Patterson, P. (2009). Toward an effective code of conduct. *OR Manager, 25,* 17–18; Rosenstein, A.H., & O'Daniel, M.O. (2008). A survey of the impact of disruptive behaviors and communication defects on patient safety. *The Joint Commission Journal on Quality and Patient Safety, 34,* 464–471; Sandlin-Leming, D. (2008). Dealing with intimidating and disruptive behaviors in the health care setting. *Journal of Perianesthesia Nursing, 23,* 434–436; The Council on Surgical & Perioperative Safety. (2007). *Statement on violence in the workplace.* Retrieved May 14, 2009 from www.cspsteam.org

the impression that the individual is unapproachable (Hughes, 2008). In some situations, the role of the FA is viewed as an extension of the surgeon. Thus, the FA may also be perceived to be at an upper level of the hierarchy. It is essential that the FA recognize this and endeavor to bridge any communication barriers that exist due to these perceived hierarchical differences.

Varying Levels of Preparation, Qualifications, Status

The role of FA presents varying levels of preparation, qualifications, and status. The FA role may be undertaken by an RNFA, NP, PA, CFA, medical student, resident, fellow, or another surgeon. Mutual respect must be communicated verbally and nonverbally among these potential assistants in surgery, to others on the surgical team, and to patients. Mutual respect manifests itself as a spirit of working together that can diminish the competition that could otherwise strangle relationships (Hughes, 2008). Accordingly, FAs must know the difference between boundary limits and turf battles. Boundaries have an important purpose, but turf battles do not. State regulations and institutional credentialing define the boundaries of practice, whereas turf battles are self-serving and destructive to a collegial, collaborative effort.

Differences in Norms

Differences in norms are another important barrier to effective collaboration. In their professional education or professional practice, nurses, physicians, PAs, CFAs, and NPs learn to use different communication styles. For example, nurses learn to be descriptive of clinical situations, whereas physicians learn to be more concise (Hughes, 2008). The Situation-Background-Assessment-Recommendation technique (SBAR) is an effective communication tool that can bridge these differences (Amato-Vealey et al., 2008) (Box 11-4). The SBAR provides a framework for communication between members of the surgical team about the patient's condition and needs. The SBAR technique can help ensure a safe surgical intervention, but it is only one method of standardizing communication. Standardized best-practice recommendations for communicating during handoffs suggest that such communication be face-to-face, take place in a quiet setting without interruption, and follow a standard format to reduce the likelihood of variability, missed information, and incomplete information (deVries et al., 2008; Kitch et al., 2008) (Box 11-5).

DEVELOPMENT OF COLLABORATIVE PRACTICE

In the early 1990s, patient-centered care expanded the scope of decentralization by recognizing the interdependence of every department in achieving quality care. Patient care came to be seen as a multifaceted, multidisciplinary endeavor. Consequently, decision making was delegated to those involved in patient care processes. At the same time, patients were increasingly seen as entitled to self-determination. A shift in decision making and authority to patients made them partners in their own care, empowering them to make decisions and influence

Box 11-4	SBAR Technique

The SBAR (Situation-Background-Assessment-Recommendation) technique provides a framework for communication between members of the health care team about a patient's condition. SBAR is an easy-to-remember mnemonic and useful for framing any conversation, especially a critical one that requires a clinician's immediate attention and action. It allows an easy and focused way to set expectations for what will be communicated and how it will be communicated between members of the team, which is essential to developing teamwork and fostering patient safety. The following is an example of the FA using SBAR communication with patient admission to the postanesthesia care unit (PACU).

Situation: This is C.P. a 61-year-old female patient of Dr. T, who had a right total hip arthroplasty this morning. She received spinal anesthesia with conscious sedation. She is still groggy, and her spinal has not yet begun to wear off. Her vital signs were stable during the procedure. There were no complications during her surgery.

Background: Her chief complaint was pain in her right hip and leg, which she had for more than a year. She has an allergy to IV contrast dye. This was an anaphylactic reaction. There is an allergy sticker on her chart and she is wearing an allergy ID band. She also has a history of hypothyroidism and stable hypertension. I'll review her meds for these conditions when we go over the postop orders. Her husband is in the family waiting room.

Assessment: She had 300 cc of blood loss, which is within normal limits. Her urinary output was 180 cc. She received 1200 ml of Plasmalyte during the procedure, and it is still running into the IV line in her left hand. At both the beginning and end of the procedure, her neurovascular assessment was normal, and she had positive pulses in her bilateral extremities. She is currently wearing knee-high antiembolic stockings and has SCDs on. She has an "On Q" pump in her operative site.

Recommendation: When you are ready, I'll review the postop orders with you and her VTE prevention protocol. Do you have any questions right now about C.P.?

their environment. Patient-centered care and patient-centric environments recognize that patients and their caregivers are part of the same system and that health care is built on the relationship between patients and clinicians (Berman, 2005). These changes have important consequences for caregivers in general and FAs in particular. Collaborative practice now includes complementary as well as collegial relationships, not only with physicians, but also with other providers of care and the recipients of that care.

The effects of these changes on perioperative practice can be seen in a health care system which values the processes of care mainly as they relate to the outcomes achieved. For example, FAs can preoperatively enhance patient outcomes and reduce costs by educating patients and families about what to expect

Box 11-5	Standardized Information to Include in Handoff Communication

Standardizing communications improves the clarity of information shared about a patient and helps communicators stay focused on the situation at hand. The following list, or one like it, can be developed by FAs to ensure that key information is shared each time they hand off a patient to another care provider:

Patient data: name/age/gender/cultural considerations important to patient-centered care.

Key information from the problem list: significant medical or surgical history, current problem.

Current status: include level of consciousness, vital signs, significant respiratory status (oxygen saturation, need for oxygen, method of delivery).

Medications: include regular medications, new medications, medications infusing.

Lines/invasive devices: location and size of IV lines, fluid running; presence of NG tube and output; presence of indwelling urinary catheter and output; endotracheal tube.

Study results/those pending: lab and radiology results.

Events during the time you were responsible for patient: this may be a shift you were covering or events during surgery that are important for the next caregiver.

Tasks remaining to be done for the patient: pending results of any tests or those that still need to be ordered (may be labs or imaging studies), consults requested or to be requested.

Source: Adapted from Berkenstadt, H., Haviv, Y., Tuval, A., Shemish, Y., Megrill, A., Perry, A., et al. (2008). Improving handoff communications in critical care: Using simulation-based training toward process improvement in managing patient risk. *Chest, 134,* 158–162; Smith, I.J. (Ed.). (2006). *Engaging physicians in patient safety: A handbook for leaders.* Oakbrook Terrace, IL: Joint Commission Resources.

before, during, and after surgery (see Chapter 9 for a discussion of the positive effects of patient education). As early as 1994, Swan described a collaborative ambulatory care model consisting of nurses and anesthesia care providers who worked together to perform preoperative assessments, obtain laboratory data, identify "at risk" individuals, and initiate the discharge-planning process. Preoperative assessment data are critical to the FA when planning intraoperative care, such as proper positioning to prevent or minimize muscle or nerve injury. Information about activities of daily living, learning needs, and psychosocial concerns obtained during the preoperative assessment can be shared by the FA with other team members to improve discharge planning and anticipate home care needs.

The FA cooperates intraoperatively with the surgical team to achieve a successful surgical intervention. Although sometimes responsible for supervising the FAs performance, the surgeon is also dependent on the FA for help with the operation. Thus, the FA assumes responsibility for his or her own performance. It is during surgery that the surgeon and FA are most closely associated and most need to rely on one another. Some of the factors necessary to accomplish this interdependence are covered extensively in previous chapters of this book and include:

- Possessing the requisite knowledge and experience related to anatomy, physiology, microbiology, pharmacology, and behavioral sciences.
- Understanding the procedure and the rationale for surgery.
- Acquiring the manual skill and dexterity to perform the required maneuvers.
- Being familiar with the individual surgeon's preferences.
- Anticipating the needs of the surgeon and the patient.
- Communicating information relevant to the procedure.
- Concentrating on the operative field throughout the procedure.
- Protecting the patient from injury.
- Maintaining flexibility and adaptability in the event of emergencies or unanticipated events.
- Possessing creativity in solving problems or dealing with difficulties during the procedure.
- Knowing one's limits as required by experience, conscience, professional ethics and responsibility, and legal and jurisdictional constraints.
- Becoming a lifelong learner.

The FAs contributions extend beyond the immediate sterile field. One of the major benefits to be derived from assisting in surgery is the knowledge gained from directly observing and participating in the surgery itself. Sharing this knowledge with other perioperative staff increases their level of participation in the patient's care and leads to a greater appreciation of potential risks and complications. Moreover, knowledgeably communicating with surgeons and other members of the health care team encourages active participation by all perioperative staff and can improve staff morale and self-esteem.

Postoperative evaluation provides an opportunity for the FA to investigate areas for improvement and to confirm the adequacy of aseptic technique, preoperative teaching, prevention of thermal, chemical, or mechanical injury, and participation in discharge planning. Teams that perform in high-risk areas such as the OR can also benefit from participation in debriefing processes for critical incidents or recurring events (Salas et al., 2008). Such participation enables FAs, members of the surgical team, and other perioperative staff to contribute to the continual improvement of clinical care.

JOINT PRACTICE COMMITTEES

Joint Practice Committees, representing FAs, perioperative staff, and physicians, and supported by the administration, can continuously monitor and recommend appropriate actions that support joint practice. Joint practice committees enable participants to communicate effectively, clarify roles, discuss questions of competence and accountability, and foster trust and mutual respect.

In the OR, committees consisting of nurses, surgeons, FAs, anesthesia providers, and other key players (e.g., materials managers, case managers) have been successful in encouraging joint practice. Specific patient care issues may include the development of critical pathways, patient care protocols, evidence-based practices, and problem solving at the level of occurrence. Other agenda items specific to the OR may include cost containment, value analysis/product selection, scheduling of procedures, new team member orientation, codes of conduct, debriefings, and assignment of specialty personnel.

FAs can provide insights into practice problems encountered in the OR. Their familiarity with the surgeons' perceived needs and the requirements specific to operative procedures are invaluable in bridging the knowledge gap and promoting understanding between the professions. The interactive roles of nurses and physicians on joint practice committees underscore the value of discussion, negotiation, and compromise.

Even with the best intentions, joint practice committees cannot succeed without administrative support. As previously noted, the workplace culture should support an environment conducive to positive relationships between clinicians and support staff to improve the quality of service. In addition, committee discussions about practice issues that focus on licensure laws and hospital policies may require professional advice from risk managers and attorneys. As new surgical techniques and technologies evolve, scope of practice issues may also arise. It is therefore essential that committees addressing the scope of practice of FAs familiarize themselves with state practice acts, governmental guidelines, regulatory rulings, and institutional policies.

Committee sessions will not always be harmonious. Complex subjects require careful exploration, frank appraisal, and sometimes reappraisal of roles and duties. This will inevitably lead to disagreements. As long as disagreements focus on issues rather than on personalities, conflicts can form the basis for better understanding and teamwork. It is important that communication remains open, frank, and ongoing. Committee members who approach difficult issues in an open-minded manner will foster trust and respect.

CLINICAL DECISION MAKING

Participative clinical decision making is essential for collegial practice. To exercise their professional skills to the fullest, members of the surgical team must be encouraged to integrate clinical decisions. Such joint decision making tests the level of trust and respect among team members. Physicians must trust and respect their FA colleagues, but so too must supervisors, administrators, patients, and peers. These attitudes originate from the recognition of clinical competence, which is the basis for any form of collaborative practice. The patient is ultimately the focus of all efforts; therefore, patients cannot afford to accept anything less than the highest level of collaborative clinical practice.

For the FA, clinical competence incorporates experience, an educational/intellectual component, and demonstrated manual skill and dexterity. Many of the technical skills demonstrated by FAs, such as suturing or exposing tissue, require additional knowledge and experience to perform safely. The potential for injury to major organs, blood vessels, or nerves during retraction, for example, necessitates a level of critical thinking and decision making that can be developed only with additional and intensive professional education and training. Even during relatively simple procedures, assisting in surgery is more than simply an "extra pair of hands" (see Chapter 4 for a discussion of retractor-holders).

A surgeon's competence is judged mainly by his or her ability to accomplish a successful operative repair. This requires mental skills in addition to manual skills to prepare and execute the procedure. The FA accepts these same dual demands. The reward is the satisfaction of participating in what can be an aesthetically pleasing creation as well as a meticulous scientific intervention that leaves the patient healed or improved. Appreciating an assistant's work from different aspects yields greater satisfaction and pride. This in turn inspires continued efforts for improvement.

Conscientious practitioners must be aware of their limitations and use extra caution in situations in which they lack experience. Understanding basic principles of anatomy and surgical technique forms the foundation for safe practice while the FA continues to develop expertise. Being aware of what one does not yet know, and practicing accordingly, is a sign of wisdom, maturity, and professional responsibility. Asking questions and requesting assistance should not be rebuked; such behavior should be encouraged and respected for the courage it implies. The FA with a secure self-image will accept such risk-taking as normal and routine for effective coordination of patient care and meaningful joint clinical decision making. Professionals who realize their limitations and seek to fill knowledge gaps can better understand the learning needs of others. The FA can provide learning experiences and foster collegiality in interactions with students by offering formal and informal educational sessions.

Neither the FA nor anyone else can fulfill all patient needs or solve all patient problems. Physicians accept this limitation and use referral systems and consultation mechanisms for problem solving. The need to consult may not always exist, but when it does, consultation should be available. This not only encourages better patient care but also creates a sense of mutual respect for the knowledge and skills that FAs offer one another. This in turn fosters pride in one's accomplishments and promotes professional growth. Turning to a colleague for professional advice reflects strength and a desire to use all resources available to provide the best possible care.

CONCLUSION

Collaborative practice between the FA and other members of the surgical team is based on trust. Such practice forms the foundation for a patient care partnership wherein the participants perceive one another as peers who mutually contribute to the same desired outcome—excellence in surgical patient care. Collaborative practice improves communication among team members, increases respect and trust, and boosts job satisfaction. The establishment of joint practice committees promotes collaborative practice, but committees in and of themselves are neither necessary nor sufficient for true teamwork. Working together in a collaborative framework brings forth a joint intellectual effort and a sharing in planning, making decisions, solving problems, setting goals, and assuming responsibility, as well as cooperation, coordination, and communication.

Gianakos (1997) listed three reasons why a collegial, unified relationship among surgical team members can improve patient care. First, collegiality is a moral imperative requiring respectful interactions that encourage sharing of information. Second, members of the surgical team should jointly advocate for patients to further the patient's best interest, especially when threatened by external pressures to maximize efficiency. Finally, collaboration allows members of the team to educate one another and thereby improve their ability to achieve patient well-being. When complex care, such as that rendered to surgical patients, is managed by a team, care is so integrated that it is difficult to attribute provider-specific outcomes to any one individual or group (Myers et al., 2008). These reasons underscore the value of teamwork for patients and caregivers. Teamwork can be achieved only when FAs and other health care providers all decide that working together in the interest of consistent quality patient and family care will bring them to their fullest professional potential.

REFERENCES

1. Adler, S.L., Bryk, E., Cesta, T.G., & McEachen, I. (1995). Collaboration: The solution to multidisciplinary care planning. *Orthopedic Nursing, 14*, 21–29.

2. Alpert, H.B., Goldman, L.D., Kilroy, C.M., & Pike, A.W. (1992). Gryzmish: Toward an understanding of collaboration. *Nursing Clinics of North America, 27*, 47–59.

3. Amato-Vealey, E., Barba, M., & Vealey, R.J. (2008). Hand-off communication: A requisite for perioperative patient safety. *AORN, 88*, 763–770.

4. Berman, S. (Ed.). (2005). *From front office to front line—essential issues for health care leaders.* Oak Terrace, IL: Joint Commission Resources, The Joint Commisson.

5. Birmingham, J. (2002). The science of collaboration. *The Case Manager,* March/April, 68–71.

6. Catchpole, K.R., Giddings, S.E.B., Wilkinson, M., et al. (2007). Improving patient safety by identifying latent failures in successful operations. *Surgery, 142*, 102–110.

7. Clapesattle, H. (1941). *The doctors mayo.* Garden City, NJ: Garden City Publishing.

8. Dellasega, C.A. (2009). Bullying among nurses. *American Journal of Nursing, 109*, 52–58.

9. deVries, E.N., Hollman, M.W., Smorenburg, S.M., Gouma, D.J., & Boermeester, M.A. (2008). Development and validation of the SURgical PAtient Safety System (SURPASS) checklist. *Journal of Quality and Safety in Health Care, 18*, 121–126.

10. Disch, J., Beilman, G., Ingbar, D. (2001). Medical directors as partners in creating healthy work environments. *AACN Clinical Issues, 12*, 366–377.

11. Duke University. (2004). *Physician assistant history center.* Retrieved May 17, 2009 from http://pahx.org/period03.html

12. Fagin, C.M. (1992). Collaboration between nurses and physicians: No longer a choice. *Academic Medicine, 6*, 295–303.

13. Gianakos, D. (1997). Physicians, nurses, and collegiality. *Nursing Outlook, 45*, 57–58.

14. Henneman, E.A., Lee, J.L., & Cohen, J.I. (1995). Collaboration: A concept analysis. *Journal of Advanced Nursing, 21*, 103–109.

15. Hughes, R.G. (2008). Patient safety and quality: An evidence-based handbook for nurses. *Agency for Healthcare Research and Quality, Advancing Excellence in Healthcare, 2*, 2–272.

16. The Joint Commission on Accreditation of Health Care Organizations. (2005). *The Joint commission guide to improving staff communication.* Oakbrook Terrace, IL: Joint Commission Resources.

17. Kitch, B.T., Cooper, J.B., Zapol, W.M., Marder, J.E., Karson, A., Hutter, M., et al. (2008). Handoffs causing patient harm: A survey of medical and surgical house staff. *The Joint Commission Journal on Quality and Patient Safety, 34*, 563–570.

18. Knaus, W.A., Draper, E.A., Wagner, D.P., & Zimmerman, J.E. (1986). An evaluation of outcome from intensive care in major medical centers. *Annals of Internal Medicine, 104*, 410–418.

19. Kneedler, J.A., & Dodge, G.H. (1994). *Perioperative patient care: The nursing*

Perspective. Boston: Jones & Bartlett Publishers.

20. Lockhart-Wood, K. (2000). Collaboration between nurses and doctors in clinical practice. *British Journal of Nursing, 9,* 276–280.

21. Marcus, L.J., Dorn, B.C., Kritek, P.B., Miller, V.G., & Wyatt, J.B. (1995). *Renegotiating Health care: Resolving conflict to build collaboration.* San Francisco: Jossey-Bass Publishers.

22. McEwen, M. (1994). Promoting interdisciplinary collaboration. *Nursing & Health Care, 15,* 304–307.

23. Myers, S.S., Clark, M.D., Russell, J.A., Graham, C.C., Stultz, M.B., & Reidy, K.M. (2008). Focusing measures for performance-based privileging of physicians on improvement. *The Joint Commission Journal on Quality and Patient Safety, 34,* 724–733.

24. Norsen, L., Opladen, J., & Quinn, J. Practice model: Collaborative practice. *Critical Care Nursing Clinics of North America, 7,* 45.

25. Patterson, P. (2009). Toward an effective code of conduct. *OR Manager, 25,* 17–18.

26. Prescott, P.P. (1993). Nursing: An important component of hospital survival under a reformed health care system. *Nursing Economic$, 11,* 192–193.

27. Rosenstein, A.H., & O'Daniel, M.O. (2008). A survey of the impact of disruptive behaviors and communication defects on patient safety. *The Joint Commission Journal on Quality and Patient Safety, 34,* 464–471.

28. Salas, E., Klein, C., King, H., Salisbury, M., Augenstein, J.S., Birnbach, D.J., et al. (2008). Debriefing medical teams: 12 evidence-based best practices. *The Joint Commission Journal on Quality and Patient Safety, 34,* 518–526.

29. Sheely, C.M., & McCarthy, M.C. (1998). *Advanced Practice nursing emphasizing common roles.* Philadelphia: F.A. Davis.

30. Stefancyk, A. (2009). One-hour, off unit meal breaks. *American Journal of Nursing, 109,* 64–66.

31. Swan, B.A. (1994). A collaborative ambulatory preoperative evaluation model. *AORN Journal, 59,* 430–437.

32. The Council on Surgical & Perioperative Safety. (2007). *Statement on violence in the workplace.* Retrieved May 14, 2009 from www.cspsteam.org

33. White, C., & Howse, E. (1993). Managing Humor: When is it funny—and when is it not? *Nursing Management, 24,* 80–96.

34. Wikipedia (2009a). *Integrity.* Retrieved May 11, 2009 from wikipedia.org/wiki/Integrity

35. Wikipedia (2009b). *Optimism.* Retrieved May 11, 2009 from en.wikipedia.org/wiki/Optimism

12 Institutional Credentialing

Jeanne K. LaFountain

INTRODUCTION

Health care services, organizations, delivery systems, and providers are changing at a rapid pace. Today, health care is provided in venues that range from ambulatory to hospital settings. In addition, health care services are provided by numerous specialized practitioners including those who assist in surgery. As health care has changed, so too has the process of credentialing.

Credentialing for these specialized practitioners, hereafter referred to as allied health professionals (AHP), is important for patient safety and to ensure that services are provided by individuals who are qualified and competent. Hospitals are obligated to protect patients from incompetent practitioners. Credentialing of AHPs is influenced by state regulation, scopes of practice, institutional policy, medical bylaws, and regulatory compliance (Pybus & Cairns, 2004). This is not a simple task and varies greatly from organization to organization and from state to state.

WHO NEEDS TO BE CREDENTIALED?

All AHPs allowed to provide patient care services within an organization should go through some type of credentialing process. This includes hospital employees, physician-employed AHPs, and contract AHPs. The extent of credentialing depends on the role of the individual and may be done through the human resources department (utilizing job descriptions) or the medical staff office (approval of clinical privileges). The scope of medical and legal risk to the patient and organization generally determines the extent of the credentialing process (Pybus & Cairns, 2004).

To guide the credentialing process, it is important to examine state laws to establish which AHPs can function as licensed independent practitioners

(LIP); credentialing of LIPs usually parallels that of the medical staff. State law and health care organization policy will determine whether the health care provider can practice independently. As with medical staff credentialing, qualification validation should be an objective evaluation of the applicant's current licensure, training and experience, competence, and ability to perform the services requested. Ultimately, each individual health care facility will determine the best method of properly credentialing applicants classified as AHPs. It is to the health care organization's advantage to standardize the credentialing process for all AHPs to mirror that of the medical staff credentialing process, thus setting the standard of patient care within the institution to ensure quality patient care (Hospital Peer Review, 2002).

WHAT IS CREDENTIALING?

As defined by the Joint Commission (2007), credentialing is the process by which an organization obtains, evaluates, and certifies qualifications of health care professionals who provide patient care services in or for a health care organization. The process, based on predetermined and standardized criteria, focuses on verification of training, experience, licensure, competence, and the validation of the credentials collected to determine if the practitioner is qualified to render the patient care services requested. Credentialing is not complete until the information is reviewed and approved by the health care organization's governing body (Deutsch & Mobley, 1999).

HISTORY OF HOSPITAL CREDENTIALING

The hospital credentialing process was instituted for the purpose of granting hospital privileges to physicians. This process became necessary as increasing numbers of physicians began using hospitals. In the early 1900s, there was a growing acceptance of hospitals as centers for treating patients with acute illnesses and for performing surgical interventions. More and more physicians wanted to use the hospital facility as a "workshop." Hospitals were eager for physicians to admit their patients, especially those patients able to pay the hospital for their care. Because physicians determined which patients were to be admitted, they were powerful in influencing how hospitals were managed and controlled.

Physicians who had obtained hospital privileges soon controlled the "credentialing process." Occasionally, other physicians were not granted hospital privileges and were unable to use the hospital for their patients. In 1907, a survey of New York physicians in the Bronx and in Manhattan found that only 10% had hospital privileges. Those physicians who had been excluded began establishing their own hospitals, and increasing competition forced hospitals to open their staff privileges to qualified physicians. By 1933, 75% of all physicians had some type of hospital privileges (Zusman, 2001).

Because of financial reasons, the authority in hospitals initially passed from the trustees to the physicians. In the 1930s and 1940s, however, hospital administrators began challenging physicians' authority over hospitals. Administrators assumed more authority, due to the increasing complexity of the hospital's internal organization and its relationship with outside agencies. Prior to 1970, hospitals did little to no formal credentialing because there was no medical staff office. A physician's license was checked, but no recordkeeping was conducted. During this time, medical staff credentialing and privileges were of no interest to the law (Zusman, 2001).

In 1975, an accrediting agency was developed to create standards for the verification of education and licensure for physicians practicing in health care institutions. Due to the malpractice crisis during the 1980s, the Healthcare Quality Improvement Act of 1986 was passed. As a result, the National Practitioner Data Bank (NPDB) was developed, and an organization that was to become the Joint Commission on the Accreditation of Healthcare Organizations (JCAHO) created standards for primary source verification (Zusman, 2001).

Over the past 20 years, these quality improvement initiatives have been influenced by JCAHO, state laws and regulations, and the requirements of inspection agencies such as the Health Care Financing Administration (HCFA). Credentialing has been standardized to include credentialing and privileging based on regulated qualification and mandatory recredentialing every two years (Zusman, 2001).

ALLIED HEALTH PROFESSIONALS (NON-PHYSICIAN PROVIDERS)

Since 1982, health care has undergone profound changes, requiring the health professions to redefine their responsibilities to respond more quickly and effectively to the needs of consumers. Health care regulation, which is intended to protect the public, has come under scrutiny. The health care workforce is regulated by each individual state. Regulatory systems, aimed at standardizing levels of care, were initiated by surgeons during an era in which there were few health professions.

In recent years, Allied Health Professionals (AHP), such as nurse practitioners, physician assistants, RN first assistants, and surgical assistants have successfully increased their efforts to obtain hospital practice privileges. Although economic independence is certainly a factor in this movement, a major force is the desire for professional autonomy. Due to reduced number of hours residents can work, there is a growing demand for qualified assistants in surgery. This has created an influx of several professions vying to fill the void. Opposition originally came from physicians concerned about the fragmentation of patient care and the competition for health care dollars. Antitrust actions were subsequently initiated by non-physician providers who were denied hospital privileges. As a result, the Department of Justice and the Federal Trade Commission have issued six statements of their antitrust enforcement policies (Federal Trade Commission, 1993). New consumer options and competitive pressures on practitioners already in the market may enhance consumer welfare in the health care field by leading to quality health care improvements and reduced costs.

Challenges have also arisen from professional rivalries or "turf battles" among PAs, NPs, nurses, surgical assistants, and technologists, especially where there is vagueness or confusion over qualifications and roles of these health care providers. Professional territorialism can defeat the building of teamwork. As the level of knowledge, skills, and experience of these AHPs improve, their professional organizations are seeking recognition for their enhanced abilities. These issues can be resolved by the credentialing process during which institutions clearly delineate the duties and skills that are specific to each profession. Credentialing thus allows each profession to maintain its unique identity (Pybus & Cairns, 2004).

Clear definitions of the role of the assistant in surgery must be established within institutional policy; policies should be explicit with regard to the knowledge and skills that an assistant in surgery should possess. The scope of practice that is permitted by licensure or certification varies from state to state. The scope of practice must be well defined and verified, according to state law, before practice privileges are granted. Institutional practice privileges can limit activities associated with practice as an assistant in surgery, but they cannot expand the assistant's practice beyond the legal parameters established by the state's regulatory board (Bischel, 2008).

"Scope of practice" is defined as health care services that are provided by health care professionals authorized through state licensure, registration, and/or certification. These scopes of practice may overlap, reflecting shared competencies among groups of health care professionals. While some practitioners are authorized through state law and regulatory and institutional policy to function independently, others are required to practice under the supervision of or in collaboration with a licensed physician. Collaboration involves the interdependent planning and implementation of patient care services by physicians and allied health professionals within the boundaries of their respective scopes of practice. This interdisciplinary process promotes shared values and mutual respect for each other's contribution to provide quality patient care (FSMB, 2005).

CREDENTIALING AND PRACTICE PRIVILEGES

Each institution establishes its own guidelines for credentialing. Although there are no national credentialing standards specifically for AHPs who function as surgical assistants, resources are available for the institution to use in establishing such a credentialing policy.

Several professional organizations representing surgical first assistants have official position statements for the first assistant. The Association of periOperative Registered Nurses (AORN) *Official Statement on RN First Assistants* (RNFA) (Appendix 12-A) addresses the need to establish practice privileges in the institution in which the RNFA is practicing (AORN, 2005). The position of the American College of Surgeons (ACS) (Appendix 12-B) is that "practice privileges of those acting as first assistant should be based on verified credentials reviewed and approved by the hospital credentialing committee" (ACS, 2004). Such requirements are part of the institution's duty toward its patients—ensuring that those persons who provide patient care services are qualified to do so. While the American Association of Surgical Physician Assistants (AASPA) does not have an official position statement, they define the surgical physician assistant as a "highly skilled clinician who has received didactic and clinical training to function in all areas of the peri-operative environment" (AASPA, 2008). The American Academy of Physician Assistants' publication (Appendix 12-C), *Competencies for the Physician Assistant Profession*, outlines the knowledge and skills required to function in the surgical setting (AAPA, 2005). Finally, the Association of Surgical Technologist's *Position Statement on First Assistant* (Appendix 12-D) states, "the Certified Surgical Technologist with additional specialized education or training may function as first/surgical assistants to the surgeon" (AST, 2008).

Whereas credentialing and granting of practice privileges is a legal process that is part of the institution's bylaws and is approved by the board of the institution, the rationale for credentialing is to ensure quality patient care (Pybus & Cairns, 2004). Practice privileges for RNFAs meet the American Nurses Association (ANA) requirement that the nursing profession provides methods of identifying and recognizing nurses with specialized skills, experience, and competence (ANA, 2008).

Thus, the right to perform certain activities within an institution is a privilege granted through a credentialing process. This process determines whether the individual is qualified to perform the activities for which the application is being made. This verification is essential for both employees and nonemployees of the institution, although the institution's credentialing process may differ for employees and nonemployees. However, in both instances, the credentialing process aims to ensure that established and accepted legal and professional standards for the AHP in the role of FA, are met. By verifying that the AHP is competent to function in the role of FA, the institution ensures that patients will receive quality care and minimizes the liability exposure for itself and its staff. The processes and criteria used to grant clinical privileges must be applied uniformly to all applicants. This is to ensure a uniform level of quality throughout the health care organization, regardless of the specialty or health care discipline of the provider. Such uniformity fulfills both legal and accreditation requirements and is part of the health care system's ethical responsibility to the patients it serves (Bischel, 2008).

THE JOINT COMMISSION

In 1918, the ACS established the Hospital Standardization Program to ensure a minimum level of care. In 1951, other organizations were asked to participate, and the JCAHO (now called The Joint Commission [TJC]) was formed. Initially, the participating organizations were the American College of Physicians, the American Medical Association, the American Hospital Association, and the Canadian Medical Association. The Canadian Medical Association withdrew in 1959 to form its own organization (Davis, 1999).

The Joint Commission's accreditation process is voluntarily accepted by health care organizations. Reimbursement by third-party payers often requires that the institution has Joint Commission approval. This economic determinant increases the use of the accreditation process. Additional benefits to the accredited institution include enhanced community confidence in the facility; recruitment of medical staff; educational tools to improve care, services, and programs; and partial or complete fulfillment of state and federal requirements for licensure and certification.

To assist facilities seeking accreditation, the Joint Commission publishes the *Comprehensive Accreditation Manual for Hospitals,* which identifies the standards to be met by the institution, specifies the characteristics of each standard, and describes the measures that the institution must implement to meet the standard. The Joint Commission standards no longer directly reference AHP credentialing, although the Joint Commission medical staff standards do require that AHPs, classified as licensed independent practitioners (LIP), go through the same credentialing process as the medical staff (Pybus & Cairns, 2004). In 2005, the Joint Commission clarified the definition of LIP to "any practitioner permitted by law and by the organization to provide care and services, without direction or supervision, within the scope of the practitioner's license and consistent with individually assigned clinical responsibilities" (Joint Commission, 2007). State law and hospital policy determine whether a health care provider can practice independently as an LIP; the Joint Commission does not make that determination. According to John Harringer of the Joint Commission Standards Interpretation Group,

"'For practitioners credentialed and privileged under the medical staff standards, organizations are required to maintain specific, ongoing data collection on practitioner performance (case logs, compliance with core measures or other clinical practice guidelines, complication rates, prescribing patterns, etc.) as part of the credentialing/re-credentialing process. The maintenance of these documents must be as specified in MS 4.40 EP.2 (MS.08.01.03 in 2009) of the Joint Commission's Medical Staff Standards, with medical staff departments defining the data to be collected and the organized medical staff approving the defined data.' A job description in lieu of privileges is never acceptable to either the Joint Commission or CMS [Centers for Medicare and Medicaid Services]". (J. Harringer, Associate Director, Joint Commission Standards Interpretation Group, personal communication, November 4, 2008)

The Joint Commission Standards do not prohibit appointment of AHPs to the medical staff, generally as associate members, although this may be regulated through state administrative codes or institutional bylaws (Hospital Peer Review, 2002). Institutions have a unique opportunity to develop their own credentialing methodology for AHPs not classified as LIPs (Pybus & Cairns 2004).

The National Committee for Quality Assurance (NCQA, 2009) is another accrediting agency that accredits managed care organizations (MCO), and preferred provider, physician, and credentials verification organizations. Their credentialing and recredentialing standards are similar to those of the Joint Commission's standards (Pybus & Cairns, 2004).

According to the Centers for Medicare & Medicaid Services (CMS), credentialing is required for all health care professionals who provide service to their members under their Medicare+Choice organizations and who are licensed to practice independently under state law. Credentialing is not required for those health care professionals who provide services only under the direct supervision of another practitioner. Compliance with Medicare laws and regulations dictates the condition of participation (Centers for Medicare & Medicaid Services [CMS], 2003).

CREDENTIALING MECHANISMS

Institutions have credentialing mechanisms, as defined in institutional or medical staff bylaws, for granting or denying practice privileges. These mechanisms are based on standards that ensure the accountability and competence of the individual in performing activities within the institution. Criteria established by the institution for the credentialing process must be substantially related to the position or function of the applicant, whether they are employed by the institution, physician-employed, or a contracted provider with a member of the medical staff serving as their sponsor (Bischel, 2008).

Institutions are required to validate the credentials and competency for all AHPs who provide direct patient services within the organization. Hospital staff employees may be credentialed through human resources or the medical staff office according to institutional policy. The validation of education, licensure, and current competence is a part of the initial process and the recredentialing process.

First Assistants Employed by the Institution

Joint Commission standards require a process or processes designed to ensure that all individuals who provide patient care services, but who are not subject to the medical staff privilege delineation process, are competent to provide such services. An institutional policy of the credentialing process for non-physician providers (AHPs) should be in place, regardless of whether the process is channeled through the human resources office or the medical staff office's medical staff bylaws (The Joint Commission, 2008).

Employee credentialing by the institution can be used to meet these requirements. This mechanism ensures that the provider is competent to function in the FA role. Not only does this improve the quality of patient care, it also gives the FA recognition for the additional education and clinical expertise needed to function in this role.

The AORN perioperative nursing credentialing model (Chart 12-1) describes a credentialing process that can be used by an institution (AORN 2005b). This model is directed toward the credentialing of nurses practicing in the operating room, although the model can be customized for other non-physician providers in the role of FA. Specific criteria regarding the employee or new employee are verified by the institution. Files maintained on each employee, updated annually, should contain documentation of the following information:

- Educational qualification (diplomas, degrees, certificate of completion of recognized first assistant program)
- Licensure (verify original and copy for file)
- Peer evaluation (references, letters of recommendation)
- Certification (CNOR, CRNFA, CFA, PA-C)
- Evidence of continuing education and in-service education
- Verification of orientation, job description, and skill list
- Performance appraisal, documentation of competence, professional development activities (professional association activity, research, publications) (see Chart 12-1)

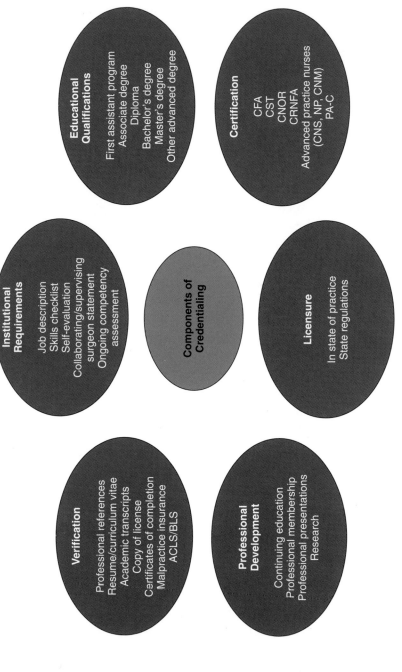

Chart 12-1

Components of Perioperative Credentialing

Institutions need to develop a job description (Chart 12-2) for the FA that identifies the specific qualifications, responsibilities, and functions of the position. The institution may wish to use the job description of the staff nurse or the surgical

---

JOB TITLE: First Assistant

SHIFT: _____   **SCHEDULE:** _____

DEPARTMENT: Surgical Services   **SUPERVISOR:** _____

JOB DESCRIPTION: Provides First Assistant services in the operating room during surgical procedures and assists surgical team as needed in any other capacity, according to established procedures. Provides services and support in the preoperative and postoperative patient care areas.

REQUIREMENTS:

Education: Graduate of an accredited school (nursing [RN], physician assistant [PA], surgical technologist [ST], and Certificate of completion from first assistant program [RN, NP, or ST]).

Experience: Minimum of 2 years OR experience (RN, ST). May be negotiated based on other similar experience (PA, NP).

Licensure/Certifications: Current licensure in the State of_____for Physician Assistant and Registered Nurse. CNOR/CST and secondary certification as First Assistant.

Duties (dependent on state and institutional regulations): Under the direction and supervision of a physician, will work as the first assistant during the patient's surgical procedure. Practices within limitations of preparation and experience.

Preoperatively:
- May perform admission evaluation on patients to include: obtaining medical information and history; review of patient's medical record noting allergies, pertinent medical history, and abnormal physical findings; performing physical exam; transcribing history and medical findings into patient medical record; and reporting deviations from normal findings to attending physician.
- Collaborates with other health team members to devolop, coordinate, and implement a preoperative plan of care unique to individual patient needs.
- Serves as a resource for patients and family regarding surgical preparation, surgical procedure, and postoperative expectations; locates and utilizes x-rays, instruments, and pertinent patient information.

Intraoperatively:
- Recognizes safety hazards and initiates appropriate corrective action.
- Applies principles of asepsis and infection control.
- Applies knowledge of surgical anatomy, physiology, and operative technique relative to operative procedures in which he/she is assisting.
- Performs positioning, prepping, and draping of the patient.
- Provides hemostasis by clamping blood vessels, electrocoagulation, and vessel ligation, as directed by the surgeon.
- Provides exposure through appropriate use of instruments, retractors, suctioning, and sponging techniques.
- Handles tissue as directed by the surgeon during the operative procedure.
- Performs wound closure of muscle, fascia, subcutaneous, and skin tissue as directed by the surgeon.
- Applies surgical dressings.
- Assists with transfer of the patient from the operating room.

Chart 12-2

Sample First Assistant Job Description

Postoperatively:
- May perform postoperative procedures to include: transcription of standard postoperative orders into patient medical records; assists physicians with evaluation and management of patient's status during recovery.
- Assists with management of postsurgical patients (i.e., dressing change, removal of drainage devices, suture removal, lab test evaluation, etc.).
- Facilitates patient discharge in collaboration with social services, pharmacy, and physical therapy.
- Dictates discharge and transfer summaries in a timely manner.

General Duties:
Demonstrates ability to develop and maintain a working relationship with patients, physicians, and other team members. Exhibits a professional manner when interacting with employees, patients, and visitors. Possesses effective verbal and written communication skills. Able to work long hours under stressful and emergent conditions. Ongoing collaboration with physician, while maintaining compliance with institutional policies.

Chart 12-2   (*Continued*)

Source: Adapted from Davis, N.B. (1999). Institutional credentialing of the RN First Assistant. In J.C. Rothrock (Ed.), *The RN First Assistant: An expanded perioperative nursing role* (p. 57). Philadelphia: Lippincott.

technologist in the operating room that relates to the scrub position and develop a separate job description for first assistant as a supplement.

A skills list (Chart 12-3) is used in conjunction with the job description. The list is based on the knowledge required to actualize the role and on the employee's ability to perform the specific tasks required. A skills list is maintained for each employee; often this will be the employee's responsibility. The skills may be incorporated into a checklist or a gradation scale that ranges from 1, "not performed," to 5, "able to teach." The skills list developed for the provider acting as a FA must address behaviors specific to that role. The behaviors might be classified as suturing, handling tissue, providing exposure, using instruments, and achieving hemostasis. Documentation of the numbers and types of operative procedures in which the provider has assisted is suggested. The skills list is useful for evaluating the FAs performance and for providing evidence of continued competence. The samples of the job description and skills checklist must be customized to the AHP in accordance with state law and institutional policy of the provider's scope of practice.

First Assistants Not Employed by the Institution

AHPs not employed by an institution, but who wish to function as first assistants within that institution, must have practice privileges. Application for privileges is usually made through the medical staff credentialing office. Non-physicians are considered "limited" health care practitioners, in contrast to physicians. Practice privileges are based on the legal scope of the applicant's professional practice and on the need for the services that the individual desires to provide within the institution.

FIRST ASSISTANT NAME: _____

EVALUATOR: _____

DATE: _____ YEARS PERIOPERATIVE EXPERIENCE: _____

YEARS FIRST ASSISTANT: _____

Key:
1 = Never   2 = Rarely   3 = Sometimes   4 = Very Often   5 = Always

		1	2	3	4	5
A.	1. Identifies normal/abnormal anatomy.					
	2. Participates in clinical decision making.					
	3. Modifies techniques based on findings.					
	4. Anticipates steps in surgical procedure.					
B.	1. Interviews patient and family preoperatively and assesses patient's needs.					
	2. Implements and evaluates plan of care.					
	3. Implements revised plan of care based on patient's outcomes.					
C.	1. Communicates relevant data to team members (physical findings, lab data, x-rays).					
	2. Discusses radiological/surgical procedures to be implemented during surgery.					
	3. Discusses unusual techniques/instruments required based on data collected.					
D.	1. Assists team members as needed.					
	2. Collaborates with surgical team members to plan perioperative patient plan of care.					
	3. Analyzes critical situations and implements appropriate action.					
E.	1. Reports safety hazards and variances in aseptic technique.					
	2. Relates changes in patient's condition.					
	3. Demonstrates CPR technique.					
	4. Reports concerns to appropriate members.					
	5. Prioritizes calmly and efficiently in stressful or emergency situations.					
F.	1. Provides appropriate retraction.					
	2. Demonstrates proper handling of tissue.					
	3. Uses appropriate suctioning techniques.					
	4. Demonstrates manual dexterity in the use of surgical instruments.					
	5. Provides hemostasis using: electrosurgery, bipolar electrocoagulation, clamps, pressure/sponging, hemostatic agents, bone wax, other (state).					
	6. Demonstrates suturing skills, tying techniques, ligating vessels, wound closure approximation, subcuticular closure, skin closure, staples, securing drains.					
	7. Demonstrates appropriate use of instruments.					

Chart 12-3
First Assistant Skills List

G.	1. Reviews postoperative orders with surgeon and team members.				
	2. Reports patient's status to PACU/OPU/ICU personnel.				
	3. Participates in patient's and family's education and discharge planning.				

First Assistants move through stages from novice to expert. Below are some characteristics of learners moving through each stage.

STAGE 1.   NOVICE
• Has no experience of the situations in which he or she is expected to perform.
• Is given context-free rules to guide actions to different attributes.
• Is unfamiliar with goals and tools of patient care.

STAGE 2.   ADVANCED BEGINNER
• Demonstrates marginally acceptable performance and has coped with enough real situations to note the recurring "aspects of the situation."
• Formulates guidelines (rather than rules) that dictate actions in terms of attributes and aspects.

STAGE 3.   COMPETENT
• Begins to see his or her actions in terms of long-range goals or plans of which he or she is consciously aware.
• Establishes a perspective and a plan based on considerable conscious, abstract, analytic contemplation of the problem and helps to achieve efficiency and organization (characteristic of this skill level).
• Has a feeling of mastery and has the ability to cope with and manage the many contingencies of clinical patient care.
• Lacks speed and flexibility of the proficient FA and does not base conclusions on salient points of the whole picture.

STAGE 4.   PROFICIENT
• Perceives situations as a whole guided by maxims, rather than in terms of aspects and attributes. Maxims reflect nuances of situations and provide directions as to what must be taken into consideration. Perception is the key. Practice is not "thought out" but "presents itself" based on experience and recent events."
• Has a holistic understanding of situations, which improves decision making.

STAGE 5.   EXPERT
• Possesses multifaceted knowledge with concrete references that cannot be put into abstract principles or explicit guidelines, but rather is based on an intuitive grasp of the situation. No longer relies on analytic principles (rules, guidelines, maxims) to connect his or her understanding of the situation, but zeros in on the accurate region of the problem without wasteful consideration of a large range of unfruitful alternative diagnoses and solutions.
• Operates from a deep understanding of the total situation. The vision of "what is possible" is one of the characteristics that separate competent from proficient and expert performance.
• Possesses an intuitive and holistic overview.
• Implements rapid decision making.

Chart 12-3   *(Continued)*

Source: Adapted from Davis, N.B. (1999). Institutional credentialing of the RN First Assistant. In J.C. Rothrock (Ed.), *The RN First Assistant: An expanded perioperative nursing role* (pp. 58–60). Philadelphia: Lippincott.

In some institutions, AHPs are considered "dependent" practitioners. When functioning as an FA, the AHP is under the supervision of the surgeon and is therefore "dependent." The AHP's practice privileges usually require a professional association and collaboration with a specific surgeon or group of surgeons. The surgeon or group of surgeons must provide a signed collaborating/supervisory statement (Chart 12-4).

This will certify that _____
                                          (Applicant's Name)

is authorized to provide services at Ohio State University Hospital and The James Cancer Hospital on behalf of and under my direction. I agree not to request the above named individual to perform any procedure or operate any equipment in The Ohio State University Hospitals that the applicant is not qualified to perform or operate by reason of training and experience and/or Board of Trustees approval.

I hereby agree that applicable professional activities of the above named individual will be under my supervision, and I will be responsible for the monitoring and evaluation of the above named individual's professional performance of applicable activities. I hereby further agree to provide such information to The Ohio State University Hospitals, the Licensed Healthcare Professionals Credentials Subcommittee, Corporate Credentials Committee, and the Medical Director, as such persons may request evaluation of the above named individual's professional performance and/or qualification for hospital privileges.

If the applicant above named is my employee, I warrant that I have secured coverage for workers' compensation for the above named applicant in accordance with the laws of the State of Ohio, and am paying required withholdings and taxes in accordance with state and federal laws in connection with all services rendered at Ohio State University Hospitals or The James Cancer Hospital.

_____   _____

_____   _____

_____   _____
Signature of Primary Collaborating or   Print Name of Physician(s)
Supervising Physician(s)

_____
Date

_____   _____
Signature of Department Chair   Date

_____
Signature of Medical Director (office use only)

Chart 12-4
Collaborating/Supervising Physician(s) Statement

Source: From *OSU Addendum Application Appendix D: Collaborating/Supervising Physician(s) Statement.* (Jan. 2008). The Ohio State University Health System. Available online at http://www.medctr.ohio-state.edu/ Departments/Credentialing; Modified with permission.

It is usually necessary for the applicant to provide the credentialing committee with information such as a description of the role of the first assistant, the legal interpretation and constraints of the practice in the particular state, historical information, national trends, and acceptance and support from professional associations (e.g., AORN, ANA, ACS, AAPA, AST, AASPA), as well as educational and certification credentials. This documentation should be gathered and submitted before applying for practice privileges.

Credentialing Process

All AHPs applying for privileges are required to complete an application and delineation of privilege form. The application process begins with the request for and submission of the application form and requisite information to the appropriate credentialing office (human resources, medical staff). From this committee, the application is usually sent to the surgical department committee, medical staff committee, executive committee of the medical staff, and then to the governing body for the final decision (Chart 12-5). Several states (Kansas, Rhode Island, Indiana, Vermont, Kentucky, Tennessee, Louisiana, Maryland, Ohio, and the District of Columbia) have implemented regulations that require hospitals, health insurance companies, and other credentialing organizations to accept the standardized, uniform credentialing form that was developed by the Council for Affordable Quality Healthcare (CAQH, 2009). This uniform credentialing form, which can be accessed online through CAQH's Universal Credentialing Datasource, provides physicians and allied health professionals with a common online database in which to update and complete the credentialing application form. Other states, such Georgia, Minnesota, North Carolina, Nevada, West Virginia, Illinois, and Iowa have state-specific uniform credentialing forms (see Chapter 13, Resources, for additional information). Due to the extensive time and expense of the credentialing process for hospitals and third party payors, the uniform credentialing form will improve efficiencies and reduce the time spent filling out numerous forms.

Before applying for practice privileges, the allied health professional should review the institutional policies that apply to practicing within that particular health care setting. If the institution does not have a policy related to non-physician assistants, such a policy should be developed and approved before the official application process begins. Institutional policies that govern the role of the non-physician assistant should cover activities that may be performed, qualifications required, and the mechanism for supervision by the surgeon. A credentialing checklist (Chart 12-6) is helpful for ensuring that the AHP applicant obtains all the required documents and signatures.

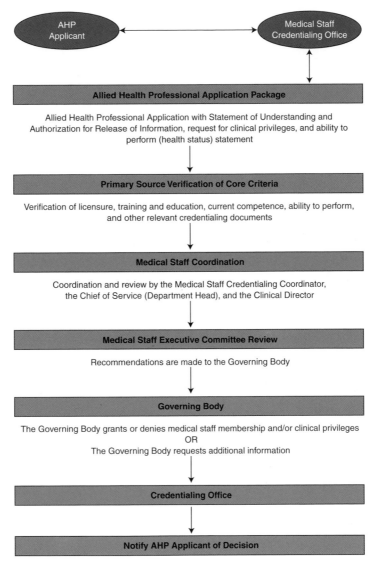

Chart 12-5

Sample Allied Health Professional Credentialing Flowsheet

Source: Developed by J.K. LaFountain.

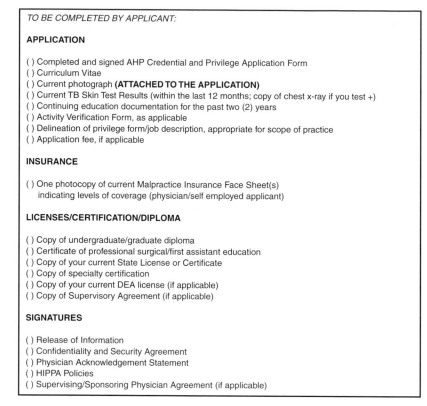

TO BE COMPLETED BY APPLICANT:

APPLICATION

( ) Completed and signed AHP Credential and Privilege Application Form
( ) Curriculum Vitae
( ) Current photograph **(ATTACHED TO THE APPLICATION)**
( ) Current TB Skin Test Results (within the last 12 months; copy of chest x-ray if you test +)
( ) Continuing education documentation for the past two (2) years
( ) Activity Verification Form, as applicable
( ) Delineation of privilege form/job description, appropriate for scope of practice
( ) Application fee, if applicable

INSURANCE

( ) One photocopy of current Malpractice Insurance Face Sheet(s)
    indicating levels of coverage (physician/self employed applicant)

LICENSES/CERTIFICATION/DIPLOMA

( ) Copy of undergraduate/graduate diploma
( ) Certificate of professional surgical/first assistant education
( ) Copy of your current State License or Certificate
( ) Copy of specialty certification
( ) Copy of your current DEA license (if applicable)
( ) Copy of Supervisory Agreement (if applicable)

SIGNATURES

( ) Release of Information
( ) Confidentiality and Security Agreement
( ) Physician Acknowledgement Statement
( ) HIPPA Policies
( ) Supervising/Sponsoring Physician Agreement (if applicable)

Chart 12-6

Checklist for Allied Health Professional Credentialing Application

Source: Developed by J.K. LaFountain.

When the AHP applies for institutional practice privileges, it is important to provide the information required by the Joint Commission. The 2007 standards specify that criteria for all applicants for medical staff privileges or delineated clinical privileges should include at least the following (Chart 12-7):

1. Evidence of current licensure
2. Relevant education and experience
3. Current competence (usually verified through references and peer recommendations)
4. Ability to perform requested privileges (TJC, 2007); see "Health status" in Glossary

Information regarding the AHP's licensure, specific educational preparation, experience, and current competence will be verified by the institution utilizing primary source verification. It is very important that the applicant provide detailed

SPECIALTY AREA: Surgical Assistant (*Please check one*) { } RNFA { } PA { } CFA	DEPARTMENT: **Surgery**

Please print:

Name _____ Dept _____
       Last   First   Middle Initial

Basic Qualifications for Printed List of Privileges:
- **PA**–Completion of an approved Physician Assistant Program.
- **RNFA**–Graduate of an approved school of nursing. Successful completion and holds a certificate from a recognized program, which shall consist of: 1) The Association of periOperative Registered Nurses, Inc, Core Curriculum for the Registered Nurse First Assistant; and 2) One (1) year of post-basic nursing study, which shall include at least 45 hours of didactic instruction and 120 hours of clinical internship or its equivalent of two college semesters.
- **CFA**–Graduate of formal training program.
- Current formal arrangement for employment/supervision by a current member in good standing, of the Active or Associate Staff, of the credentialing institution.
- Current, unrestricted nursing license as required by the state.
- Malpractice Liability Coverage in the amount of $1,000,000/$3,000,000.

✓= Check Privileges Requesting and submit letter from physician documenting current clinical experience
Please check only those procedure(s) in which you are proficient:
A = Approved, T = Tabled, D = Denied

R	LEVEL 1 CFA/RNFA/PA PRIVILEGE DESCRIPTION	CRITERIA for PRIVILEGES (Education/Training/ Experience)	APPLIES TO: (setting/ age group)	*A/T/D	RESTRICTIONS 1–Direction 2–Supervision 3–Direct Supervision
	Establish and maintain sterile field	See Basic Qualifications	__Adult __Peds		
	Assist in draping prepped surgical site	See Basic Qualifications	__Adult __Peds		
	Pass needed instruments, sutures, supplies and other equipment	See Basic Qualifications	__Adult __Peds		
	Provide hemostasis by coagulating bleeding points	See Basic Qualifications	__Adult __Peds		
	Provide exposure through appropriate use of instruments, retractors, suctions, and sponging techniques	See Basic Qualifications	__Adult __Peds		
	Agrees to follow departmental/hospital applicable policies/procedures including all surgical required counts	See Basic Qualifications	__Adult __Peds		
	Tie sutures	See Basic Qualifications	__Adult __Peds		
	Subcutaneous closure	See Basic Qualifications	__Adult __Peds		
	Skin Closure	See Basic Qualifications	__Adult __Peds		

Chart 12-7

Clinical Privilege Delineation Description Surgical Assistant

contact information to expedite this process. Additional information, such as current professional liability insurance, will likely be requested as well. Medical staff bylaws or policies will also require:

1. Information related to involvement in professional liability actions
2. Information related to any challenges (previously successful or currently pending) to licensure or registration or voluntary relinquishment of licensure or registration

R	LEVEL 2 RNFA/PA PRIVILEGE DESCRIPTION	CRITERIA for PRIVILEGES (Education/Training/ Experience)	APPLIES TO: (setting/ age group)	*A/T/D	RESTRICTIONS 1–Direction 2–Supervision 3–Direct Supervision
	Positioning, prepping, and draping of the patient	See Basic Qualifications	__Adult __Peds		
	Provide hemostasis by clamping blood vessels, coagulating bleeding points, ligating vessels, and by other means as directed by surgeon	See Basic Qualifications	__Adult __Peds		
	Perform wound closure as directed by the surgeon, suture the peritoneum, fascia, subcutaneous tissue, and skin	See Basic Qualifications	__Adult __Peds		
R	LEVEL 3 PA, NP PRIVILEGE DESCRIPTION	CRITERIA for PRIVILEGES (Education/Training/ Experience)	APPLIES TO: (setting/ age group)	*A/T/D	RESTRICTIONS 1–Direction 2–Supervision 3–Direct Supervision
	Take/perform a complete, detailed and accurate history and physical (under supervision of sponsor). **Authenticated & Countersigned by Physician**	See Basic Qualifications	__Adult __Peds		
	Perform local blocks as directed by surgeon. **Authenticated & Countersigned by Physician**	See Basic Qualifications	__Adult __Peds		
	Write orders. **Authenticated & Countersigned by Physician**	See Basic Qualifications	__Adult __Peds		
	I&D of superficial skin infections	See Basic Qualifications	__Adult __Peds		
	Debridment or suturing of superficial wound after surgeon has examined patient	See Basic Qualifications	__Adult __Peds		
	Removal of foreign body from external surface	See Basic Qualifications	__Adult __Peds		
	Removal of sutures	See Basic Qualifications	__Adult __Peds		
	Removal of drains	See Basic Qualifications	__Adult __Peds		
	Removal of cast	See Basic Qualifications	__Adult __Peds		
	Application of splints and cases as directed by surgeon	See Basic Qualifications	__Adult __Peds		

Chart 12-7 *(Continued)*

3. Any limitation, reduction, or loss of privileges at another institution (voluntary or involuntary)
4. A criminal background check and/or a drug screening test (depending on institution policy)

Information related to professional liability action and licensure issues may be obtained through the National Practitioner Data Bank (NPDB, 2009), although the information found there may not be complete for non-physician providers, due to the lack of reporting requirements for adverse events involving AHPs.

1–**Direction** means following the attending surgeon's verbal or written orders. The surgeon does not have to be physically present while tasks are being performed.

2–**Supervision** means the attending surgeon must be physically present in the operation room suite and is available to answer questions and respond to an emergency until the patient is released from the operating room.

3–**Direct supervision** means the attending surgeon is physically present in the operating room with the patient and observes the tasks delegated to the non-physician surgical assistant during the surgical procedure.

All activities of Allied Health Professionals who may provide care under the supervision or direction of a Physician shall be under the direct supervision of a Medical Staff member, but such supervision shall not always require the physical presence of the Medical Staff member unless otherwise required by law. If any other Hospital employee questions the authority or instructions of an Allied Health Professional either to act or to issue instructions outside of the presence of the supervising Staff member, the Hospital employee may delay acting until the supervising Physician has validated the order or instructions of the Allied Health Professional. (Medical Staff Rules & Regulations for Allied Health Professionals) Each direct patient care service provided by the RNFA, PA, or CFA must be documented as such in the patient's medical record either by the supervising physician or by the assistant him/herself. All entries by the RNFA, PA, or CFA must be countersigned by the supervising physician within 24 hours. Under no circumstance may the surgical assistant write or dictate the operative note or report or the discharge summary.

Applicant's Signature   Date

I have reviewed the entire delineation of privileges and agree that the functions specific above constitute the functions which the surgical assistant applicant will perform while under my supervision.

Sponsoring Physician's Signature   Date

Reviewed by Department Chairman – Signature   Date

BOARD APPROVAL: _____

Chart 12-7 *(Continued)*

Source: From *Clinical Privilege Delineation Description, Frankfort Regional Medical Center/HCA Healthcare,* Frankfort, KY. Available online at http://www.frankfortregional.com/CPM/Surgical%20Asst.pdf; Modified with permission.

AORN's official statement on RNFAs provides additional information regarding the credentialing process. It calls for mechanisms for the following:

- Assessing individual qualifications for practice
- Assessing continuing proficiency
- Evaluating performance annually
- Assessing compliance with relevant institutional and departmental policies
- Defining lines of accountability
- Retrieving documentation of participation as first assistant and establishing a system for peer review (AORN, 2005a & b)

The ACS's position statement on qualifications of the FA in the operating room addresses the application for practice privileges by non-physician assistants. The criteria outlined for practice privileges include the following:

- Outline of qualifications and credentials
- Request to "assist in a surgeon's practice including assisting at the operating table"
- Identity of the surgeon responsible for the applicant's performance
- Requirement that the qualifications be reviewed and approved by the hospital (institutional) board (ACS, 2004)

When an application for practice privileges is submitted, the institution usually requests specific information related to first assistant activities. The request may be a narrative description of the first assistant's role or for a checklist (see Chart 12-3). The non-physician assistant may apply for privileges in all surgical specialties or in a specific surgical area (or areas), such as cardiovascular or orthopedics. The privileges will be granted only in those specialty areas designated by the applicant. Examples of activities to include on the application are:

- Preoperative assessment of the patient
- Preoperative education of the patient, family, and significant others
- Assisting with patient positioning, prepping, and draping
- Providing exposure by suctioning, sponging, and retracting
- Providing hemostasis by applying hemostatic clamps or clips, coagulating bleeding points, and ligating bleeding vessels
- Suturing
- Performing postoperative activities, which may include:
  - Removing sutures, chest tubes, drains, or pacing wires
  - Performing postoperative evaluation
  - Providing discharge instructions

It is important to state that intraoperative activities will be performed in collaboration with the operating surgeon and to delineate the nature of the surgeon's supervisory functions.

STEPS TO THE CREDENTIALING PROCESS
Request for Application:
1. Application for permission to practice at the designated health care facility must be submitted in writing to the credentialing office.

2. The Allied Health Professional (AHP) requesting an application for permission to practice shall be sent a letter detailing specific eligibility criteria to practice within the designated health care facility with the appropriate application forms.

Authorization to Obtain Information from Third Parties:

The AHP applying for privileges to practice at the designated health care facility will authorize the health care facility's credentialing office:

1. To seek information from any third party who may have information on the AHP's professional qualifications, credentials, clinical competence, character, ability to perform safely and competently, ethics, behavior, and any other information which may have an impact on the applicant's qualifications for permission to practice at the health care facility, and

2. The AHP will sign a release of information to these third parties to release appropriate information, including criminal background checks, to the health care facility and its authorized representatives upon request.

Initial Review of Application:

1. The completed application, with copies of all required documents, must be submitted to the credentialing office within the designated time frame. An application processing fee may be required, which should be submitted at this time.

2. The application will be reviewed by the credentialing office for completeness and that all criteria have been met. Attention to detail is paramount during this process as incomplete applications will delay the process or will result in a rejected application.

3. The health care facility's credentialing office shall validate relevant information, references, and other requested materials.

Department Chair Procedure:

1. The credentialing office will submit the complete application and all supporting documents to the appropriate department chair. The department chair shall notify the credentialing office, in writing, whether the applicant has satisfied all of the criteria for permission to practice and the clinical privileges approved.

Credentials Committee Procedure:

1. The Credentials Committee shall evaluate the department chair's report.

2. After validating the applicant's references and supporting documents, the Credentials Committee shall review the applicant's Clinical Privileges/Scope

of Practice Requested form to determine if there is any question about the applicant's ability to perform within the scope of practice or privileges requested. In case of a discrepancy between the facility and the state's scopes of practice, the scope of practice outlined by state regulatory agencies will supercede those of the facility.

Medical Executive Committee Procedure:

1. After receipt of the written findings and recommendation of the Credentials Committee, the Medical Executive Committee shall:
    a. approve the findings and recommendations of the Credentials Committee; or
    b. refer the documents back to the Credentials Committee for further consideration and/or responses to specific inquiries raised by the Medical Executive Committee; or
    c. recommend dissent, with supporting documentation and rationale for its disparity with the Credentials Committee's recommendation.
2. Medical Executive Committee must submit its recommendation to the health care facility's governing body. The Medical Executive Committee's decision must specifically address the clinical privileges or scope of practice requested by the applicant, and any related restriction or prohibitions to requested clinical privileges requested.

Governing Body Procedure:

1. The health care facility's governing body, upon receipt of the Medical Executive Committee's recommendation, may:
    a. grant the applicant permission to practice, and clinical privileges or scope of practice as recommended; or
    b. refer the matter back to the Credentials Committee or Medical Executive Committee for additional research or information; or
    c. reject or modify the recommendation.

Renewal of Permission to Practice:

1. Permission to practice at the health care facility as an AHP is approved by the Board and shall be for a period not to exceed two years. Renewal of clinical privileges or scope of practice shall be granted only upon submission of a completed renewal application.
2. Failure to submit a complete application in the designated time period prior to the expiration of the individual's privilege term shall result in termination of clinical privileges or scope of practice at the expiration of the current credentialing period.

3. Upon completion and submission of the application for renewal of practice privileges to the Credentialing Office, the application shall be evaluated in the same manner and procedure as initial applications.
4. The renewal of clinical privileges will include the following factors:
    a. The competency of the practitioner as assessed by the appropriate department chair and documented on a biennial evaluation form (Chart 12-8).
    b. A recommendation from a peer in the same or similar specialty.
5. Renewal of a practitioner's scope of practice will include the annual competency assessments performed by the supervising physician(s) and applicable hospital department heads. These evaluation forms, along with other reasonable indicators of continuing qualifications, including professional continuing education and surgical case logs, shall be factors for the renewal of practitioners' continued permission to practice
        (Adapted from *St. Ann's Medical Staff Policy on Allied Health*, 2009).

Reappointment or renewal of practice privileges will be determined in relation to competence. Information concerning professional performance, clinical judgment and decision making, interpersonal skills, and clinical or technical skills will be requested during the reappointment process. Peer recommendations are part of the basis for reappointment; these, as well as documentation of continuing education activities, should be submitted. Also required are recommendations from the department or major clinical service where the AHP functions.

For applicants who are denied clinical privileges or who receive adverse decisions, the Joint Commission requires that institutions offer a mechanism for appropriate action, including a fair hearing and an appeal process. Sex, race, creed, and national origin are not bases for decisions on granting or denying appointment or clinical privileges. The institution must abide by antitrust laws that prohibit restraint of trade or attempts to monopolize by excluding certain providers from access to the institution. The bylaws of the medical staff must define the criteria for admission to or denial of medical staff privileges within the institution. Decisions or recommendations cannot be made on the basis of competitive considerations (Pybus & Cairns, 2004).

Applying for Privileges as an Assistant Intern

The importance of educational preparation for assisting in surgery is well documented. In its official statement on RNFAs, AORN clearly states that "the RN first assistant practices perioperative nursing and must have acquired the necessary knowledge, skills, and judgment specific to clinical practice … through completion

Allied Health Professional
Annual Performance/Competency Evaluation

Name: _____

Supervising or Sponsoring Physician

Name: _____
                                    (please print)

The following annual performance/competency evaluation form is forwarded to you as a current sponsoring or supervising physician of the above-named Allied Health Professional (AHP). Joint Commission now requires that accredited facilities evaluate AHPs on an annual basis. We would appreciate your assistance in evaluating the above-named AHP by completing this form. Each competency has several definitions that help explain it. It is not necessary to address each definition. It is possible some may not be applicable.

	Does not meet basic expectations; may still be on the learning curve.	Meets expectations; meets all objectives; exceeds some; is recognized as a solid performer.	Exceeds expectations on most objectives; is recognized as exceptional.	NA—Not Applicable; this competency does not apply.
COMPETENCY				
Integrity: Behaves ethically and honestly; communicates openly in all directions; fosters trust in relationships; uses and allocates resources effectively and ethically; accepts responsibility for own decisions and actions.				
Teamwork: Promotes cooperation; actively contributes to team efforts; supports team decisions; puts aside self interest; works with diversity; treats others with dignity and respect.				
Customer & Quality Focus: Monitors quality and customer satisfaction; delivers to high standards; exercises good judgment in meeting customer needs; meets all compliance and regulatory requirements pertinent to privileges.				
Job Knowledge (Professional/technical knowledge): Working knowledge of other related jobs/functions; plans and organizes work well; practices priority management; work quality is good.				
Development: Provides timely and candid feedback; coaches and supports others.				

Chart 12-8

Sample of AHP Annual Performance/Competency Evaluation

Leadership: Sets a living example; shares and promotes Organization's Code of Conduct, Mission, and Values.				
SAFETY AND PREVENTION				
Infection Control: Uses standard precautions with all patients; uses appropriate protective measure if there is a risk of exposure to patient blood or body fluid; reduces the risk of health-care-associated infections; applies principles of aseptic technique and reports any discrepancies.				
HIPAA Guidelines: Maintains confidentiality, security and integrity of patient data; follows all HIPAA guidelines related to Protected Health Information (PHI).				
Environmental Safety: Identifies and reports safety hazards; monitors changes in patient's condition and reports issue to appropriate surgical team members.				
POSITION SPECIFIC COMPETENCIES				
Medical/Clinical knowledge: Demonstrates knowledge of surgical procedures, anatomy, surgeon preferences.				
Technical and clinical skills: Provides appropriate exposure, tissue handling, hemostatic, and suturing techniques.				
Clinical judgment: Utilizes critical thinking skills to assess, plan, implement, and evaluate patient care needs pre-, intra-, and postoperatively.				
Interpersonal skills: Collaborates with surgical team members to provide optimal patient outcomes.				
Communication skills: Communicates relevant data to surgical team members, (e.g., lab results, x-rays, diagnostic tests, instrumentation, equipment, etc.).				
Professionalism: Maintains standards; performs competently; engages in ongoing learning; practices in ethical manner.				

Chart 12-8   *(Continued)*

of an RNFA program that meets the AORN Recommended Education Standards for RN First Assistant Programs" (AORN, 2005a & b, p. 1). The AORN Recommended Education Standards for RN First Assistant Programs further clarify the nature of the didactic and supervised clinical learning required to develop the cognitive, psychomotor, and affective behaviors necessary for role assumption as an RNFA.

QUESTIONS		
1. Have you worked with this AHP in the last 12 months?	Yes	No
2. What is your association with this AHP?		
3. Does this AHP have any mental or physical health problems that might affect the ability to exercise the prerogatives requested? (If "yes", please explain.)	Yes	No

RECOMMENDATION (check one)

_____ I believe this AHP has satisfactory qualifications and competencies necessary for the privileges requested.

_____ I do not believe this AHP has satisfactory qualifications and competencies necessary the privileges requested.

_____ I do not have adequate information available with regards to this AHP's job-related performance in order to make a recommendation.

Comments (optional):

_____

_____

_____

_____

Signature (original signature only – no stamps)   Date

Please return this form to the (Healthcare Organization's Name) Credentialing Office in the enclosed envelope or fax to XXX-XXX-XXXX.

Chart 12-8   *(Continued)*

Source: From *Peer Recommendation.* (August 2007). The Ohio State University Health System. Available online at http://www.medctr.ohio-state.edu/Departments/Credentialing; Modified with permission.

Educational programs for many first assistants require a clinical internship, during which the intern builds on a knowledge base acquired through classroom instruction. The internship is supervised by faculty or a surgeon. These internships require acquisition of a depth and breadth of clinical skills. To engage in such internship activities, the first assistant student may need to apply for privileges as a first assistant intern. The delineation of privileges may vary from institution to institution and is often based on the specific clinical requirements of the educational program. The institution in which the first assistant interns intend to obtain their clinical hours may require Training Agreements or Memorandum of Understanding. The FA intern should contact the surgical department to determine current institutional policy prior to beginning their FA program to avoid any delay in clinical training.

CONCLUSION

The ultimate purpose of credentialing is for the benefit and safety of patients. Credentialing is the institution's method of scrutiny to ensure that patient care is provided by only qualified health care providers. A credentialing process provides a system within the institution for identifying and validating the individual AHP's knowledge and skill. This is important as a competency assessment and quality improvement mechanism. With credentialing, the institution has a method to evaluate each AHP and assign specific aspects of patient care based on the AHP's qualifications, thus ensuring patient safety and contributing to quality of care, increased productivity, and efficiency.

GLOSSARY

Accreditation: process whereby a healthcare accrediting agency determines that specific standards are met in an eligible healthcare organization.

Allied health professionals (AHP): non-physicians whose training, experience, and current competence comply with the policies of the hospital's governing body to practice that discipline in that facility. AHPs may be employed by a physician or the hospital, or may be independent practitioners with a sponsoring physician who is a member of the medical staff (Hospital Peer Review, 2002). There are two categories of AHPs:

- Independent AHP has a recognized but limited scope of practice and is licensed and permitted to provide services independently in the hospital without the direction of or immediate supervision of a physician. The healthcare organization, as well as the licensing agency, may determine which practitioners will be categorized as allied health and the degree of their independence to provide services.
- Non-independent AHP or physician-directed AHP functions in a medical support role to a physician. These may have a job description rather than privileges.

Certification: process by which an authorized certifying body, governmental or nongovernmental, evaluates and awards an official designation to an individual as having met predetermined criteria.

Clinical competence: current clinical competence is the practitioner's actual clinical performance and technical skills for the scope of practice. At appointment, clinical competence is based on training and experience. For reappointment, it is based on results of performance improvement activities and recommendations from peers and the department chairperson.

Clinical privileges: authorization granted to an individual to perform specific patient care functions, within the healthcare delivery system, as governed by his/her licensure, certification, or registration and in accordance with the bylaws of the organization.

Competency: qualifying an individual's skills, knowledge, and capability to meet predetermined expectations.

Contracted provider: healthcare provider who has a contractual agreement to provide specific services to a healthcare organization.

Core components: core components of appointment and reappointment are:

- Licensure
- Education/training
- Clinical competence
- Health status or the ability to perform requested privileges

Credential: documentation that demonstrates qualifications, i.e., certificate, license, training, case logs, and other experiential records.

Credentialing: process by which an organization obtains, evaluates and certifies qualifications, based on predetermined and standardized criteria, of healthcare professionals to provide patient care services in or for a health care organization.

Credentials verification organization (CVO): agency that gathers data and verifies credentials of health care providers.

Delineation of privileges: clinical privileges, which are provider-specific and extended to each practitioner based on his or her training and experience.

Health status: the Americans with Disabilities Act (ADA) prohibits employers from inquiring about an applicant's health status. To comply with ADA requirements, health status is not mentioned in the current Joint Commission standards. Instead, the ability to perform requested privileges is addressed.

Licensed independent practitioners (LIP): practitioners permitted by law and by the organization to provide patient care services, without direct supervision, within the scope of the individual's license, and consistent with individually granted clinical privileges. Definition may vary from state to state.

Licensure: mandatory process by which a governmental agency grants time-limited permission to an individual to engage in a given occupation after verifying that he/she has met predetermined and standardized criteria, and offers title protection for those who meet the criteria.

Peer review: review, evaluation, and assessment of the quality and efficiency of care by a practicing peer.

Primary source verification: verification by the original source of the accuracy of a health care practitioner's reported credential. This may be done by direct correspondence, telephone verification, internet verification, or reports from the organization verifying credentials.

Recredentialing: abbreviated process of renewing privileges that occurs at least every two (2) years. The process includes quality performance assessment and peer review with information related to judgment, performance, and skills.

Secondary source verification: verification of credentials by a means other than direct contact with the issuing source. This form of verification includes the original credential, notarized copy of the credential, or a copy of the credential made by a staff member of the facility. LIP credentialing also requires secondary source verification of the following:

1. Government issued picture identification
2. Drug Enforcement Administration (DEA) registration (as applicable)
3. Immunization and tuberculosis skin test (PPD) status
4. Life support training (as applicable)

Source: Migrant Clinicians Network. *Sample health center credentialing and privileging policy.* Retrieved April 7, 2009 from http://www.migrantclinician.org/files/resourcebox/CredentialingPolicy.pdf

REFERENCES

1. American Academy of Physician Assistants (AAPA). (2005). *Competencies for the Physician Assistant profession.* Retrieved October 17, 2008 from http://www.aapa.org/gandp/competencies-competencies.pdf

2. American Association of Surgical Physician Assistants (AASPA). *Specialty practice areas.* Retrieved October 3, 2008 from http://www.aaspa.com/page.asp?tid=95&name=The-Surgical-PA&navid=18

3. American College of Surgeons (ACS). (2004). *Qualifications of the responsible surgeon.* Retrieved October 3, 2008 from http://www.facs.org/fellows_info/statements/stonprin.html#anchor129977

4. American Nurses Association (ANA). (2008). *Professional role competence.* Retrieved October 3, 2008 from http://www.nursingworld.org/MainMenuCategories/HealthcareandPolicyIssues/ANA-PositionStatements/practice/Position StatementProfessionalRoleCompetence.aspx

5. Association of periOperative Registered Nurses (AORN). (2005a). *AORN Official Statement on RN First Assistants.* Retrieved October 3, 2008 from http://www.aorn.org/PracticeResources/AORNPositionStatements/Position_RNFA

6. Association of periOperative Registered Nurses (AORN). (2005b). *RN First Assistant guide to practice* (2nd ed.). Denver: AORN.

7. Association of periOperative Registered Nurses (AORN). (2006). *Allied health*

care providers and support personnel in the perioperative practice setting. Retrieved October 3, 2008 from http://www.aorn. org/PracticeResources/AORNPosition-Statements/Position_HealthCareProvidersAndSupportPersonnel

8. Association of Surgical Technologists (AST). (2008). *AST position statement on first assisting.* Retrieved October 3, 2008 from http://www.ast.org/pdf/Standards_of_Practice/Position_First_Assisting.pdf

9. Bischel, M.D., & Margaret, D. (2008). *Credentialing and privileges manual* (3rd ed.). Santa Barbara, CA.: Apollo Managed Care Consultants.

10. Centers for Medicare & Medicaid Services (CMS). (2003). *CMS Medicare Manual System Pub. 100-16 Managed Care Chap 6. Sec. 60.3.* Washington DC: Government Printing Office.

11. Council for Affordable Quality Healthcare (CAQH) (2009). http://www.caqh.org/ Universal Credentialing Datasource available at http://www.caqh.org/search.php?query=universal+credentialing+ datasource

12. Davis, N.B. (1999). Institutional Credentialing of the RN First Assistant. In J.C. Rothrock (Ed.), *The RN First Assistant: An expanded perioperative nursing role* (3rd ed., pp. 49–74). Philadelphia: Lippincott.

13. Deutsch, S., & Mobley, C.S. (1999). *The credentialing handbook.* Gaithersburg, MD: Aspen Publishers, Inc.

14. Federal Trade Commission. (1993). *Department of Justice and Federal Trade Commission statements of antitrust enforcement policy in health care.* Retrieved October 30, 2008 from http://www.ftc.gov/bc/healthcare/industryguide/policy/intro.htm

15. Federation of State Medical Boards (FSMB). (2005). *Assessing scope of practice*

in health care delivery: critical questions in assuring public access and safety.* Retrieved October 28, 2008 http://www.fsmb.org/pdf/2005_grpol_scope_of_practice.pdf

16. Joint Commission. (2007). *Comprehensive accreditation manual for hospitals: The official handbook.* Oakbrooke Terrace, IL: Joint Commission Resources, Inc (JCR).

17. The Joint Commission. (2008). *Credentialing non-medical staff member licensed independent practitioners who order tests and treatments from a Joint Commission Accredited Organization.* Retrieved April 30, 2009, from http://www.jointcommission.org/AccreditationPrograms/CriticalAccessHospitals/Standards/09_FAQs/MS/Credentialing_Non_Medical_Staff.htm

18. Mt. Carmel St. Ann's. (2009). *St. Ann's medical staff policy on allied health professionals.* Retrieved August 24, 2009 from http://www.mountcarmelhealth.com/pdf/AHP%20Policy%20-%20FINAL%204-27-2009.pdf

19. National Council of State Boards of Nursing (NCSBN). (2005). *Meeting the ongoing challenge of continued competence.* Retrieved October 31, 2008 from https://www.ncsbn.org/Continued_Comp_Paper_TestingServices.pdf

20. Pybus, B.E. & Cairns, C.S. (2004). *A guide to AHP credentialing.* Marblehead, MA: HCPro.

21. Spath, P. (2002). Credential your allied health professionals. *Hospital Peer Review. 27,* 13–6. Retrieved October 17, 2008 from http://www.accessmylibrary.com/coms2/summary_0286-24926600_ITM

22. Zusman, J. (2001). *The credentialing desk reference.* Marblehead, MA: Opus Communications, Inc.

Additional resources can be found in Chapter 13, Resources.

APPENDIX 12-A   AORN OFFICIAL STATEMENT ON RN FIRST ASSISTANTS

PREAMBLE

Perioperative nursing practice historically has included the role of the registered professional nurse (RN) as assistant at surgery. As early as 1977, documents issued by the American College of Surgeons supported the appropriateness for qualified RNs to first assist.

The Association of periOperative Registered Nurses (AORN) officially recognized this role as a component of perioperative nursing in 1983 and adopted the first "Official statement on RN first assistants (RNFA)" in 1984. AORN's official statement delineates the definition, scope of practice, educational requirements, and qualifications that must be met and suggests clinical privileges for the perioperative RN who practices as an RNFA. AORN supports appropriate compensation/reimbursement for RNs who fulfill this role.

DEFINITION OF RN FIRST ASSISTANT

The RNFA is a perioperative registered nurse who works in collaboration with the surgeon and health care team members to achieve optimal patient outcomes. The RNFA must have acquired the necessary knowledge, judgment, and skills specific to the expanded role of RNFA clinical practice. Intraoperatively, the RNFA practices at the direction of the surgeon and does not concurrently function as a scrub nurse.

SCOPE OF PRACTICE

All state boards of nursing recognize the role of the RNFA as being within the scope of nursing practice. Perioperative nursing is a specialized area of practice. Registered nurses practicing as first assistants in surgery are functioning in an expanded perioperative nursing role. Activities included in first assisting are further refinements of perioperative nursing practice and are executed within the context of the nursing process. First assisting behaviors are based on an extensive body of scientific knowledge. Certain of these behaviors include delegated medical functions that are unique to the perioperative RN qualified to practice as an RNFA. Registered nurse first assistant behaviors may vary depending on patient populations, practice environments, services provided, accessibility of human and fiscal resources, institutional policy, and state nurse practice acts. Examples of RNFA behaviors in the perioperative arena include:

- Preoperative patient management in collaboration with other health care providers, including but not limited to,
  - performing preoperative evaluation/focused nursing assessment,
  - communicating/collaborating with other health care providers regarding the patient plan of care, and
  - writing preoperative orders according to established protocols;
- Intraoperative surgical first-assisting, including but not limited to,
  - using instruments/medical devices,
  - providing exposure,
  - handling and/or cutting tissue,
  - providing hemostasis, and
  - suturing; and
- Postoperative patient management in collaboration with other health care providers in the immediate postoperative period and beyond, including but not limited to,
  - writing postoperative orders/operative notes according to established protocols,
  - participating in postoperative rounds, and
  - assisting with discharge planning and identifying appropriate community resources as needed.

PREPARATION OF THE RNFA

The complexity of knowledge and skill required to effectively care for recipients of perioperative nursing services compels nurses to be specialized and to continue their education beyond generic nursing programs. Perioperative nurses who wish to practice as RNFAs should develop a set of cognitive, psychomotor, and affective behaviors that demonstrate accountability and responsibility for identifying and meeting the needs of their perioperative patients.

Development of this set of behaviors begins with and builds upon the education program leading to licensure as an RN, which teaches basic knowledge, skills, and attitudes essential to the practice of perioperative nursing. Further preparation for the RNFA includes perioperative nursing practice with diversified experience culminating in the nurse achieving certified nurse operating room (CNOR) certification through the Competency and Credentialing Institute (CCI).

Additional preparation is then acquired through completion of an RNFA program that meets the "AORN standards for RN first assistant education programs" and is accepted by CCI. These programs should be equivalent to one academic year of formal, post-basic nursing study; consist of curricula that address all of the modules in the *Core Curriculum for the RN First Assistant;* and award college credits and degrees or certificates of RNFA status upon satisfactory completion of all requirements. The RNFA programs should be associated with schools of nursing at universities or colleges that are accredited for higher education by an accrediting agency that is nationally recognized by the Secretary of the US Department of Education. The registered nursing program should be approved by a state licensing jurisdiction for nursing programs at the university, college, or community college level or by another national or regional agency that is nationally recognized by the Secretary of the US Department of Education as a specialized accrediting agency for nursing programs.

Each RNFA demonstrates behaviors that progress on a continuum from basic competency to excellence. When educational and experiential requirements have been met, the RNFA is encouraged to achieve and maintain certification status (CRNFA) through CCI, an independent entity.

QUALIFICATIONS FOR ENTRY INTO RNFA PRACTICE

AORN believes the minimum qualifications to practice as a RN first assistant are as follows:

- Certification in perioperative nursing (CNOR);
- Successful completion of an RNFA program that meets the "AORN standards for RN first assistant education programs" and is accepted by CCI; and
- Compliance with statutes, regulations, and institutional policies relevant to RNFAs.

CLINICAL PRIVILEGING FOR THE RNFA

To determine if the RN qualifies for clinical privileges as a first assistant, an approval process should be established by the facility(ies) in which the individual will practice. The process of granting clinical privileges should include mechanisms for

- Assessing individual qualifications for practice,
- Assessing continuing proficiency,
- Evaluating annual performance,
- Assessing compliance with relevant institutional and departmental policies,
- Defining lines of accountability,
- Retrieving documentation of participation as first assistant, and
- Establishing systems for peer review that include a process for incorporating continuing education/contact hours relevant to RNFA practice.

Documentation of competency should be maintained within the facility.

The decision by an RN to practice as a first assistant must be made voluntarily and deliberately, with an understanding of the professional accountability that the role entails. For additional sources of information, refer to the following AORN publications:

- *Perioperative Standards and Recommended Practices*
- *RN First Assistant Guide to Practice*
- *Core Curriculum for the RN First Assistant*

These publications are available from AORN's Perioperative Bookstore, (800) 755–2676, ext. 1, or online at http://www.aorn.org

For additional information regarding CRNFA certification, contact the Competency and Credentialing Institute (CCI), (888) 257–2667 or online at http://www. http://www.cc-institute.org

Sources: American Colleges of Surgeons. (1977). Statement and qualifications for surgical privileges in approved hospitals. *Bulletin of the American College of Surgeons, 62,* 12–13; AORN. Task force defines first assisting. (1984). *AORN Journal,* 403–405.

Submitted in March 1984; adopted by the House of Delegates, Atlanta, March 5, 1984; proposed revision to Board of Directors in September 1992; adopted by the House of Delegates, Anaheim, Calif, March 4, 1993; proposed revision to Board of Directors in November 1997; adopted Nov 17, 1997; ratified by the House of Delegates, Orlando, April 1998; proposed revision to Board of Directors in November 2003, ratified by the House of Delegates, San Diego, March 2004. Revised; approved by the House of Delegates in December 2005. Sunset review: March 2010.

Note: Reprinted with permission from http://www.aorn.org/PracticeResources/AORNPositionStatements/Position_RNFA Copyright © 2005 AORN, Inc., 2170 South Parker Road, Suite 300, Denver, CO 80231. All rights reserved.

APPENDIX 12-B AMERICAN COLLEGE OF SURGEONS

STATEMENTS ON PRINCIPLES

(These statements were collated, approved by the Board of Regents, and initially published in 1974. They were last revised in March 2004.)

G. SURGICAL ASSISTANTS

The first assistant during a surgical operation should be a trained individual who is able to participate in and actively assist the surgeon in completing the operation safely and expeditiously by helping to provide exposure, maintain hemostasis, and serve other technical functions. The qualifications of the person in this role may vary with the nature of the operation, the surgical specialty, and the type of hospital or ambulatory surgical facility.

The American College of Surgeons supports the concept that, ideally, the first assistant at the operating table should be a qualified surgeon or a resident in an approved surgical education program. Residents at appropriate levels of training should be provided with opportunities to assist and participate in operations. If such assistants are not available, other physicians who are experienced in assisting may participate.

It may be necessary to utilize non-physicians as first assistants. Surgeon's assistants (SAs) or physician's assistants (PAs) with additional surgical training should meet national standards and be credentialed by the appropriate local authority. These individuals are not authorized to operate independently. Formal application for appointment to a hospital as a PA or SA should include:

Qualifications and Credentials of Assistants

- Specification of which surgeon the applicant will assist and what duties will be performed.
- Indication of which surgeon will be responsible for the supervision and performance of the SA or PA.
- The application should be reviewed and approved by the hospital's board.
- Registered nurses with specialized training may also function as first assistants. If such a situation should occur, the size of the operating room team should not be reduced; the nurse assistant should not simultaneously function as the scrub nurse and instrument nurse when serving as the first assistant. Nurse assistant practice privileges should be granted based upon

the hospital board's review and approval of credentials. Registered nurses who act as first assistants must not have responsibility beyond the level defined in their state nursing practice act.

Surgeons are encouraged to participate in the training of allied health personnel. Such individuals perform their duties under the supervision of the surgeon.

Note: From American College of Surgeons (ACS), (2004). Copyright 1974, revised Sept. 2008 by ACS. Retrieved October 3, 2008 from http://www.facs.org/fellows_ info/statements/stonprin.html#anchor129977 Reprinted with permission.

APPENDIX 12-C   COMPETENCIES FOR THE PHYSICIAN ASSISTANT PROFESSION

PREAMBLE

In 2003, the National Commission on Certification of Physician Assistants (NCCPA) intiated an effort to define physician assistant (PA) competencies in response to similar efforts being conducted within other health care professions and growing demand for accountability and assessment in clinical practice. The following year, representatives from three other national PA organizations, each bringing a unique perspective and valuable insights, joined NCCPA in that effort. Those organizations were the Accreditation Review Commission for Education of the Physician Assistant (ARC-PA), the body that accredits PA educational programs; the Association of Physician Assistant Programs (APAP), the membership association for PA educators and program directors; and the American Academy of Physician Assistants (AAPA), the only national membership association representing all PAs.

The resultant document, *Competencies for the Physician Assistant Profession*, is a foundation from which each of those four organizations, other physician assistant organizations, and individual physician assistants themselves can chart a course for advancing the competencies of the PA profession.

INTRODUCTION

The purpose of this document is to communicate to the PA profession and the public a set of competencies that all physician assistants, regardless of specialty or setting, are expected to acquire and maintain throughout their careers. This document serves as a map for the individual PA, the physician-PA team, and organizations that are committed to promoting the development and maintenance of these professional competencies among physician assistants.

The clinical role of PAs includes primary and specialty care in medical and surgical practice settings. Professional competencies[1] for physician assistants include the effective and appropriate application of medical knowledge, interpersonal and communication skills, patient care, professionalism, practice-based learning and improvement, systems-based practice, as well as an unwavering commitment

---

[1] In 1999, the Accreditation Council for Graduation Medical Education (ACGME) endorsed a list of general competencies for medical residents. NCCPA's Eligibility Committee, with substantial input from representatives of AAPA, APAP and ARC-PA, has modified the ACGME's list for physician assistant practice, drawing from several other resources, including the work of Drs. Epstein and Hundert; research conducted by AAPA's EVP/CEO, Dr. Steve Crane; and NCCPA's own examination content blueprint.

to continual learning, professional growth, and the physician-PA team, for the benefit of patients and the larger community being served. These competencies are demonstrated within the scope of practice, whether medical or surgical, for each individual physician assistant as that scope is defined by the supervising physician and appropriate to the practice setting.

PHYSICIAN ASSISTANT COMPETENCIES
Vers. 3.5 (3/22/05)

The PA profession defines the specific knowledge, skills, and attitudes required and provides educational experiences as needed in order for physician assistants to acquire and demonstrate these competencies.

MEDICAL KNOWLEDGE

Medical knowledge includes an understanding of pathophysiology, patient presentation, differential diagnosis, patient management, surgical principles, health promotion, and disease prevention. Physician assistants must demonstrate core knowledge about established and evolving biomedical and clinical sciences and the application of this knowledge to patient care in their area of practice. In addition, physician assistants are expected to demonstrate an investigatory and analytic thinking approach to clinical situations. Physician assistants are expected to:

- understand etiologies, risk factors, underlying pathologic process, and epidemiology for medical conditions
- identify signs and symptoms of medical conditions
- select and interpret appropriate diagnostic or lab studies
- manage general medical and surgical conditions to include understanding the indications, contraindications, side effects, interactions, and adverse reactions of pharmacologic agents and other relevant treatment modalities
- identify the appropriate site of care for presenting conditions, including identifying emergent cases and those requiring referral or admission
- identify appropriate interventions for prevention of conditions
- identify the appropriate methods to detect conditions in an asymptomatic individual
- differentiate between the normal and the abnormal in anatomic, physiological, laboratory findings, and other diagnostic data
- appropriately use history and physical findings and diagnostic studies to formulate a differential diagnosis
- provide appropriate care to patients with chronic conditions

INTERPERSONAL & COMMUNICATION SKILLS

Interpersonal and communication skills encompass verbal, nonverbal, and written exchange of information. Physician assistants must demonstrate interpersonal and communication skills that result in effective information exchange with patients, their patients' families, physicians, professional associates, and the health care system. Physician assistants are expected to:

- create and sustain a therapeutic and ethically sound relationship with patients
- use effective listening, nonverbal, explanatory, questioning, and writing skills to elicit and provide information
- appropriately adapt communication style and messages to the context of the individual patient interaction
- work effectively with physicians and other health care professionals as a member or leader of a health care team or other professional group
- apply an understanding of human behavior
- demonstrate emotional resilience and stability, adaptability, flexibility, and tolerance of ambiguity and anxiety
- accurately and adequately document and record information regarding the care process for medical, legal, quality, and financial purposes

PATIENT CARE

Patient care includes age-appropriate assessment, evaluation, and management. Physician assistants must demonstrate care that is effective, patient-centered, timely, efficient, and equitable for the treatment of health problems and the promotion of wellness. Physician assistants are expected to:

- work effectively with physicians and other health care professionals to provide patient-centered care
- demonstrate caring and respectful behaviors when interacting with patients and their families
- gather essential and accurate information about their patients
- make informed decisions about diagnostic and therapeutic interventions based on patient information and preferences, up-to-date scientific evidence, and clinical judgment
- develop and carry out patient management plans
- counsel and educate patients and their families
- competently perform medical and surgical procedures considered essential in the area of practice
- provide health care services and education aimed at preventing health problems or maintaining health

PROFESSIONALISM

Professionalism is the expression of positive values and ideals as care is delivered. Foremost, it involves prioritizing the interests of those being served above one's own. Physician assistants must know their professional and personal limitations. Professionalism also requires that PAs practice without impairment from substance abuse, cognitive deficiency, or mental illness. Physician assistants must demonstrate a high level of responsibility, ethical practice, sensitivity to a diverse patient population and adherence to legal and regulatory requirements. Physician assistants are expected to demonstrate:

- understanding of legal and regulatory requirements, as well as the appropriate role of the physician assistant
- professional relationships with physician supervisors and other health care providers
- respect, compassion, and integrity
- responsiveness to the needs of patients and society
- accountability to patients, society, and the profession
- commitment to excellence and on-going professional development
- commitment to ethical principles pertaining to provision or withholding of clinical care, confidentiality of patient information, informed consent, and business practices
- sensitivity and responsiveness to patients' culture, age, gender, and disabilities
- self-reflection, critical curiosity, and initiative

PRACTICE-BASED LEARNING AND IMPROVEMENT

Practice-based learning and improvement includes the processes through which clinicians engage in critical analysis of their own practice experience, medical literature, and other information resources for the purpose of self-improvement. Physician assistants must be able to assess, evaluate, and improve their patient care practices. Physician assistants are expected to:

- analyze practice experience and perform practice-based improvement activities using a systematic methodology in concert with other members of the health care delivery team
- locate, appraise, and integrate evidence from scientific studies related to their patients' health problems
- obtain and apply information about their own population of patients and the larger population from which their patients are drawn

- apply knowledge of study designs and statistical methods to the appraisal of clinical studies and other information on diagnostic and therapeutic effectiveness
- apply information technology to manage information, access on-line medical information, and support their own education
- facilitate the learning of students and/or other health care professionals
- recognize and appropriately address gender, cultural, cognitive, emotional and other biases; gaps in medical knowledge; and physical limitations in themselves and others

SYSTEMS-BASED PRACTICE

Systems-based practice encompasses the societal, organizational, and economic environments in which health care is delivered. Physician assistants must demonstrate an awareness of and responsiveness to the larger system of health care to provide patient care that is of optimal value. PAs should work to improve the larger health care system of which their practices are a part. Physician assistants are expected to:

- use information technology to support patient care decisions and patient education
- effectively interact with different types of medical practice and delivery systems
- understand the funding sources and payment systems that provide coverage for patient care
- practice cost-effective health care and resource allocation that does not compromise quality of care
- advocate for quality patient care and assist patients in dealing with system complexities
- partner with supervising physicians, health care managers, and other health care providers to assess, coordinate, and improve the delivery of health care and patient outcomes
- accept responsibility for promoting a safe environment for patient care and recognizing and correcting systems-based factors that negatively impact patient care
- apply medical information and clinical data systems to provide more effective, efficient patient care
- use the systems responsible for the appropriate payment of services

Note: From "Competencies for the Physician Assistant," American Academy of Physician Assistants. Copyright © 2005, AAPA. Retrieved Nov. 15, 2008 from http://www.aapa.org/gandp/competencies-competencies.pdf Reprinted with permission.

APPENDIX 12-D   AST POSITION STATEMENT ON FIRST ASSISTING

As defined by the American College of Surgeons, the first assistant provides aid in exposure, hemostasis, and other technical functions that will help the surgeon carry out a safe operation with optimal results for the patient. This role will vary considerably with the surgical operation, specialty area, and type of facility.

The Association of Surgical Technologists, Inc., recognizes the first assistant and scrub technologist roles are differentiated by education. First assistants must be educated in the use of surgical instruments on tissues versus the handling of instruments.

Certified Surgical Technologists with additional specialized education or training may function as first/surgical assistants to the surgeon at the operating table in those situations or facilities where more completely trained assistants are not available.

Practice privileges of those acting as first/surgical assistants should be based upon verified credentials reviewed and approved by the appropriate credentialing committee.

Footnote: The second assistant retracts and suctions.

Note: From AST Position Statement on the First Assistant, Association of Surgical Technologists (AST). Copyright © 2008 by AST. Retrieved Nov. 13, 2008 from http://www.ast.org/pdf/Standards_of_Practice/Position_First_Assisting.pdf Reprinted with permission.

13 Resources

NOTE: All references were current and correct as of June 2009.

CHAPTER 1. PATIENT POSITIONING

- INJURY

  McPeck, P. (2006). Watching our backs—RNs get a lift from 'no lift' policies. *NurseWeek* Magazine. www2.nurseweek.com/Articles/article.cfm?AID=22078

  Nelson, A., & Baptiste, A.S. (2004). Evidence-based practices for safe patient handling and movement. *Online Journal of Issues in Nursing*, 9, 3. nursingworld.org/MainMenuCategories/ANAMarketplace/ANAPeriodicals/OJIN/TableofContents/Volume92004/No3Sept04/EvidenceBasedPractices.aspx

- PRESSURE INJURY

  National Pressure Ulcer Advisory Panel. (2007). Pressure ulcer stages revised by NPUAP. www.npuap.org/pr2.htm

  Wound Ostomy and Continence Nurses Society. (2007). *Position statement: Pressure ulcer staging.* www.wocn.org/

  Institute for Healthcare Improvement. *Relieve the pressure and reduce harm.* www.ihi.org/IHI/Topics/PatientSafety/SafetyGeneral/Improvement Stories/FSRelievethePressureandReduceHarm.htm
  The Centers for Medicare and Medicaid Services. (2007). *Hospital-acquired conditions (present on admission indicator).* www.cms.hhs.gov/HospitalAcqCond

Association of periOperative Registered Nurses (AORN). (2008). Recommended practices for positioning the patient in the perioperative setting. In *Perioperative Standards and Recommended Practices* (p. 497–520). Denver, CO: AORN, Inc.

- PRODUCTS

Association of periOperative Registered Nurses (AORN). (2009). *OR Product Directory*. www.orpd.org/search.php

CHAPTER 2. PREPPING AND DRAPING

- DRAPE STANDARDS

Association for the Advancement of Medical Instrumentation. (2009). AAMI Press Release. *New Sterilization Books Issued; Major Updates Included.* www. aami.org/news/2009/042209.press.sterbooks.html

Association for the Advancement of Medical Instrumentation. (2005). AAMI TIR11:2005. *Selection and use of protective apparel and surgical drapes in health care facilities, 2ed.* www.aami.org/subscriptions/cdchart. html

Association for the Advancement of Medical Instrumentation. (1998). AAMI TIR21:1998. *Systems used to forecast remaining pacemaker battery service life, 1ed.* www.aami.org/subscriptions/cdchart.html

Association for the Advancement of Medical Instrumentation. (2008). ANSI/AAMI ST65:2008. *Processing of reusable surgical textiles for use in health care facilities.* www.aami.org/applications/search/details. cfm?webid=P1043_D5052

Association for the Advancement of Medical Instrumentation. (2008). AAMI Press Release: December 15, 2008. *AAMI Translates Popular Standard into Spanish.* www.aami.org/news/2008/121508.press.translate. html

Association for the Advancement of Medical Instrumentation. (2009). AAMI Standards Program (active projects only): May 1, 2009. *Selection and use of protective apparel and surgical drapes in health care facilities, 05-Feb-06. Final (Due for review. 10/17/2008).* www.aami.org/Applications/CommitteeCentral-app/Documents/AAMIActStds.pdf

Association for the Advancement of Medical Instrumentation. (2009). *Sterilization in Health Care Facilities. New guidance on processing of surgical textiles (ST65), including surgical gowns and drapes.* www.aami.org/publications/standards/ster.book1.html

Association for the Advancement of Medical Instrumentation. (2008). *AAMI Hospital Sterilization Collection Revised for 2009. ST65: Processing of reusable surgical textiles for use in health care. TIR11: Selection of surgical gowns and drapes in health care facilities.* www.aami.org/news/2008/121508.press.ster1.html

Association of periOperative Registered Nurses (AORN). (2009). Recommended Practice for the Selection and Use of Gowns and Drapes. In *AORN Standards and Recommended Practices.* Denver, CO: AORN.

Cardinal Health, Inc. (2005). *Finally, an industry standard that eliminates the guesswork.* www.cardinal.com/mps/brands/convertors/aami/2366AAMIREV.pdf

World Intellectual Property Organization (WIPO). (1998). *WO/1998/056304: Absorbent surgical drape.* www.wipo.int/pctdb/en/wo.jsp?wo=1998056304

• PRODUCTS

Association of periOperative Registered Nurses (AORN). (2009). *OR Product Directory.* www.orpd.org/search.php

CHAPTER 3. TISSUE HANDLING

Covidien Surgical Education. (2009). *Surgical Education.* www.covidien.com/covidien/pageBuilder.aspx?topicID=108982&page=Education: Introduction

eMedicine (Medscape). (2009). *eMedicine results: Tissue handling.* http://search.medscape.com/emedicine-search?newSearch=1&queryText=tissue+handling

Fundamentals of Laparoscopic Surgery. (2008). *What is FLS.* www.flsprogram.org/

Surgeons-Net. (2009). *Welcome to the Surgeons Net Surgical Education site.* www.surgeons.org.uk/

CHAPTER 4. PROVIDING EXPOSURE

Association of periOperative Registered Nurses (AORN). (2009). *OR Product Directory.* www.orpd.org/search.php

Vesalius: The internet source for surgical education. (2009). www.vesalius.com/welcome.asp

CHAPTER 5. METHODS FOR ASSURING SURGICAL HEMOSTASIS

Association of periOperative Registered Nurses (AORN). (2009). *OR Product Directory.* www.orpd.org/search.php

Covidien Energy-based Professional Education. (2008). *Programs recommended for nurses.* www.valleylabeducation.org/pages/list-nurse.html

Covidien Energy-based Professional Education. (2008). *Programs recommended for physicians.* www.valleylabeducation.org/pages/list-doc.html

Covidien Energy-based Professional Education. (2008). *Electrosurgical safety.* www.valleylabeducation.org/

eMedicine (Medscape). (2008). *eMedicine results: On hemostasis.* Retrieved June 2009 from http://search.medscape.com/emedicine-search?queryText=hemostasis

CHAPTER 6. SUTURING MATERIALS AND TECHNIQUES

- EDUCATION ABOUT SUTURES AND NEEDLES

  Lai, S.Y. (2009). Sutures and Needles. http://emedicine.medscape.com/article/884838-overview

- PRODUCTS

  Association of periOperative Registered Nurses (AORN). (2009). *OR Product Directory.* www.orpd.org/search.php

- SUTURE MANUAL

  Dunn, D.L. (Ed.). (2004). *Ethicon Wound Closure Manual.* www.orthonurse.org/portals/0/wound%20closure%20manual.pdf

  Additional Web sites: www.jnjgateway.com, www.syneture.com

CHAPTER 7. THE ASSESSMENT AND DIAGNOSTIC PROCESS

- DIAGNOSTIC TOOLS

  Diagnostic Tools available at:

  - ePocrates (pharmacopeia). www.epocrates.com
  - UpToDate. http://uptodate.com
  - DynaMed. www.dynamicmedical.com

- PHARMACOLOGY

ePocrates. (2009). *Premium product for mobile devices. PDA/iPhone version (free)*. www.epocrates.com/products/

Pfizer for Professionals. (2009). *Scientific literature (Pfizer)*. www.pfizerpro.com/content/home.jsp?tabname=Scientific%20Literature

Pfizer for Professionals. (2009). Online resources. www.pfizerpro.com/content/home.jsp?tabname=Product%20Centers

Pfizer for Professionals supports nurse practitioners and physician assistants. Information available at: www.pfizerpro.com

CHAPTER 8. PLANNING AND PROVIDING CARE

- INFECTION PREVENTION

Institute for Healthcare Improvement (IHI). (2005). *What you need to know about infections after surgery: A fact sheet for patients and their family members*. www.ihi.org/NR/rdonlyres/0EE409F4-2F6A-4B55-AB01-16B6D6935EC5/0/

Kinetics Concepts, Inc. (2008). *KCI nurse's page. Online Resources*. www.kci1.com

Noskins, G.A. (2009). *Methicillin-Resistant Staphylococcus aureus (MRSA Perspectives on Safety)*. http://webmm.ahrq.gov/perspective.aspx?perspectiveID=57

Torpy, J.M., Burke, A., & Glass, R.M. (2005). *Wound infections. Journal of the American Medical Association, 294,* 2122. http://jama.ama-assn.org/cgi/reprint/294/16/2122

- PAIN

International Association for the Study of Pain. www.iasp-pain.org

- PHARMACOLOGY

Moss, R., & Smart, T. (2009). *Perioperative pharmacology reference book.* Denver: CCI.

ePocrates. (2009). *Premium product for mobile devices. PDA/iPhone version (free)*. www.epocrates.com/products/

- PRESSURE INJURY

Centers for Medicare and Medicaid Services. (2006). *Stage 3 or 4 pressure ulcers acquired after admission to a healthcare system*. www.cms.hhs.gov/apps/media/press/release.asp?Counter=1863facility

- SAFETY

Agency for Healthcare Research and Quality. (2009). *Patient Safety Primers.* http://psnet.ahrq.gov/primerHome.aspx

Three new Patient Safety Primers have recently been added to AHRQ PSNet:

- Adverse Events after Hospital Discharge
- Safety Culture
- Teamwork Training

Agency for Healthcare Research and Quality. (2008). *Patient Safety and Quality: An Evidence-Based Handbook for Nurses.* Washington, DC: AHRQ. www.ahrq.gov/qual/nurseshdbk/

Centers for Medicare and Medicaid Services (CMS). (2009). *Healthcare Acquired Conditions, known as "Never Events."* www.cms.hhs.gov/HospitalAcqCond

Institute for Healthcare Improvement (IHI). (2009). *Continuous Improvement.* Issue #93, June 2009. See "The Alert Mind and Patient Safety." To subscribe to *Continuous Improvement* (free of charge), go to the link on IHI's homepage: www.ihi.org *Listen Up!* Join WIHI for *The Alert Mind and Patient Safety*

The Joint Commission. (2008). *The Joint Commission Perspectives on Patient Safety*, Volume 8, Issue 1. www.jointcommission.org/NR/rdonlyres/677EC466-DD6D-43FE-945E-83B8FDD0BC5B/0/StrategiesforPreventingPressureUlcers.pdf

The Joint Commission. (2009). *"Speak Up"*™ *campaign.* www.jointcommission.org/PatientSafety/SpeakUp

United States Department of Labor, OSHA. (2009). *Surgical Suite Module. Common Safety and Health Topics.* www.osha.gov/SLTC/etools/hospital/surgical/surgical.html

- SCIP

Colorado Foundation for Medical Care. (2007). *Surgical Care Improvement Project (SCIP).* www.cfmc.org/hospital/hospital_scip.htm. See also Premier Website www.premierinc.com/safety/topics/scip/index.jsp

Oklahoma Foundation for Medical Quality. (2006). *Tips for safer surgery. Questions to ask your doctors and nurses before surgery.* www.ofmq.com/Websites/ofmq/Images/FINALconsumer_tips2.pdf

- WOUND HEALING

  Kinetics Concepts, Inc. (2008). *Challenges in management of the lower extremities vascular surgery wounds.* www.kci1.com/KCI_VAC_LowerExtremity_Wounds_Training_31Jul08.ppt

CHAPTER 9. PATIENT EDUCATION

- HEALTH LITERACY

  Agency for Healthcare Research and Quality (AHRQ). (2004). *Literacy and Health Outcomes: Summary of Evidence Report, Technology Assessment No. 87.* www.ahrq.gov/clinic/epcsums/litsum.htm

  American Medical Association (AMA). (2007). Health Literacy Program video *"Health literacy and patient safety: Help patients understand."* Retrieved March 2, 2009 from www.ama-assn.org/ama/no-index/about-ama/8035.shtml

  American Medical Association literacy kit (with DVD and written materials) can be purchased for $35 from www.ama-assn.org/ama/pub/about-ama/our-people/affiliated-groups/ama-foundation/our-programs/public-health/health-literacy-program/health-literacy-kit.shtml

  National Network of Libraries of Medicine. (2007). *Consumer Health Manual.* www.nnlm.gov/outreach/consumer

  Joint Commission: Speak Up™ Understanding your doctor and other caregivers; see "Speak Up" campaign literature (free and available in Spanish). www.jointcommission.org/NR/rdonlyres/58522693-0927-42B5-8860-B12004CFBEF0/0/speakup_understanding

  Murphy, P.W. (1993). Rapid Estimate of Adult Literacy in Medicine (REALM). *Journal of Reading, 37,* 124–130. www.blackwell-synergy.com/doi/suppl/10.1111/j.1475-6773.2006.00532.x/suppl_file/HESR532sm.doc. Search under REALM

  National Reading Campaign. (2009). *Readability—how to test how easy a text is to read.* www.literacytrust.org.uk/campaign/SMOG.html

  Nurss, J.R., Parker, R.M., Williams, M.V., & Baker, D.W. (1995). *Short Test of Functional Health Literacy in Adults (S-TOFHLA).* www.nmmra.org/resources/Physician/152_1485.pdf

  Pfizer for Professionals. (2009). *Pharmaceutical patient education materials from Pfizer.* www.pfizerpro.com/patient_education/patient_education.jsp

- SAFETY

  Agency for Healthcare Research and Quality (AHRQ). (2009). *Patient Safety Primers.* http://psnet.ahrq.gov/primerHome.aspx

  Safety Target
  - Adverse Events after Hospital Discharge
  - Diagnostic Errors
  - Handoffs and Signouts
  - Health Care-Associated Infections

  Error Types
  - Adverse Events after Hospital Discharge
  - Never Events

  Approach to Improving Safety
  - Computerized Provider Order Entry
  - Handoffs and Signouts
  - Medication Reconciliation
  - Never Events
  - Patient Disclosure
  - Rapid Response Systems
  - Root Cause Analysis
  - Safety Culture
  - Teamwork Training

- SURGICAL SITE INFECTIONS

  Association for Professionals in Infection Control and Epidemiology (APIC). www.apic.org

  Consumer-related information is available at www.preventinfection.org

  Institute for Healthcare Improvement. (2009). *What you need to know about infections after surgery: A fact sheet for patients and their family members.* www.ihi.org/NR/rdonlyres/0EE409F4-2F6A-4B55-AB01-16B6D6935EC5/0/

Oklahoma Foundation for Medical Quality. (2006). *Tips for safer surgery. Questions to ask your doctors and nurses before surgery.* www.ofmq.com/Websites/ofmq/Images/FINALconsumer_tips2.pdf

Torpy, J.M., Burke, A., & Glass, R.M. (2005). Wound Infections. *Journal of the American Medical Association, 294,* 2122. http://jama.ama-assn.org/cgi/reprint/294/16/2122

CHAPTER 10. ANESTHESIA

- PATIENT EDUCATION (see also Chapter 9 Patient Education)

American Society of Anesthesiologists (ASA). (2009). *Patient Education Brochures.* www.asahq.org

- Anesthesia & Me © Checklist
- Anesthesia and You
- Anesthesia for Ambulatory Surgery
- Anesthesia for Ambulatory Surgery *(Spanish Version)*
- Be Smoke-Free for Surgery
- Know Your Anesthesiologist
- Know Your Anesthesiologist *(Spanish Version)*
- The Management of Pain
- The Medical Specialty of Anesthesiology
- Office-Based Anesthesia and Surgery
- Pain Relief During Labor and Delivery
- Pain Relief During Labor and Delivery *(Spanish Version)*
- Patient Awareness
- Patient Awareness *(Spanish Version)*
- Patient Awareness *(Portuguese Version)*
- Sedation Analgesia
- The Senior Citizen as a Patient
- Sleep Apnea
- What You Should Know About Herbal Use and Anesthesia
- When Your Child Needs Anesthesia

CHAPTER 11. THE FIRST ASSISTANT AND COLLABORATION PRACTICE

- ACCREDITING AGENCY

  The Joint Commission. (2008). *Behaviors that undermine a culture of safety.* Retrieved Aug. 21, 2008 from www.jointcommission.org/SentinelEvents/ SentinelEventAlert/sea_40.htm

- MULTIDISCIPLINARY ORGANIZATIONS

  Council on Surgical and Perioperative Safety (CSPS). A multidisciplinary coalition of professional organizations whose members are involved in the care of surgical patients. www.cspsteam.org/education/education8.html

  Agency for Healthcare Research and Quality (AHRQ). (2006). TeamSTEPPS™ Program developed by AHRQ and Department of Defense to promote collaboration and improved teamwork. http://teamstepps.ahrq.gov/

- MEDICAL JOURNALS

  American College of Surgeons
  Journal of the American College of Surgeons
  www.facs.org/jacs/index.html

  American Medical Association (www.ama-assn.org/)
  Journal of the American Medical Association
  http://jama.ama-assn.org

  American College of Emergency Physicians (www.acep.org)
  Annals of Emergency Medicine
  www.annemergmed.com/

  Association of American Medical Colleges (www.aamc.org)
  Academic Medicine
  http://journals.lww.com/academicmedicine/

- MEDICAL ASSOCIATIONS

  Massachusetts Medical Society (www.massmed.org)
  New England Journal of Medicine
  http://content.nejm.org

  Texas Medical Association (www.texmed.org/)
  Texas Medicine
  www.texmed.org/Template.aspx?id=487

- NURSING

  American Association of Critical Care Nurses. (2005). White paper on healthy work environments: AACN standards for establishing and sustaining healthy work environments: A journey to excellence. *American Journal of Critical Care, 14*, 187–197.

  Kaiser Permanente: Evergreen, CO. (2009). *SBAR Technique for Communication: A Situational Briefing Model*. Retrieved June 2009 from www.ihi.org/IHI/Topics/PatientSafety/SafetyGeneral/Tools/ SBARTechniqueforCommunicationASituationalBriefingModel.htm

CHAPTER 12. INSTITUTIONAL CREDENTIALING

- AGENCIES

  Council for Affordable Quality Healthcare (CAQH). A nonprofit alliance of health plans and trade associations offering programs that simplify and streamline healthcare administration for health plans and providers. The CAQH credentialing process provides a universal credentialing system for healthcare providers. www.caqh.org

  Centers for Medicare/Medicaid Services (CMS). Federal Government's Health and Human Services agency responsible for administering the Medicare and Medicaid programs. www.cms.gov

  Joint Commission (JC), previously known as Joint Commission on Accreditation of Healthcare Organizations (JCAHO). An independent, not-for-profit organization which evaluates, accredits, and certifies health care organizations who comply with state-of-the-art standards that improve quality and safety of patient care. www.jointcommission.org

  National Practitioner Data Bank (NPDB). An information clearinghouse to collect and release information related to the professional competence and conduct of physicians, dentists, and other health care practitioners. Other health care practitioners are defined as licensed or otherwise authorized (certified or registered) by a State to provide health care services (i.e., Physician's Assistant, Registered Nurse or Licensed Practical Nurse). www.npdb-hipdb.com

  Universal Provider Datasource (UPD). Online database provided by CAQH that collects all provider information necessary for credentialing. https://upd.caqh.org

  National Committee for Quality Assurance (NCQA). A private, not-for-profit organization which sets credentialing and recredentialing standards for credentials verification organizations (CVO), managed care organizations (MCO) and preferred provider organizations (PPO). www.ncqa.org

- ALLIED HEALTH PROFESSIONAL POLICIES

Baylor Regional Medical Center at Grapevine. (2001). *Policy on Credentialing Allied Health Professionals.* www.baylorhealth.com/SiteCollectionDocuments/ Medical_Staff/Baylor_Grapevine_Allied_Health_Professional_Manual.pdf

Grady Memorial Hospital, Ohio Health. (2004). *Allied Health Professionals Policy.* www.ohiohealth.com/documents/orb_grady/ah_professionals_policy. pdf

New Hanover Regional Medical Center. (2007). *Allied Health Professionals Policy and Procedure.* www.nhhn.org/documents/Physician%20Website/ Allied%20Health%20Professionals%20Policy%20and%20Procedure%20%20 Revised%206%2007.pdf

Stanford Hospital and Clinics/Lucile Packard's Children's Hospital. (2008). *Authorization for Individuals to Provide Services as Allied Health Practitioners Policy.* https://medicalstaffservices.stanfordhospital.com/PDF/ policiesProcedures/AHP_Policy_Jan_08.pdf

- CREDENTIALING AND PROFESSIONAL ORGANIZATIONS

American Academy of Physician Assistants (AAPA). National organization representing Physician Assistants. www.aapa.org

American Association of Surgical Physician Assistants (AASPA). National organization that represents PAs that work in the preoperative, intraoperative, and postoperative settings. www.aaspa.com

American Board of Surgical Assistants (ABSA). A national credentialing/ certification organization for physicians (U.S. or foreign trained), licensed and nonlicensed allied health professionals who have completed ABSA approved surgical assisting programs (CAAHEP programs, American Center for Excellence in Surgical Assisting or Elite School of Surgical First Assisting. www.absa.net

American Nurses Credentialing Center. National credentialing association affiliated with American Nurses Association. www.nursecredentialing.org

Association of periOperative Registered Nurses (AORN). International association representing perioperative nurses. www.aorn.org

Association of Surgical Assistants (ASA). Organization representing nonphysician surgical assistants. http://surgicalassistant.org

Association of Surgical Technologists (AST). National organization representing surgical technologists. www.ast.org

Competency and Credentialing Institute (CCI). International organization whose focus is on competency, credentialing, assessment and education for nursing healthcare practitioners working in surgical environments. www.cc-institute.org

National Board of Surgical Technologist and Surgical Assisting (NBSTSA). Certifying agency for surgical technologists (CST) and first assistants (CST/CFA). www.nbstsa.org

National Commission on Certification of Physician Assistants (NCCPA). National credentialing organization for Physician Assistants. www.nccpa.net

National Surgical Assistant Association (NSAA). A national organization offering surgical assistant certification to graduates of CAAHEP-approved Surgical Assistant Training programs, Medical Graduates, Allied Health Professionals and Military Trained individuals (surgical assisting emphasis). www.nsaa.net

- ORGANIZATIONAL STATEMENTS

American College of Surgeons. (2008). *Statement on Surgical Assistants.* www.facs.org//fellows_info/statements/stonprin.html#anchor 129977

Association of periOperative Registered Nurses (AORN) (2008). *Official Statement on RN First Assistants.* www.aorn.org/SearchResults/?Search=RNFA&x=13&y=5

Other AORN documents include:

RNFA Guide to Practice.

AORN Position Statement on RN First Assistants.

Information about the role of the RN First Assistant.

RNFA Specialty Assembly (RNFASA). Dedicated to the role of the RN First Assistant

- STATE AND NATIONAL CREDENTIALING ORGANIZATIONS

Alabama
www.bcbsal.org/webapps/upa/Dispatch?application=org.bcbsal.uniprovapp.UniProvApplication

CAQH
www.caqh.org/pdf/CAQH_Provider_Applicationv5_2006-10-31.pdf

Colorado
www.cdphe.state.co.us/op/bh/cohealthcareprofessionalcredentialsapp.html

Competency and Credentialing Institute (CCI)
www.cc-institute.org

District of Columbia
www.credentialingapplicationdc.org/
Georgia
www.georgiacredentialing.org/applications.htm

Illinois
www.idph.state.il.us/about/IDPH_credentialing_form_97_pro.doc

Iowa
www.uihealthcare.com/depts/clinicalstaffoffice/applications/pdf/
isupa.pdf

Minnesota
www.mamss-mn.org/MN%20Uniform%20App%207-05%20Form%20Fillable.
doc

Nevada
www.doi.state.nv.us/CI-LH-Index-Credential-7-1-04.htm

New Hampshire
www.nhha.org/fhc/initiatives/system/uniformcredentialing.php

North Carolina
www.ncdoi.com/LH/Documents/Licensing/Credentialing
Application.pdf

Oklahoma
www.health.state.ok.us/program/condiv/ucapp.pdf

Texas
www.tdi.state.tx.us/hmo/crform.html

Vermont
www.bishca.state.vt.us/HcaDiv/Uniform_Credentialing/uniform_
credentialing.htm

West Virginia
www.wvinsurance.gov/credentialing/uniform_cred_instructions.htm

PHYSICIAN ASSISTANT (PA)

- American Academy of Physician Assistants
  300 Washington St.
  Alexandria, VA 22314-1552
  (703) 836-2272
  www.aapa.org

- American Association of Surgical Physician Assistants
  PMB 201 4267 NW Federal Highway
  Jensen Beach, FL 34957
  (888) 882-2772 • 772-388-3457 (fax)
  E-Mail: aaspa@aaspa.com
  www.aaspa.com/

- American College of Clinicians (Membership available to NPs and PAs)
  841 Worcester Road #344
  Natick, MA 01760
  (862) 926-8315
  www.amcollege.org (Publish *Clinician's Advocate Newsletter*)

- Physician Assistant Education Association
  300 N. Washington St., Ste. 505
  Alexandria, VA 22314-2544
  (703) 548-5538
  www.paeaonline.org

- Physician Assistant Job Description
  www.hsfvirginia.edu/HRD/HR/Jobs/C1022.pdf

- Physician Assistants and Protocols
  www.aapa.org/gandp/protoc.html

- Physician Assistant Careers
  http://careers.stateuniversity.com/pages/491/Physician-Assistant.html

- Publications
  Journal of the American Academy of Physician Assistants (JAAPA)
  www.aapa.org/news/publications/jaapa and http://jaapa.com/

  Sutureline
  www.aaspa.com/Publications.asp

Clinician Reviews
www.clinicianreviews.com

Journal of Physician Assistant Education
http://jpae.msubmit.net/cgi-bin/main.plex

PA Professional
www.aapa.org/news/publications/pa-professional

Clinician's Advocate Newsletter
www.amcollege.org

Perspective on Physician Assistant Education
http://medspace.mc.duke.edu/vital/access/manager/Repository/dumca:4780

- PA Education

  Verification of PA education (Delaware)
  http://dpr.delaware.gov/boards/medicalpractice/documents/
  paeducver.pdf
  http://careers.stateuniversity.com/pages/491/Physician-Assistant.html

  Physician Assistant Job Description
  www.hsfvirginia.edu/HRD/HR/Jobs/C1022.pdf

  Physician Assistants and Protocols
  www.aapa.org/gandp/protoc.html

  New York State problems related to communication
  www.health.state.ny.us/press/releases/2002/mtsinai.htm

  Additional references and reading on PAs. Retrieved June 8, 2009 from
  www.aaspa.com/SurgInfo.asp

REGISTERED NURSE (RN)

- Association of periOperative Registered Nurses (AORN)
  2170 S. Parker Road, Suite 300
  Denver, CO 80231
  (800) 755-2676
  www.aorn.org

- *AORN Organizational Units*
  RN First Assistant (RNFA) Specialty Assembly

www.aorn.org/Community/SpecialtyAssemblies/SpecialtyAssemblyGroups/RNFASA

Advanced Practice Specialty Assembly

www.aorn.org/Community/SpecialtyAssemblies/SpecialtyAssemblyGroups/APNSA

- *AORN publications*
  AORN Journal
  www.aornjournal.org

  Association of periOperative Registered Nurses (AORN). (2007). *RN First Assistant Guide to Practice (3rd ed.).* Denver: AORN, Inc.

  Association of periOperative Registered Nurses (AORN). (2009). *AORN Standards for RNFA Education.* Retrieved June 2009 from http://ems.aorn.org/docs_assets/55B250E0-9779-5C0D-1DDC8177C9B4C8EB/C469FC4E-FBB8-0DBD-7731AE8F298A4847/RNFA_ED_STDS.pdf

- *AORN* Tool Kits

  Retrieved June 8, 2009 from www.aorn.org/PracticeResources/ToolKits/
  - Correct Site Surgery
  - Fire Safety
  - Human Factors in Health Care
  - Just Culture
  - Organizational Leadership
  - Patient "Hand-Off"
  - Safe Medication Administration
  - Surgical Smoke Evacuation

- *Additional Nursing Publications*

  American Academy of Nurse Practitioners
  Journal of the American Academy of Nurse Practitioners
  www.aanp.org/AANPCMS2/Publications/Journal%28JAANP%292/

  American Association of Nurse Anesthetists
  AANA Journal
  www.aana.com/Resources.aspx?ucNavMenu_TSMenuTargetID=12&ucNavMenu_TSMenuTargetType=4&ucNavMenu_TSMenuID=6&id=8724&terms=Journal

American College of Nurse Practitioners

The Journal for Nurse Practitioners

www.acnpweb.org/i4a/pages/index.cfm?pageid=1

American Nurses Association
8515 Georgia Avenue, Suite 400
Silver Spring, MD 20910-3492
www.nursingworld.org

American Nurses Credentialing Center. Nurse Practitioner and other Advanced Nursing Practice certifications. Subsidiary of the American Nurses Association. www.nursecredentialing.org/Certification.aspx

National Association of Clinical Nurse Specialists

CNS: The Journal for Advanced Nursing Practice
www.nacns.org/journal.shtml

National Association of Pediatric Nurse Practitioners
Journal of Pediatric Health Care
http://journals.elsevierhealth.com/periodicals/ymph/content/pcarticles

Competency & Credentialing Institute (CCI). (2004). *CRNFA Study Guide and Practice Resource.* Denver: CCI (www.cc-institute.org)

SURGICAL TECHNOLOGIST (ST)

- Association of Surgical Technologists
  6 West Dry Creek Circle, Suite 200
  Littleton, CO 80120-8031
  800-637-7433 AST Toll Free
  (303) 694-9130 AST Main Local
  (303) 694-9169 AST Main Fax
  www.ast.org

- Publications

  Core Curriculum for Surgical Technology and *Core Curriculum for Surgical Assisting*

  AST Recommended Standards of Practice.

APPENDIX I

Laboratory Studies and Their Clinical Significance

TABLE OF CONTENTS:

Note: The values listed provide an overview of some common laboratory studies. First Assistants (FAs) and other clinicians should consult their institutional laboratory manual for values which may be affected by the reagents used and the specific testing procedures performed.

A. ABBREVIATIONS

CONVENTIONAL UNITS		SI UNITS (International System of Units)
kg = kilogram	kM = millimole	g = gram
g = gram	nM = nanomole	L = liter
mg = milligram	mOsm = milliosmole	d = day
µg = microgram	mm = millimeter	h = hour
µµg = micromicrogram	µ = micron or micrometer	mol = mole
ng = nanogram	mm Hg = millimeter mercury	mmol = millimole
pg = picogram	U = unit	µmol = micromole
dl = 1 deciliter or 100 milliliters	mU = milliunit	nmol = nanomole
	µU = microunit	pmol = picomole
ml = milliliter	mEq = milliequivalent	
cu mm = cubic millimeter	IU = International Unit	
fL = femtoliter	ImU = International milliunit	

B. HEMATOLOGY*

Determination	Conventional Units	SI Units	Clinical Significance
I. Complete Blood Count with Differential (CBC with diff)			
Red Blood Cell Count (RBC)	$RBC \times 10^6$ / µl	$RBC \times 10^{12}$ / L	*Increased* in severe diarrhea and dehydration, polycythemia vera, acute poisoning, pulmonary fibrosis.
			Decreased in all anemias, in leukemia, and after hemorrhage when blood volume has been restored.
	Adult:		
	Male: 4.7–6.1×10^6 / µl	4.7–6.1×10^{12} / L	
	Female: 4.2–5.4×10^6 / µl	4.2–5.4×10^{12} / L	
	Children:		
	Newborn: 4.8–7.1×10^6 / µl	4.8–7.1×10^{12} / L	
	2–8 weeks: 4.0–6.0×10^6 / µl	4.0–6.0×10^{12} / L	
	2–6 months: 3.5–5.5×10^6 / µl	3.5–5.5×10^{12} / L	
	6 months – 1 year: 3.5–5.2×10^6 / µl	3.5–5.2×10^{12} / L	
	1–6 years: 4.0–5.5×10^6 / µl	4.0–5.5×10^{12} / L	
	6–18 years: 4.0–5.5×10^6 / µl	4.0–5.5×10^{12} / L	

(continued)

Determination	Conventional Units	SI Units	Clinical Significance
Hemoglobin (Hgb)			Possible critical values: <5.0 g/dl or >20 g/dl
			Increased in polycythemia vera, chronic obstructive pulmonary disease, congenital heart disease, dehydration.
			Decreased in anemia, hemorrhage, hemolysis, lymphoma, kidney disease.
	Adult: Male: 14–18 g/dl	8.7–11.2 mmol/L	
	Female 12–16 g/dl	7.4–9.9 mmol/L	
	Pregnant female >11g/dl		
	Elderly: Values may be slightly decreased		
	Children: Newborn: 14–24 g/dl		
	0–2 weeks: 12–20 g/dl		
	2–6 months: 10–17 d/dl		
	6 months-1 year: 9.5–14 g/dl		
	1–6 years: 9.5–14 g/dl		
	6–18 years: 10–15.5 g/dl		

Determination	Conventional Units	SI Units	Clinical Significance
Hematocrit (Hct)			Possible Critical Values: <15% or >60%
			Increased in polycythemia vera, chronic obstructive pulmonary disease, congenital heart disease, severe dehydration, eclampsia, burns.
			Decreased in anemia, hemorrhage, hyperthyroidism, hemolysis, leukemia, kidney disease, normal pregnancy.
	Adult: Male: 42%–52%	0.42–0.52 volume fraction	
	Female: 37%–47%	0.37–0.47 volume fraction	
	Pregnant female: >33%		
	Elderly: Values may be slightly decreased		
	Children: Newborn: 44–64%		
	2–8 weeks: 39–59%		
	2–6 months: 35–50%		
	6 months-1 year: 29–43%		
	1–6 years: 30–40%		
	6–18 years: 32–44%		

(continued)

Determination	Conventional Units	SI Units	Clinical Significance
Red Blood Cell Indices			
Mean Corpuscular Volume (MCV)	Adult/elderly/child: 80–95 µg^3	80–90 fL	*Increased* in liver disease, alcoholism, pernicious anemia. *Decreased* in iron deficiency anemia, Thalassemia.
	Newborn: 96–108 µg^3		
Mean Corpuscular Hemoglobin (MCH)	Adult/elderly/child: 27–31 pg	27–32 pg	*Increased* in macrocytic anemia. *Decreased* in microcytic anemia.
	Newborn: 32–34 pg		
Mean Corpuscular Hemoglobin Concentration (MCHC)	Adult/elderly/child: 32–36 g/dl (or 32%–36%)	Concentration fraction: 0.33–0.38	*Increased* in intravascular hemolysis, cold agglutinins. *Decreased* in iron deficiency anemia.
	Newborn: 32–33 g/dl (or 32%–33%)		
Red Blood Cell Distribution Width (RDW)	Adult: 11%–14.5%		*Increased* in iron deficiency anemia, folate deficiency anemia, hemolytic anemias.
Reticulocytes	Adult/elderly/child: 0.5%–2%		Immature red blood cell; normally few cells in bloodstream. *Increased* levels seen in hemolytic anemia, sickle cell anemia, leukemias. *Decreased* levels seen in pernicious anemia, aplastic anemia, bone marrow failure, anterior pituitary hypofunction.

Determination	Conventional Units	SI Units	Clinical Significance
	Infant: 0.5%–3.1%		
	Newborn: 2.5%–6.5%		
White Blood Cell Count (WBC)			
			Possible critical values: WBCs <2500 or >30,000 mm^3
			WBCs *increased* in infection, trauma, stress, inflammation, tissue necrosis.
			WBCs *decreased* in drug toxicity, bone marrow failure, overwhelming infections, autoimmune disease.
Total WBC	Adult/child >2 years: 5000–10,000/mm^3	5–10 × 10^9 /L	
	Child ≤ 2 years: 6200–17,000 /mm^3		
	Newborn: 9000 – 30,000 /mm^3		
Differential Count	Per cent (%)	Absolute (per mm^3)	
Neutrophils (Granulocytes)	55–70	2500–8000	*Increased* in infection.
Lymphocytes	20–40	1000–4000	*Increased* with certain leukemias, Graves disease, respiratory viral diseases.
			Decreased with tuberculosis, Hodgkin's disease, aplastic anemia.

(*continued*)

Determination	Conventional Units	SI Units	Clinical Significance
Monocytes	2–8	100–700	*Increased* in collagen diseases, parasitic infections, hematologic disorders.
			Decreased with prednisone treatment, rheumatoid arthritis, HIV.
Eosinophils	1–4	50–500	*Increased* in allergies, parasitic diseases.
Basophils (Mast cells)	0.5–1	25–100	*Increased* in granulocytic and basophilic anemia.
			Decreased in allergic reactions, prolonged steroid therapy, hyperthyroidism.
2. Platelets			Possible critical values: <50,000 or >1 million/mm^3
			Increased in malignancy, polycythemia vera, rheumatoid arthritis, iron deficiency anemia.
			Decreased with prolonged aspirin use, hypersplenism, hemorrhage, leukemias, thrombotic thrombocytopenia, disseminated intravascular coagulation (DIC), various anemias.
	Adult/elderly: 150,000–400,000/mm^3		
	Premature infant: 10,000–300,000/mm^3		

Determination	Conventional Units	SI Units	Clinical Significance
	Newborn: 150,000–300,000/mm^3	15–400 × 10^9/L	
	Infant: 200,000–475,000/mm^3		
	Child: 150,000–400,000/mm^3		

3. Arterial Blood Gases (ABGs)

Determination	Conventional Units	SI Units	Clinical Significance
pH (arterial) (Reflects acidity and alkalinity of blood)	Adult/child: 7.35–7.45		Possible critical value: <7.25, >7.55
	Newborn: 7.32–7.49		
	2 months-2 years: 7.34–7.46		
	pH (venous) 7.31.–7.41		
PCO$_2$ (Partial pressure of carbon dioxide)	Adult/child: 35–45 mm Hg		Possible critical value: <20, >60
	Child <2 years: 26–41 mm Hg		
	PCO$_2$ (venous): 40–50 mm Hg		
HCO$_3$ (Bicarbonate)	Adult/child: 21–28 mEq/L		Possible critical value: <15, >40
	Newborn/infant: 16–24 mEq/L		
PO$_2$ (Oxygen tension/pressure in blood)	Adult/child: 80–100 mm Hg		Possible critical value: <40
	Newborn: 60–70 mm Hg		
	PO$_2$ (venous): 40–50 mm Hg		
O$_2$ saturation (Per cent hemoglobin saturated with oxygen)	Adult/child: 95%–100%		Possible critical value: 75% or lower
	Elderly: 95%		
	Newborn: 40%–90%		

(continued)

Determination	Conventional Units	SI Units	Clinical Significance
O_2 content (Amount of oxygen in the blood)	Arterial: 15–22 vol % Venous: 11–16 vol %		Possible critical value: similar to PO_2
Base excess (Amount of buffers in the blood)	0 ± 2 mEq/L		Possible critical value: ±3 mEq/L

4. Coagulation Factors

Determination	Conventional Units	SI Units	Clinical Significance
			Increased in certain inflammatory disorders; stress, smoking. *Decreased* in certain liver diseases, anticoagulation use, congenital deficiencies, vitamin K deficiency.
I (Fibrinogen)	Adult: 200–400 mg/dl	2–4 g/L	
II (Prothrombin)	80–120 (% of "normal")		Vitamin K- dependent; inactivated by heparin
III (Tissue factor or thromboplastin)	Not applicable		
IV (Calcium)	*Total calcium* (adult): 9.0–10.5 mg/dl;	2.25–2.75 mmol/L	
	Ionized calcium (adult): 4.5–5.6 mg/dl	1.05–1.3 mmol/L	
V (Proaccelerin)	50–150 (% of "normal")		
VII (Proconvertin [stable factor])	65–140 (% of "normal")		
VIII (Antihemophilic factor)	55–145 (% of "normal")		
von Willebrand factor (second component of factor VIII)	See factor VIII		

Determination	Conventional Units	SI Units	Clinical Significance
IX (Christmas factor)	60–140 (% of "normal")		Vitamin K- dependent
X (Stuart factor)	45–155 (% of "normal")		Vitamin K -dependent
XI (Plasma thromboplastin antecedent)	65–135 (% of "normal")		
XII (Hageman factor)	50–150 (% of "normal")		
XIII (Fibrin stabilizing factor)	No quantitation of minimum hemostatic level.		

5.Coagulation Tests

Determination	Conventional Units	SI Units	Clinical Significance
Prothrombin Time (PT); (Results dependent on reagent used)	11.0–12.5 seconds	85%–100%	With full anticoagulant therapy: PT >1.5–2 times control value. *Increased* in prothrombin deficiency, vitamin K deficiency, hemorrhagic disease in newborn, liver disease, anti-coagulant therapy.
International Normalized Ratio (INR)	0.8–1.1 (ratio)		Possible critical value: >5.5
Activated Clotting Time (ACT)	70–120 seconds		Therapeutic range for heparin anticoagulation: 150–210 seconds (longer during cardiopulmonary bypass)
Activated Partial Thromboplasin Time (APTT)	30–40 seconds		Possible critical value: >70 seconds

(continued)

Determination	Conventional Units	SI Units	Clinical Significance
Partial Thromboplasin Time (PTT)	60–70 seconds		Possible critical value: >100 seconds.
			Increased in hemophilia, vitamin K deficiency, liver disease, presence of circulating anticoagulants.
			Decreased in extensive cancer, immediately after hemorrhage, very early DIC.
Fibrin Split Products (FSPs)	<10mcg/ml	>10mg/L	Commonly performed to support the diagnosis of DIC.

C. BASIC METABOLIC PANEL

Determination	Conventional Units	SI Units	Clinical Significance
Sodium (Na+)	Adult/elderly: 136–145 mEq/L	136–145 mmol/L	Possible critical value: <120 or >160 mEq/L. May be *increased* by trauma, surgery or shock. May be *decreased* by drugs: diuretics, sodium-free intravenous fluids, and ACE inhibitors.
Potassium (K+)	Adult/elderly: 3.5–5.0 mEq/ L	3.5–5.0 mmol/L	Possible critical value: (adult) <2.5 or >6.5 mEq/L. *Increased* in acute or chronic renal failure, hypoaldosteronism, hemolysis, infection, acidosis, dehydration. *Decreased* in burns, diuretics, diarrhea, vomiting, trauma, surgery.
Chloride (Cl⁻) (blood)	Adult/elderly: 98–106 mEq/L	98–106 mmol/L	Possible critical value: <80 or >115 mEq/L. *Increased* in dehydration, renal tubular acidosis, excessive saline infusion, metabolic acidosis, respiratory alkalosis. *Decreased* in overhydration, heart failure, vomiting, Addison's disease, hypokalemia, respiratory acidosis.
CO_2 Content (blood)	Adult/elderly: 23–30 mEq/L	23–30 mmol/L	Possible critical value: <6 mEq/L. *Increased* in severe diarrhea, starvation, severe vomiting, aldosteronism, emphysema. *Decreased* in renal failure, diabetic ketoacidosis, shock.

(continued)

Determination	Conventional Units	SI Units	Clinical Significance
Blood Urea Nitrogen (BUN)	Adult: 10–20 mg/dl (Elderly may have slightly higher values)	3.6–7.1 mmol/L	Possible critical value: >100 mg/dl (indicates seriously impaired renal function)
			Increased in advanced pregnancy, gastrointestinal bleeding, drugs (e.g., cephalosporins, furosemide, aspirin, gentamicin, vancomycin).
			Decreased with overhydration, drugs (e.g., streptomycin, chloramphenicol).
	Child: 5–18 mg/dl		
	Infant: 5–18 mg/dl		
	Newborn: 3–12 mg/dl		
	Cord blood: 21–40 mg/dl		
Creatinine (serum)	Adult: Female: 0.5–1.1 mg/dl	44–97µmol/L	Possible critical value: >4 mg/dl (indicates seriously impaired renal function)
	Male: 0.6–1.2 mg/dl	53–106 µmol/L	
	Elderly: decreased muscle mass may cause decreased values.		*Increased* in glomerulonephritis, pyelonephritis, acute tubular necrosis, reduced renal blood flow (related to, e.g., heart failure, atherosclerosis), acromegaly.
			Decreased in debilitation, decreased muscle mass.
	Adolescent: 0.5–1.0 mg/dl		
	Child: 0.3–0.7 mg/dl		
	Infant: 0.2–0.4 mg/dl		
	Newborn: 0.3–1.2 mg/dl		

Determination	Conventional Units	SI Units	Clinical Significance
Glucose (blood)			*Increased* (*hyperglycemia*) in diabetes mellitus, chronic renal failure, acute stress response, pheochromocytoma.
			Decreased (*hypoglycemia*) in insulinoma, hypothyroidism, Addison's disease, extensive liver disease, starvation.
	Child >2 years to adult:	<6.1 mmol/L	*"Fasting"* refers to no caloric intake for 8 hours or more.
	Fasting: 70–110 mg/dl	<11.1 mmol/L	
	Casual: ≤ 200 mg/dl		*"Casual"* refers to any time of day regardless of food intake.
	Elderly: increase in normal range after 50 years.		Possible critical values:
			Adult male: <50 and >400 mg/dl. Adult female:
	Child < 2 years: 60–100 mg/dl	3.3–5.5 mmol/L	<40 and >400 mg/dl.
	Infant: 40–90 mg/dl	2.2–5.0 mmol/L	Possible critical values: <40 mg/dl
	Newborn: 30–60 mg/dl	1.7–3.3 mmol/L	Possible critical values: <30 and >300 mg/dl
	Premature infant: 20–60 mg/dl	1.1–3.3 mmol/L	
	Cord Blood: 45–96 mg/dl	2.5–5.3 mmol/L	
Additional tests:			
Calcium (Ca++)	Total calcium: Adult: 9.0–10.5 mg/dl	2.25–2.75 mmol/L	*Increased* in hyperparathyroidism, metastatic tumor to the bone, prolonged immobilization, lymphoma, Addison's disease.
			Decreased in hypoparathyroidism, renal failure, rickets, vitamin D deficiency, pancreatitis, alkalosis.

(*continued*)

Determination	Conventional Units	SI Units	Clinical Significance
	Ionized calcium: Adult: 4.5–5.6 mg/dl	1.05–1.3 mmol/L	
Magnesium (Mg++)	Adult: 1.3–2.1 mEq/L	0.65–1.05 mmol/L	Possible critical values: <0.5 mEq/L or >3 mEq/L
			Increased in renal insufficiency, uncontrolled diabetes, Addison's disease, hypothyroidism.
			Decreased in malnutrition, malabsorption, alcoholism, diabetic acidosis, chronic renal disease.
	Child: 1.4–1.7 mEq/L		
	Newborn: 1.4–2 mEq/L		
Phosphorus (P) and Phosphate (PO$_4$); names used interchangeably.	Adult: 3.0–4.5 mg/dl Elderly values slightly *lower* than adult	0.97–1.45 mmol/L	Possible critical values: <1 mg/dl
			Increased in renal failure, acromegaly, bone metastasis, increased intake of phosphorus, hypoparathyroidism, sarcoidosis, liver disease, acidosis, advanced lymphoma.
			Decreased in inadequate dietary intake of phosphorus, chronic antacid ingestion, hypercalcemia, hyperparathyroidism, vitamin D deficiency, diabetic acidosis, sepsis.
	Child: 4.5–6.5 mg/dl	1.45–2.1 mmol/L	
	Newborn: 4.3–9.3 mg/dl	1.4–3.0 mmol/L	

Determination	Conventional Units	SI Units	Clinical Significance
Lipids			
Cholesterol	Adult/elderly: <200mg/dl	<5.20 mmol/L	The main lipid associated with atherosclerotic vascular disease.
			Increased in hypercholesterolemia, hyperlipidemia, uncontrolled diabetes mellitus, nephrotic syndrome, pregnancy, hypertension, high-cholesterol diet, stress.
			Decreased in severe liver disease, malabsorption, malnutrition, hyperthyroidism, cholesterol-lowering medication (statins), sepsis, stress, acute myocardial infarction.
	Child: 120–200 mg/dl		
	Infant: 70–175 mg/dl		
	Newborn: 53–135 mg/dl		
Lipoproteins			
High-density lipoprotein (HDL)	Male: >45 mg/dl	>0.75 mmol/L	25% of cholesterol bound to HDL.
	Female: >55 mg/dl	>0.91 mmol/L	
			Increased in familial HDL, excessive exercise, lipoproteinemia.
			Decreased in metabolic syndrome, familial low HDL, hepatocellular disease, hypoproteinemia.
Low-density lipoprotein (LDL)	60–100 mg/dl	<3.37 mmol/L	75% of cholesterol bound to LDL.

(continued)

Determination	Conventional Units	SI Units	Clinical Significance
			Increased in familial LDL, nephrotic syndrome, hypothyroidism, chronic liver disease, hepatoma, Cushing's syndrome.
			Decreased in familial hypolipoproteinemia, severe burns, malnutrition, hyperthyroidism.
Very-low-density lipoprotein (VLDL)	7–32 mg/dl		(see LDL above)

D. CARDIAC / SKELETAL MUSCLE, BRAIN ENZYMES

Determination	Conventional Units	SI Units	Clinical Significance
Creatine kinase (CK), creatine phosphokinase (CPK)	Adult/elderly: Male: 55–170 units/L Female: 30–135 units/L	55–170 Units/L 30–135 units/L	*Increased* after exercise, intramuscular injections, certain drugs (e.g., statins, anticoagulants, aspirin, lidocaine, propranolol), and in disease or injury to heart or skeletal muscle and brain. *Decreased* in some early pregnancies.
	Newborn:	68–580 units/L	
Isoenzymes:	CPK-MM (CPK3): 100%		*Increased* in skeletal muscle injury, convulsions, recent surgery, muscular dystrophy, crush injuries, shock, intramuscular injections.
	CPK-MB (CPK2): 0%		Specific to myocardial cells. *Increased* in myocardial ischemia, myocardial infarction, cardiac defibrillation, myocarditis, renal failure.
	CPK-BB (CPK1): 0%		Found predominantly in brain and lung. *Increased* in cerebral or pulmonary injury.
Troponins (Cardiac)			More specific marker than CK/CPK for myocardial injury; results usually *normal* in *non-cardiac* muscle disease. *Increased* in myocardial injury/infarction.
Cardiac-specific troponin T (cTnT)	<0.2 ng/ml		*Severe* skeletal muscle injury may cause false elevation of cTnT.
Cardiac-specific troponin I (cTnl)	<0.03 ng/ml		

E. KIDNEY (RENAL) FUNCTION STUDIES

Determination	Conventional Units	SI Units	Clinical Significance
Blood Urea Nitrogen (BUN) (See also above)	Adult: 10–20 mg/dl (Elderly may have slightly higher values)	3.6–7.1 mmol/L	(see BUN above)
Creatinine (serum)			(see creatinine above)
BUN/Creatinine Ratio	Adult: 6 to 25 (15.5 optimal adult value)		Measure of kidney and liver function

F. LIVER FUNCTION STUDIES

Determination	Conventional Units	SI Units	Clinical Significance
Hepatitis virus studies (blood)			*Increased* levels found in hepatitis A, B, C; in chronic carrier state for hepatitis B and in hepatitis B.
Hepatitus A virus (HAV)	Negative		
Hepatitus B virus (HBV)	Negative		
Hepatitus C virus (HCV)	Negative		
Hepatitus D virus (HDV)	Negative		
Hepatitus E virus (HEV)	Negative; No antigen or antibody tests widely available at present.		

G. URINE STUDIES

Determination	Conventional Units	SI Units	Clinical Significance
Urinalysis:			Not necessarily a clean-catch specimen unless infection suspected; in this case, a midstream clean-catch specimen is obtained.
Appearance	Clear		Cloudy urine suggests pus, RBCs or bacteria.
Color	Amber yellow		Concentrated urine is dark amber. Dark red urine may suggest bleeding from the kidneys; bright red urine may be from lower urinary tract. Green urine may be from the presence of *Pseudomonas*. Certain drugs or foods may also cause color changes.
Odor	Aromatic		Strong, sweet acetone smell may reflect diabetic ketoacidosis. A foul odor may be present in patients with a urinary tract infection.
pH	4.6–8.0 (average 6.0)		Alkaline pH is common after eating. Acidic urine most common. Urine should be kept alkalotic to prevent urinary calculi. *Increased* in respiratory alkalosis, metabolic alkalosis, vegetarian diet, renal failure, gastric suction, vomiting, urinary tract infection. *Decreased* in metabolic acidosis, diabetes mellitus, diarrhea, respiratory acidosis, starvation, sleep.

(continued)

Determination	Conventional Units	SI Units	Clinical Significance
Protein	None or up to 8mg/dl		*Increased* in glomerulonephritis, renal disease, preeclampsia, diabetes mellitus, heart failure, malignant hypertension, amyloidosis, systemic lupus erythematosus.
	50–80 mg/24 hr (at rest)		
	<250 mg/24 hr (exercise)		
Specific gravity	Adult: 1.005–1.030 (usually 1.010–1.025)		*Increased* in concentrated urine, dehydration, pituitary tumor, decreased urinary blood flow, fever, excessive sweating, vomiting, diarrhea, X-ray contrast dye.
			Decreased in dilute urine, renal disease, overhydration, diabetes insipidus, hypothermia.
	Elderly: values decrease with age.		
	Newborn: 1.001–1.020		
Leukocyte esterase	negative		Positive test suggests urinary tract infection.
Nitrites	negative		Positive test suggests urinary tract infection.
Ketones	negative		Positive test suggests poorly controlled diabetes, hyperglycemia, acute febrile illnesses (especially in children).
Crystals	negative		Presence suggests renal stone formation.
Casts	None present		Presence associated with proteinuria

Determination	Conventional Units	SI Units	Clinical Significance
Glucose	Fresh specimen: negative		*Increased* in diabetes mellitus, pregnancy, renal glycosuria, nephrotoxic chemicals (e.g., carbon monoxide, mercury, lead), hereditary defects.
	24-hour specimen: 50–300 mg/day	0.3–1.7 mmol/ day	
White blood cells	0–4 per low-power field		Presence of 5 or more WBCs may suggest urinary tract infection involving the bladder and/or kidney.
White blood cells casts	negative		When present, most commonly found in kidney infections.
Red blood cells	≤2		Presence may suggest disruption of blood-urine barrier, cystitis, nephritis.
Red blood cell casts	none		Presence may suggest glomerulonephritis, renal infarct, vasculitis.

H. CEREBROSPINAL FLUID

Determination	NORMAL ADULT REFERENCE RANGE		CLINICAL SIGNIFICANCE	
	Conventional Units	*SI Units*	*Increased*	*Decreased*
Albumin	15–45 mg/dl	150–450 mg/L	Certain neurological disorders	
			Lesion in the choroid plexus or blockage of the flow of CSF	
			Damage to the blood-central nervous system (CNS) barrier	
Cell count	0–5 mononuclear cells per cu mm	$0–5 \times 10^6$/L	Bacterial meningitis	
			Neurosyphilis	
			Anterior poliomyelitis	
			Encephalitis lethargica	
Chloride	700–750 mEq/L	700–750	Uremia	Acute generalized meningitis
				Tuberculous meningitis
Glucose	50–75 mg/dl	2.75–4.13 mmol/L	Diabetes mellitus	Acute meningitis
			Diabetic coma	Tuberculous meningitis
			Epidemic encephalitis	Insulin shock
			Uremia	
Glutamine	6–15 mg/dl	0.41–1 mmol/L	Hepatic encephalopathies, including Reye's syndrome	
			Hepatic coma	
			Cirrhosis	
IgG	0–4.5 mg/dl	0–4.5 mg/L	Damage to the blood-CNS barrier	
			Multiple sclerosis	

Determination	NORMAL ADULT REFERENCE RANGE		CLINICAL SIGNIFICANCE	
	Conventional Units	*SI Units*	*Increased*	*Decreased*
			Neurosyphilis	
			Subacute sclerosing panencephalitis	
			Chronic phases of CNS infections	
Lactic acid	10–25 mg/dl	10–25 mmol/L	Bacterial meningitis	
			Hypocapnia	
			Hydrocephalus	
			Brain abscesses	
			Cerebral ischemia	
			CNS disease	
			Acute meningitis	
Lactic dehydrogenase	≤40 units/L (Adults)	150–450 mg/L	Tubercular meningitis	
			Neurosyphilis	
		150–250 mg/L	Poliomyelitis	
		50–150 mg/L	Guillain-Barré syndrome	
Protein electrophoresis (cellulose acetate)	% of total:	Fraction:	An increase in the level of albumin alone can be the result of a lesion in the choroid plexus or a blockage of the flow of CSF. An elevated gamma	
Prealbumin	2–7	0.03–0.07		
Albumin	56–76	0.56–0.74		
Alpha$_1$ globulin	2–7	0.02–0.065		
Alpha$_2$ globulin	4–12	0.03–0.12		

(continued)

Determination	NORMAL ADULT REFERENCE RANGE		CLINICAL SIGNIFICANCE	
	Conventional Units	*SI Units*	*Increased*	*Decreased*
Beta globulin	8–18	0.08–0.185	globulin value with a normal albumin level has been reported in multiple sclerosis, neurosyphilis, subacute sclerosing panencephalitis, and the chronic phase of CNS infections. If the blood–CNS barrier has been damaged severely during the course of these diseases, the CSF albumin level may also be elevated.	
Gamma globulin	3–12	0.04–0.14		

I. GENETIC TESTING

Specimens may be obtained from blood (lavender-top tube), buccal mucosa swab, amniotic fluid, chorionic villus sampling, placental tissue, or other body parts required or available for sampling.

Type of Genetic Test	Genetic Mutation	Clinical Significance
Breast cancer	**Br**east **Ca**ncer (BRCA) genes: BRCA1 mutation – on chromosome 17. BRCA2 mutation – on chromosome 13.	BRCA1 and BRCA2 encode tumor suppressor proteins; over ½ of women who inherit mutations will develop breast cancer by age 50 (vs 2% of women without mutation)
		BRCA genes also increase susceptibility for ovarian cancer.
		Men with BRCA genetic mutations at increased risk for breast, prostate and colon cancer.
Colon cancer	Familial adenomatous polyposis (FAP) caused by mutation in the 5q 21–22 (APC) gene – on chromosome 5.	Genes encode tumor suppression proteins.
	Hereditary nonpolyposis colorectal cancer (HNPCC) is associated with mutations of MLH1, MLH2, and MSH6.	HNPCC associated with endometrial, gastric and ovarian cancer.
Cutaneous melanoma	Tumor suppressor gene CDKN2A encoding the p16 protein on chromosome 9 p21 (more common). Tumor suppressor gene CD K4 on chromosome 12 q13.	Multiple primary melanomas at an early age. Atypical or dysplastic nevi (moles). P16 carriers at increased risk for pancreatic cancer.
Cystic fibrosis (CF)	Mutation in the cystic fibrosis transmembrane conductance regulator (CFTR) gene on chromosome 7. Currently more than 1000 mutations are known to cause CF; most common mutation is Delta F508.	Mutation alters cell's ability to transport chloride. Disease involves exocrine glands (especially those secreting mucus), resulting in pancreatic insufficiency, chronic pulmonary disease, high sweat electrolyte levels, and in some cases, cirrhosis of the liver.

(continued)

Type of Genetic Test	Genetic Mutation	Clinical Significance
Hemochromatosis	Mutation analysis of the hemochromatosis-associated HFE gene is performed to determine presence of hereditary hemochromatosis (HH). Mutation called C282 Y accounts for almost 85% of mutations causing disease.	Causes iron overload, increased intestinal iron absorption and intracellular iron accumulation; can lead to progressive damage of the liver, heart, pancreas, joints, reproductive organs, and endocrine glands. Most common inherited disease in Caucasians.
Tay-Sachs Disease	Hexosaminidase A gene mutation on chromosome 15. Gene mutation impedes synthesis of hexosaminidase (HEX) which normally breaks down fatty substances called GM2 gangliosides.	Causes severe developmental and mental retardation in early life. No treatment for the disease; blood sample or amniocentesis testing performed.
Thyroid cancer	RET proto-oncogene on chromosome subband10 q11.2 encodes a receptor tyrosine kinase expressed in tissues and tumors originating from the neural crest.	Testing for RET germline mutations shows 100% sensitivity and specificity for identifying those at risk for developing inherited or familial medullary thyroid cancer. Surgically curable before spreading to regional lymph nodes.
Other genetic tests		
• Paternity tests	Compares DNA variants among mother, child, and male subject.	Proves/excludes paternity of biological father; determines if twins are identical or fraternal.
• Forensic tests	Performed on any body part, cadaver, or live person.	Collection of evidence to be used in reconstruction of event, usually in a court of law.

Source: Cundy, J.A.B. (2004). Assessment techniques: Nursing assessment skills. In S.L. Allen, *RNFA study guide & practice resources.* Denver: Certification Board Perioperative Nursing; Mann, B.D. (2009). *Surgery: A competency-based companion.* Philadelphia: Elsevier Saunders; Pagana, K.D.S., & Pagana, T.J. (2009). *Mosby's diagnostic and laboratory test reference* (9th ed.). St. Louis: Mosby.

J. PULMONARY FUNCTION TESTS

Test	Purpose	Clinical Significance
Spirometry	Air flow volumes and flow rates	Diminished: reduced airflow due to obstruction or restriction of airflow; test may be repeated after administration of bronchodilators. Normal is 80% or better

VOLUMES

Test	Purpose	Clinical Significance
Forced vital capacity (FVC)	Amount of air that can be forcefully expelled	Decreased: in obstructive and restrictive pulmonary disease
Forced expiratory volume in 1 second (FEV$_1$)	Volume of air expelled during the first second of FVC	Decreased (80% or less): less air expelled secondary to narrower airway and less air originally inhaled
Maximal volume ventilation (MVV), formerly called maximal breathing capacity	Maximal volume of air that can be breathed in and exhaled within1 minute.	Decreased in restrictive and obstructive pulmonary disease
Tidal volume (TV)	Volume of air inspired and expired during each normal respiration	Reduced in pulmonary disease
Inspiratory reserve volume (IRV)	Maximal volume of air that can be inspired from the end of a normal inspiration; reflects forced inspiration over and above TV	Reduced in pulmonary disease
Expiratory reserve volume (ERV)	Maximal volume of air that can be exhaled after a normal inspiration	Reduced in pulmonary disease
Residual volume (RV)	Volume of air in the lungs after forced expiration	Increased in pulmonary disease

CAPACITIES

Test	Purpose	Clinical Significance
Inspiratory capacity (IC)	Maximal amount of air inspired after a normal expiration (IC=TV+IRV)	
Functional residual capacity (FRC)	Amount of air left in lungs after expiration (FRC=ERV+RV)	
Vital capacity (VC)	Maximal amount of air expired after a maximal inspiration (VC=TV+IRV+ERV)	

(continued)

Test	Purpose	Clinical Significance
Total lung capacity (TLC)	Volume to which the lungs can be expanded with the greatest inspiratory effort (TLC=TV+IRV+ERV+RV)	
Minute volume (MV); also known as minute ventilation	Volume of air inhaled and exhaled per minute	
Dead space	Part of the TV that is not part of alveolar gas exchange; includes air within trachea	
Forced expiratory flow$_{200-1200}$ (FEF)	Airflow rate of expired air between 200 ml and 1200 ml during FVC;	most affected by airway obstruction
Forced expiratory Flow$_{25-75'}$ (FEF)	Airflow rate of expired air between 25% and 75% of the flow during FVC	This part of airflow curve most affected by airway obstruction
Peak inspiratory flow rate (PIFR)	Flow rate of inspired air during maximal inspiration	Used to indicate tracheal and bronchial airway disease
Peak expiratory flow rate (PEFR)	Maximum airflow rate during forced expiration	

Source: Cundy, J.A.B. (2004). Assessment techniques: Nursing assessment skills. In S.L. Allen, *RNFA study guide & practice resources.* Denver: Certification Board Perioperative Nursing; Mann, B.D. (2009). *Surgery: A competency-based companion.* Philadelphia: Elsevier Saunders; Pagana, K.D.S., & Pagana, T.J. (2009). *Mosby's diagnostic and laboratory test reference* (9th ed.). St Louis: Mosby; Rothrock, J.C. (1999). *The RN First Assistant: An expanded perioperative nursing role* (3rd ed.). Philadelphia: Lippincott.

The following list reviews common diagnostic imaging procedures and testing examples with which the First Assistant should be familiar.

Arteriogram (Angiogram): Serial x-ray imaging of the vascular system utilizing a contrast media. With the use of *digital subtraction angiography*, bony structures can be removed from the picture.
Examples: Abdominal aortogram, carotid arteriogram, renal angiography, lower extremity arteriography.

Arthrogram: X-ray study involving injection of contrast medium into a joint cavity allowing visualization of joint structures.
Example: Arthrogram of knee.

Barium enema: X-ray study of the colon involving injection of barium into the colon allowing visualization of tumors, polyps, and diverticula.
Example: Barium enema of the terminal ileum for Crohn's disease or colonic tumors.

Barium swallow: X-ray study of the esophagus involving injection of barium into the upper gastrointestinal tract allowing visualization of tumors, polyps, and diverticula.
Examples: Barium swallow to visualize esophageal tumors, reflux, or strictures.

Bone densitometry: Accurate means of measuring bone mass and predicting risk of fracture. Utilizes low-dose x-ray.
Example: Bone density study.

Bone scan: See *Nuclear imaging.*

Bone x-ray: Single exposure radiographic film to evaluate bone. Films vary by density and anatomic location. Films may be taken from different angles: anterior, posterior, lateral, or oblique.
Examples: Fracture, tumor, infection, or congenital bone abnormalities.

Breast scintigraphy: Nuclear scan of breast with sestamibi in patients whose tissue is too dense for conventional mammography studies.
Example: Cancer lesions in patients with dense breast tissue.

Breast sonogram: Ultrasound examination of breast useful for differentiating cystic from solid tumors.
Example: Monitor changes in size of breast cyst.

Capsule endoscopy (Virtual endoscopy): Endoscopy uses scopes to visualize the interior aspects of an organ. Capsule endoscopy employs a vitamin pill-sized camera containing a radiofrequency transmitter and batteries that records images of the entire digestive tract, especially the small intestine. The capsule is swallowed and expelled after 6 to 10 hours (the capsule does not need to be retrieved).
Examples: Bleeding from the small intestine, polyps, Crohn's disease, tumors.

Cardiac catheterization: Method of studying and diagnosing defects in heart chambers, valves, and blood vessels. Utilizes fluoroscopy and arterial and venous catheters that deliver contrast material into chambers and vessels of the heart.
Examples: Coronary arteriography, left ventriculogram, mitral valve regurgitation.

Cardiac Stress Test: The heart is stressed (with exercise or drugs) and electrocardiographically monitored to evaluate heart function. A treadmill or bicycle may be used if the patient is able to perform physical exercise.
Examples: Monitor for coronary occlusive disease, heart rate, blood pressure.

Carotid artery duplex scanning: Test employing both Doppler and B-mode ("duplex") ultrasound to study vertebral and extracranial carotid artery stenoses or occlusions. Color Doppler may be added.
Example: Monitor for transient ischemic attacks (TIAs), hemiparesis, and speech or visual deficits.

Chromosome karotyping: Analysis of the chromosomal arrangement of cells.
Examples: Determination of fetal sex, prenatal chromosomal disorders. (See *Genetic Testing* in Appendix I, H.)

Colonoscopy: Direct visualization of the colon from anus to cecum with fiberoptic colonoscope. Visualization is enhanced by insufflating air to distend the bowel.
Examples: Polyps, tumors, inflammatory bowel disease, bleeding.

Colposcopy: Direct visualization of the cervix with a binocular microscope. May be accompanied by biopsy testing.
Example: Cervical cancer.

Computed tomography (CT): Cross-sectional radiographs of a portion of the body performed with or without contrast media.
Examples: CT of head, brain, sinuses, abdomen.

Cytology studies: Pathology study that examines cell structure for abnormal cellular changes, growth, and cell type.
Example: Urine cytology, surgical specimen cytology to determine pathology of tumor.

Discogram: X-ray study that involves injection of a contrast medium into the nucleus pulposa allowing visualization of intervertebral disk abnormalities.
Example: Lumbar discogram.

Doppler echocardiography: In addition to using pulsed high frequency sound waves to evaluate the position, size, and movement of the heart and blood vessels, *Doppler echocardiography* also measures turbulence and velocity. With the addition of *color*, the direction of a given stream of blood can be determined; the hue of the color (dull to bright) represents the varying blood velocities. *Tissue Doppler imaging* (TDI) is a more recent echocardiographic technique that is used to evaluate longitudinal myocardial function and systolic and diastolic dysfunction.
Examples: Blood turbulence, velocity, and direction of intracardiac and intravascular blood flow; adequate collateral flow to the hand (when considering removal of radial artery for use as a conduit during coronary artery bypass grafting).

Echocardiogram: Uses pulsed high-frequency sound waves to evaluate the position, size, and movement of heart walls, valves, and great vessels, and to observe the directional flow of blood within the heart. Studies may be *M-Mode* (one dimensional linear tracings), *two-dimensional* (2-D picture of organ), or *three-dimensional* (3-D picture). The probe may be placed over the chest (transthoracic echocardiogram/ TTE) or inserted into the esophagus (transesophageal echocardiogram/TEE); TEE images are not obscured by the sternum and rib cage.
Examples: Valvular stenosis, valvular regurgitation, pericardial effusion, myxoma, septal defects, endocarditis, ventricular hypertrophy, ventricular or atrial mural thrombus.

Electrocardiogram (ECG): Recording of the electrical impulses that stimulate the heart to contract. Indicates cardiac rhythm and dysfunctions that influence conduction of the myocardium.
Examples: Heart block, bradycardia, tachycardia, ST segment changes.

Electroencephalography (EEG): Recording of the electrical impulses from the cortex of brain to determine brain activity. Utilizes scalp electrodes.
Examples: Brain tumor, intracranial hemorrhage, cerebral infarct, encephalitis.

Electromyography (EMG) and electromyoneurography: Skin and needle electrodes are used to measure and record nerve conduction and electrical properties of skeletal muscle. Used to detect neuromuscular abnormalities.
Examples: Muscular dystrophy, myopathy, traumatic injury, hypothyroidism, hyperadrenalism, spinal cord injury, sarcoidosis, Guillain-Barre syndrome, amyotrophic lateral sclerosis.

Electrophysiology (EP) study: Invasive procedure used to diagnose atrial and ventricular dysrhythmias. Measures properties of the electrical conduction system of the heart via solid catheters placed in the heart under fluoroscopy. Purpose is to reproduce dysrhythmias in a controlled environment leading to determination of therapy.
Examples: Re-entrant tachydysrhythmias, atrial fibrillation, Wolff-Parkinson-White syndrome.

Endoscopy: Utilization of scopes to visualize the interior aspects of an organ.
Examples: Cystoscopy, gastroscopy, thoracoscopy, laparoscopy, bronchoscopy.

Esophageal manometery, Esophageal motility studies: Tests for normal esophageal contractility by measuring pressures within the esophagus and measuring acid levels during the exam.
Examples: gastroesophageal reflux disease (GERD), diffuse esophageal spasm.

Exercise Stress Test: Measures the efficiency of the heart during a dynamic exercise stress session on a motor-driven treadmill or ergometer. Evaluates symptoms suggestive of ischemic heart disease, measures functional capacity and function of devices such as physiologic responsive pacemakers.
Examples: Coronary ischemia, heart rate response to exercise.

Fluoroscopy: Radiology technique that allows real-time visualization; may or may not involve use of intravenous or oral contrast media.
Examples: Intravenous pyelogram, fluoroscopy for placement of pacemaker leads or implantable cardiac defibrillator, upper GI study, cholecystography.

Lung scans: Nuclear studies used to determine the percentage of normal functioning lung, diagnose and locate pulmonary emboli, and assess the pulmonary vascular supply by estimating regional blood flow. Ventilation scans evaluate air movement or lack of air-flow. Perfusion scans demonstrate blood flow. Inhalation scans are similar to perfusion scans; however, they provide improved visualization of the trachea and major airways.
Examples: Pulmonary embolus, tuberculosis, bronchitis, tumor.

Magnetic resonance angiography (MRA): Enhanced scanning with MRI to examine vascular structures. Can be performed with the use of a dye medium that is not excreted via the kidneys.
Examples: MRA of carotid arteries.

Magnetic resonance imaging (MRI): Enhanced scanning that uses radio frequency waves and a magnetic field to produce images from multiple planes or axes; often used to examine areas of soft tissue; performed with or without contrast media.
Examples: MRI of knee to examine cartilage, MRI of spine.

Mammography, Mammogram: X-ray examination of the breast to identify cancer and other diseases of the breast. Mammograms usually include two views of each breast: cranial to caudal dimensions and the medial to lateral dimension. Preoperative mammogram localization may be performed before surgical biopsy of suspected lesions. Non-operative stereotactic needle (or mammotomy probe) biopsy provides tissue for study.
Examples: Breast cancer, fibroadenoma, cysts, abscess.

Nuclear imaging: Uses intravenous injection of a radionuclide material (such as technetium [Tc]-99m), which emits gamma rays that provide an image of organs systems and evaluate function.
Examples: Kidney scan, bone scan, brain scan, thyroid scan, liver scan, myocardial perfusion.

Nuclear stress test: Study utilizes the existence of detectable differences in the concentrations of administered radioactive materials in normal and abnormal tissue to evaluate cardiac properties and function. This test achieves desired cardiac stress and maximum cardiac dilatation equivalent to exercise and is used for patients unable to exercise. Gated stress test evaluates heart wall motion and ejection fraction.
Example: cardiac response to pharmacologic stress.

Positron emission tomography (PET scan): Measures the metabolic activity of tissue (mainly heart and brain) to assess cell damage or death utilizing a radioactive compound.
Examples: Myocardial infarction, brain tumor, dementia, Alzheimer's disease, Parkinson's disease, epilepsy.

Radioisotope scanning: Visualization of specific organs or tissue using radioisotope media.
Examples: Bone scan, lung perfusion scan.

Scintography: Nuclear study (see *Nuclear imaging*) using an intravenous injection of a radionuclide material (such as technetium [Tc]-99m), which emits gamma rays. A scintillator camera is placed over the target organ to record the radiation emitted and provide an image of organ under study.
Examples: Breast scintography for hyperplasia, breast cancer.

Single Photon Emission Computed Tomography (SPECT): A two-dimensional nuclear imaging test that shows blood flow through tissues and organs. A SPECT scan integrates computed tomography (CT) and a radioactive tracer that emits gamma rays. A computer collects the information from the gamma rays. The test differs from the PET scan in that the chemical remains in the bloodstream rather than being absorbed by surrounding tissues.
Example: Cerebral blood flow.

Sinogram: Involves taking an x-ray after a contrast medium has been injected into a sinus tract allowing visualization of the areas involved.
Example: Sinogram of wound fistula.

Ultrasound: Recording of the reflection of high-frequency sound waves against organs and structures. Utilizes a conductive gel applied to body. (See also *Echocardiogram*)
Examples: Carotid ultrasound, ultrasound of abdomen.

Urodynamic, Uroflowmetry study: Identifies abnormal voiding patterns in patients by determining sphincter and muscle function and assessing neuroanatomic connections related to bladder function.
Examples: Urethral stricture, prostatic hypertrophy, prostate cancer.

Venogram (Phlebography, Venography): X-ray study to identify thrombi in the venous system. Dye is injected into the venous extremity and x-rays are taken at timed intervals.
Examples: Acute deep vein thrombosis, obstructed venous system.

X-ray: Single exposure radiographic film that evaluates bone and soft tissue. Films vary by density and anatomic location. May be taken from different angles: anterior, posterior, lateral or oblique.

Examples: Chest x-ray, cardiac size, lung tumors, pneumonia, pulmonary edema, extremity film, abdominal flat plate film.

Source: Adapted from Cundy, J.A.B. (2004). Assessment techniques: Nursing assessment skills. In S.L. Allen (Ed.), *RNFA Study Guide & Practice Resources*. Denver: Competency and Credentialing Institute.; Mann, B.D. (2009). *Surgery: A Competency-based Companion*. Philadelphia: Elsevier Saunders; Pagana, K.D.S., & Pagana, T.J. (2009). *Mosby's Diagnostic and Laboratory Test Reference* (9th ed.). St Louis: Mosby; Mayfield Clinic. (2009). *Spect Scan*. Retrieved June 6, 2009 from www.mayfieldclinic.com/PE-SPECT.htm

Index